AF790486

American Body Snatchers

Also by Richard S. Ross III
and from McFarland

Before Salem: Witch Hunting in the Connecticut River Valley, 1647–1663 (2017)

Contagion in Prussia, 1831: The Cholera Epidemic and the Threat of the Polish Uprising (2015)

American Body Snatchers

Merchandising the Dead in 19th Century New England and Washington, D.C.

Richard S. Ross III

McFarland & Company, Inc., Publishers
Jefferson, North Carolina

ISBN (print) 978-1-4766-9501-3
ISBN (ebook) 978-1-4766-5262-7

Library of Congress and British Library
cataloguing data are available

Library of Congress Control Number 2024017241

Printed in the United States of America

McFarland & Company, Inc., Publishers
Box 611, Jefferson, North Carolina 28640
www.mcfarlandpub.com

Table of Contents

Acknowledgments

I would like to thank the following for their invaluable contribution to this work: Countway Library of Medicine, Harvard University, Boston, Massachusetts; Rauner Special Collections Library, Dartmouth College, Hanover, New Hampshire; Library of Congress, Washington, D.C.; Massachusetts Historical Society, Boston, Massachusetts; Massachusetts Supreme Judicial Court Archives and Records Preservation Department, Boston, Massachusetts; National Library of Medicine, Bethesda, Maryland; Trinity College Library, Hartford, Connecticut; Wellcome Library, London, United Kingdom; and Manuscripts and Archives, Yale University, New Haven, Connecticut.

I also want to also acknowledge the librarians I have known over the years, especially the interlibrary loan librarians and their staff who were tireless in obtaining resources for me. The same thanks and respect go to the following individuals who were especially helpful in writing this book: Elizabeth Bouvier, head of archives, Massachusetts Supreme Judicial Court Archives and Records Preservation Department; Scout Noffke, reference and administrative specialist, Rauner Special Collections Library; Hannah Elder, assistant reference librarian for rights and reproductions, Massachusetts Historical Society; and Jessica Dooling and Jessica Becker, Public Services, Manuscripts and Archives, Yale University Library. I am also especially indebted to the interlibrary loan staff at Trinity College who have never failed me in my request for resources.

Finally, I would like to acknowledge my son Richard and daughter Nicole, my grandchildren Mitzi and Billy, and my late wife Christine who believed in my work and whose patience and advice spurred me on to complete my first two books. Christine's memory and belief in my work remain to inspire me to continue my historical research and writing.

Preface

This book grew out of my long-term interest in the interaction of medical history as it relates to social and economic history in the nineteenth century. This was to be my second foray into this topic, as my first book, *Contagion in Prussia, 1831: The Cholera Epidemic and the Threat of the Polish Uprising* (2015), required familiarity with not only the political and social history of several European countries but also their medical establishments and organizations.

The worldwide experience with Covid-19 caused me to return again to thoughts on the interaction of the medical community with society in general. What had been piquing my interest were the continuous reports on the trade and smuggling of human tissue and body parts both legal and illegal. The conflict and certitude on the part of each constituency reminded me of the body-snatching activities I read about in nineteenth-century America, especially but not limited to before the Civil War.

During the nineteenth century, the dead body had become a commodity to be bought and sold. Once again at the close of the twentieth century and into the twenty-first century, human body parts, because of medical progress, were being obtained illegally and bought and sold on the black market because of a worldwide limited supply and increasing global demand.

Reading the literature, I found a host of books and articles that described for the lay public the history of body snatching in the United Kingdom starting with the trial of the notorious body snatchers William Burke and William Hare in 1829 in Edinburgh, Scotland, and the consequences of the Parliamentary Warburton Act in 1832 in England. Although the act did not completely stop body snatching, it did much to resolve the practice. I quickly found that there were fewer books that addressed body snatching directly in nineteenth-century America, and although there were several good articles buried in the medical literature, none completely answered the questions for which I was interested in finding answers.

Some of these questions included the following: What were the religious, moral, and social objections? What was the genesis of the state anatomy laws passed throughout the nineteenth century? How did the needs of physicians in proposing anatomy laws affect the social cohesion of antebellum American society? Why was there such conflict between the local communities and the medical schools at that time? What role did the doctors and their students play in this conflict? How were doctors perceived at this time, and what was the popular view of nineteenth-century medicine and the seemingly insatiable need for bodies to dissect? What did physicians want from the proposed anatomy laws, and what were their requirements? Why and how did the poor become victims of the post–Civil War anatomy laws?

On a side note, I know from previous research and what was brought out during the Covid-19 epidemic the reluctance of Blacks to obtain new treatments such as the mNRA vaccine. Blacks had a long history of being exploited by the medical community for medical research, such as the Tuskegee syphilis experiments starting in 1932 and lasting for forty years. This resistance is not new and went back to the late eighteenth and nineteenth centuries, when even Blacks feared they would be used for medical experiments and thousands of dead bodies were removed from Black graveyards and cemeteries and sold for dissection to medical schools throughout the states.

I decided to limit my primary research to New England, as many of the issues that would later come to dominate the discussion at a national level were first addressed here. My inclusion of Washington, D.C., was for two reasons: there was a definite New England connection in the founding of the first medical school in Washington and following the Civil War, the District of Columbia gave rise to professional body snatchers who supplied the district's three medical schools as well as medical schools in the Northeast, the South, and the Midwest.

The research for this book included the examination of many nineteenth-century newspapers, medical articles, and university archives for information about body snatching. I found the issue much more complex than I originally thought but also compelling and fascinating. I hope you find it the same.

Introduction

The American people of the nineteenth century were confronted with the issues that went to the heart of their existence, including religious upheaval, slavery, the Civil War, and something as fundamental as a natural threat, diseases such as the all-consuming tuberculosis, also known as consumption, phthisis, and scrofula, a leading cause of death throughout the nation in the nineteenth century.

Along with these concerns, Americans were engaged in a *danse macabre*. In some isolated areas of New England, Michael Bell has identified cultural and physical evidence of fears of vampirism that led to the exhumation of individuals suspected of these activities and actions taken intended to keep the undead from harming the living.[1]

By the mid-nineteenth century, Americans were made conscious of premature burial, covered in popular books, magazines, and newspapers articles. The fear took off from there.[2] The authors of the book *Premature Burial and How It May Be Prevented* blamed premature burial on "the system of medical examination ... in the United States where there is usually no examination at all—there is often a reckless haste in interment."[3] The book was criticized by the English physician David Walsh, who argued that "the whole theory of premature burial is unsupported by a single scientifically proved instance.... [This] popular belief is nothing more than legend." He was especially critical of reports of premature burials from America.[4]

If the latter two beliefs were nothing more than legend, the fear of body snatching in America's burying grounds was not. The wholesale removal of the dead as subjects for dissection in the newly emerging medical schools of nineteenth-century America was a fact, and the fear and anxiety of losing a loved one to this practice was omnipresent and real for the people of America throughout the nineteenth century.[5]

In Massachusetts prior to 1831, an article in the *Boston Medical and Surgical Journal* argued that in New York and Philadelphia "hundreds of bodies are every year stolen from their places of burial." In Massachusetts "the same violation of graves was notoriously carried on, until the passage by the Legislature of what is commonly called the anatomy law" in 1831.[6]

In 1945 the medical historian Frederick C. Waite estimated that between 1820 and 1840 medical students in Vermont "used at least 400 cadavers." Almost all the cadavers were "secured illegally," and almost all were acquired within the boundary of Vermont. For New England in the nineteenth century, he estimated that if taking into account the number of physicians graduating from medical schools between 1801 and 1900 that required dissections, many grave robberies went undetected, and "there must be in cemeteries, churchyards, and private burial plots" throughout New England far more empty graves than anyone suspected.[7]

Compared to Washington, D.C., grave robbing in New England was significantly reduced. Estimates at the end of the nineteenth century for the District of Columbia ranged from more than thirty thousand empty graves in the poor house cemetery, with thousands more in the other public and private cemeteries including the Congressional Cemetery.[8]

Throughout the nineteenth century and the early twentieth century, there were few books but many newspaper reports and articles written about body snatching and the progress of anatomy laws in the various states in America. Body snatching by doctors, medical students, and "resurrection men" was seen by the medical profession as a necessary evil to provide subjects for the dissection tables until anatomy laws could be passed to ensure sufficient cadavers for instruction.

Times have indeed changed, and in the latter part of the twentieth century and today the commodification of the human body has increased exponentially. Today, not only are parts and organs harvested from dead bodies for scientific research, but there is also a brisk trade in fetal parts and the harvesting of human organs both legal and illegal, and there are reports of people being murdered for their organs.[9]

Interest has also been generated in the actions and phenomenon of body snatching in the nineteenth century by medical historians investigating body snatching in the development of medical education.[10] Their research has expanded into the relationship between medical progress, the anatomy laws, immigrants, the poor, and Black people. Other historians have begun to look at the role of the many prestigious medical institutions in the United States and their exploitation of Black bodies used for dissection on the road to scientific medical progress.[11]

In the arc of history, a gruesome endeavor such as body snatching could not remain neglected for long. In this book I have written a social history of this phenomenon by focusing primarily on the response of the people in New England and the nation's capital. During much of the nineteenth-century antebellum period, America was primarily agricultural and rural. Death and burial were as much "a community as a family matter, when the community consisted of a closely knit, geographically isolated groups of families. Occupations were less diverse than later, and unusual events were treated as community responsibilities." The "death of an individual was a deprivation of customary social give and take to a large proportion of the total group, and a matter of common knowledge and discussion. The loss of one life was a distinctly felt diminution of the total community."[12]

Body snatching for most of the nineteenth century was viewed as an egregious exploitation of the dead at a time when religious values as well as codes of behavior and customs were more strictly adhered to; when these values and codes were flouted, punishment was meted out by the community with banishment, severe reprisals, and in some instances rioting and destruction of property. The resistance to this practice can be found, first, in the legacy of a legal system that for centuries reserved dissection for convicted murderers, carrying with it the burden of shame and disgust on the part of the family, and second, in the religious belief in the liminal body and its actual resurrection. Finally, communitarian comity and neighborliness, with long-standing religious, political, and social principles, was the hallmark of antebellum nineteenth-century America.

Evidence of these values is seen in the earlier anatomy laws passed in New England that were repealed or modified to ensure that the poor were not subject to dissection (except the Massachusetts Anatomy Act of 1831 with some unique characteristics). For physicians who themselves abhorred the body trade, reform was a necessity, but where they could obtain the subjects for dissection if not in the cemeteries was a problem. The solution was to look to the poor who had lived off of the charity of society. Prior to the Civil War for the reasons noted above, this option was considered irreligious and socially unsound.

Following the Civil War, besides urbanization and increased social mobility, new values of individualism, materialism, and unbridled capitalism began to dominate American society. This gave rise to a breakdown in older institutions that previously gave a community intimate knowledge of its poor and permitted the passage of new anatomy acts that conflicted with the deeply held religious and communitarian beliefs of the earlier part of the nineteenth century. As one historian has written concerning the English experience in regard to the passage of the Anatomy Act in England in 1832, "Pauper's feelings were to be sacrificed in order that the rest of society could rest peacefully in their graves."[13] The same could be said for many of the poor in America with the passage of new state anatomy laws in the last quarter of the nineteenth century.

Even with the passage of these anatomy laws, many officials did not approve or cooperate with them. This intransigence occurred both before and after the Civil War. Examples include "a personal aversion to dissection" and "criticism from those who had known the dead person in life," and even the "decision that sent someone's body to the dissection table" might be used as a threat to inhibit an official from deciding to seek "elective office."[14]

Body snatching and, at its most visceral level, the intense opposition to it by the public was founded on not only theft of the dead but also sacrilegious treatment of the body after death. "The formalized custom of bereavement, depending as it often did on the integrity of the corpse and the respect shown it, were brutally violated by the practice of dissection."[15]

In the following chapters I evaluate several episodes that I believe contribute to a more thorough context and understanding of the public reaction to these body-snatching incidents in New England and the nation's capital. Body snatching cannot be justified only as a medical necessity to provide subjects for dissection in medical education in the nineteenth century, was antithetical to deeply held social and religious customs, and was handily resisted by the public, who opposed elites willing to transform social cohesion in society by exploiting the dead. The elites proposed doing this at first by tolerating the stealing of bodies from graveyards. The subjects came from the lowest level of society, the bodies of the destitute, immigrants, and Black people whose bodies were taken from potter's fields, Black graveyards, and cemeteries. These provided most of the corpses for the dissection tables during the nineteenth century. To forestall body snatching and expand the acquisition of legal subjects, the elites later proposed that the poor who received charity from the state should "repay society by letting their bodies be used for scientific research after their death."[16]

In Chapter 1 I evaluate a serial body-snatching case in 1818 in the parish of Chebacco, then part of Ipswich, Massachusetts. Eight bodies had been secretly removed from their graves. These outrageous body snatchings in the town burying ground created intense anxiety due to the missing bodies, the betrayal of the townspeople's deeply held religious beliefs, and the indignity over the likely dissection of their loved ones. Evidence is provided to show the reaction of the victims and their friends; the betrayal by the town doctor, Thomas Sewall; and the long-term effects of this treachery on the comity of the town.

Additionally, Robert Crowell, the town minister, preached a sermon on the interment of the empty coffins of the town victims on the issue of body snatching. His sermon is investigated and is a reliable touchstone for many of the arguments developed against this practice throughout nineteenth-century America.

In Chapter 2 I provide information on Dr. Sewall's background and medical training, his trial for body snatching, and his removal from Essex, Massachusetts (Chebacco Parish in Ipswich became Essex, Massachusetts, in 1819), to Washington, D.C.

In Chapter 3 I cover Manchester, Massachusetts, which, coincident with fallout from the body-snatching episode in neighboring Ipswich, was in an uproar due to the perceived betrayal by another elite, the town's congregational minister, Reverend James Thurston. He was accused of inviting a younger physician to Manchester to replace the town doctor by convincing him that there would be opportunities for "private dissection" and that he would have no trouble acquiring subjects in the town. The turmoil caused by the ensuing accusations and countercharges is examined.

Chapter 4 follows the path of the distinguished nineteenth-century doctor Nathan Smith, founder of the Dartmouth Medical School, the Yale Medical School, the Medical School of Maine at Bowdoin, and the Medical Department of the University of Vermont. I focus on his trials and tribulations at Dartmouth, his involvement in the body-snatching episode at Dartmouth in 1809, and its effect on the community and the consequences for the college and for himself.

In Chapter 5 I provide new information on a series of earlier events that led to the first attempt to legislate an anatomy law in 1819 in Connecticut based on earlier ordinances passed in the town of Southbury, Connecticut; a detailed analysis of events leading up to the Yale Medical School riot; the riot itself; the trial of the accused body snatcher and his punishment; and the significance of the riot.

Chapter 6 continues with the consequences of the Yale Medical School riot as well as the genesis of the Connecticut Anatomy Act of 1824, the importance and drawbacks of which are discussed. Further information is given on the development of Connecticut's Anatomical and Medical Sciences Act of 1833 and the underlying, political, social, and economic rationale for its repeal in 1834.

In Chapter 7 I discuss the founding of three medical schools in Vermont between 1817 and 1827. As a result of this embarrassment of medical riches, body snatching became rampart in Vermont during the first half of the nineteenth century. The infamous Hubbardton Raid on the Castleton Medical Academy in 1830 is investigated. The long-term effects of this raid on the town of Hubbardton continued to haunt the people of Vermont, as shown in the town of Hubbardton's visceral reaction to the epic poem "Song of Hubbardton Raid," published in Vermont nearly fifty years after the event.

In Chapter 8 I provide detailed information on Dr. Thomas Sewall who, having left Essex, Massachusetts, in disgrace for Washington, D.C., did so at the invitation of Daniel Webster. On his arrival Sewall found a newly organized city with a small medical establishment, no medical school, and no hospital to administer to the public. In this chapter I describe how Sewall was instrumental in organizing the Columbian College Medical Department, part of Columbian College (today George Washington University). At first, with one medical school, there was a limited body-snatching environment in Washington, D.C. With the establishment of the Georgetown College School of Medicine, the competition for corpses escalated and is discussed up to the beginning of the Civil War.

Other significant events are noted as they pertain to Dr. Sewall and the Columbian

College Medical Department including the scandal and trial in 1829 of William Burke and William Hare, body snatchers and murderers in Edinburgh, Scotland; the passage of the Massachusetts Anatomy Act in 1831; the cholera epidemic in 1832 in Washington, D.C.; the establishment of the Washington Infirmary in 1844; the first public hospital in the District of Columbia; and Sewall's death in 1845. The chapter concludes with the mixed legacy of his life for the people of Essex, Massachusetts, and Washington, D.C.

In Chapter 9 the diary of George Christian, a body snatcher, is introduced. It is a remarkable work and gives us the inner workings of Christian's body-snatching operation, including the expansion of his activities beyond D.C. and trafficking bodies to Virginia and the Midwest. In the context of the diary, additional information is supplied on his body-snatching operation in D.C., the doctors who assisted him, the exploitation of the Washington Asylum burying ground, and the Black and white cemeteries and burying grounds of Washington, D.C. Information is also provided on Christian's attempts to rob the graves of a local celebrity, Beau Hickman, and the "colored desperado" Thomas Wright, hanged for murder.

Chapter 10 covers the medical schools in Washington, D.C., turning to the notorious resurrectionist Vigo Jansen Ross for their supply of bodies after the arrest of George Christian. The consequences of his arrest led to an attempt to pass an anatomy law by Congress for the District of Columbia. The controversy over the attempt to pass an anatomy law is discussed along with how the consequences of its delay led to Washington, D.C., becoming not only the nation's political capital but also during the 1880s and 1890s the nation's capital for body snatching.

In Chapter 11 I discuss the role of Black people, the poor, and immigrants in the body-snatching activities of the late eighteenth century and the nineteenth century. Initially, Black people had little power to resist the exploitation of their burying grounds. I discuss an early trial in Massachusetts of a doctor sued by a free "colored man" for digging up the body of his deceased wife for dissection. Wandering afield, there is the extraordinary but unsuccessful attempt in 1787 by free Blacks and slaves to petition New York City's common council to stop private doctors and the Columbia College Medical School from acquiring their cadavers from the "Negroes Burying Grounds." Also noted is the body-snatching episode at Lebanon Cemetery, a Black cemetery, in Philadelphia that ultimately led to Pennsylvania's innovative Anatomy Act of 1883 and its national impact. The chapter concludes with a discussion of the role of native whites and immigrants who outside the South made up most residents of almshouses.

Chapter 12 concludes the book with an overview of the impact of body snatching in nineteenth-century New England and the nation's capital, the rationale for the support and passage of new anatomy laws in various states, and the reasons for the decline of body snatching by the end of the nineteenth century. However, while body snatching was in decline across America toward the end of the century, this was not the case in Washington, D.C. I discuss how and why at this time the nation's capital inaugurated a heyday of body snatching.

1

Merchandising the Dead

Americans in the late eighteenth century and a good part of the nineteenth century faced many issues that caused great anxiety in society, including premature burial and the fear that either they or their loved one's bodies might be brutally removed from the grave and sold to a doctor or a medical school to be dissected before an audience of callow beardless youths. Generally, most historians of anatomy (in which body snatching played an important part), have been sympathetic to doctors and others who recognized that the bodies were obtained unlawfully and loathed the trade. They justified these early activities of the "heroic age" of anatomy because body snatching was for the greater good of society. Also, under the prevailing felony laws at the time, there were never enough criminal bodies to meet the growing need of the physicians and the newly founded medical schools that began to offer courses in anatomy that required human dissection.

"Body snatching," "resurrection," "grave robbing," and "disturbing the dead" were terms used in the nineteenth century for stealing bodies from cemeteries. Resurrection was the preferred term used by the medical profession, and one cannot help but think that it was employed as an inside joke that was insulting to the more religiously minded citizens who were appalled by this activity. Nevertheless, it originated as a slang expression that had its origin around the time of the trial of the notorious grave robbers and murderers William Burke and William Hare in Edinburgh, Scotland.[1]

The method of grave robbing was generally a three-man affair and required following specific instructions to avoid detection. The example here is likely taken from the Northeast but undoubtedly was similar throughout the United States. First, knowledge of an upcoming burial was necessary. There were multiple ways this might be obtained. One example is given for a medical school. A former student would send a coded message to an officer at the school. The message would include the time and place of the burial and would be sent to an intermediary, who would forward the information to the school. The next step was to locate the grave in the daylight hours. One approach was to have someone disguised as a hunter. While "strolling through the cemetery, hunting for game he noted the position of the open grave and its relation to the entrance of the cemetery and to some landmark observable in the dark, such as a large monument…." A few hours later he could return and easily find the fresh grave.

Three men would arrive later that evening with a carriage. One man remained with the carriage and drove it away immediately, as a "conveyance standing in front of a cemetery at night would arouse suspicion…. Two strong men were needed to disinter the corpse. The surface of the grave was examined with a shaded lantern because often a friend of the deceased would "arrange on the closed grave a pattern of stones, shells, sticks, or flowers in order to detect disturbance. The pattern had to be mapped so that it could be restored exactly after the disinterment."

Additional equipment included two large tarpaulins that were placed beside the grave. The soil from the grave was put on one of the tarpaulins. This was necessary to avoid having any soil on the surrounding grass. The position of the head of the corpse was easily determined by looking at the position of the other gravestones. "An excavation approximately three feet square was made at the head end of the grave until the rough box was reached. The depth of the excavation was four feet or less so that not over thirty-five cubic feet of soil needed to be handled." Because the dirt was loose, it was easily removed unless other impediments such as stone or straw were in the grave, making the digging more difficult. "The head end of the rough box was removed by boring a row of holes with an auger." Neither a saw, hatchet nor ax were used as they made too much noise. The "removal of the cover of the frail coffin was a simple matter."

The next order of business was to remove the body from the coffin. This was done with a hook, a "strong iron bar five feet in length; one end was turned up into a blunt hook of about two inches, while the other end had a cross bar handle. The hooked end was placed under the chin of the body and two able bodied men could draw the body from the coffin onto the second tarpaulin previously laid at the head of the grave." Unfortunately, the hook did much damage to the upper and lower portions of the mouth. An alternative to the hook was a harness "strapped under the arms of the body, with a ring in the back to which a rope was tied." The body was laid on the tarpaulin. The shroud and other items were stripped from the body and thrown back in the grave. Clothing was difficult to get rid of because it was easily recognized.[2]

The body was now tightly wrapped to avoid anything falling to the ground, as any objects near or on the grave would be a sure sign that the burial site had been disturbed. The soil was returned to the grave, and the surface of the grave was restored to the "exact conditionin in which it had been found." What remained were two bundles that two men could easily carry to the returned conveyance. Finally, it was important that the lantern used in the excavation was a "dark lantern." This was achieved by using the hook to hold the lantern while

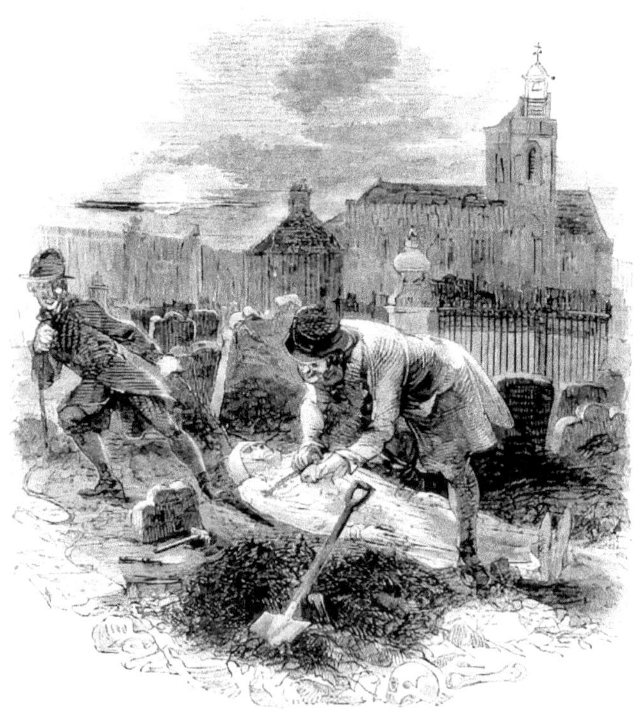

Illustration of a grave robbery. Image from "The Exhumation." George Reynolds, *Mysteries of London*, Vol. 1 (London: George Vickers, 1846), 329.

one of the tarpaulins was thrown over the excavation site, creating a tent. "Failure to protect the lantern led to many an interrupted disinterment" because "light in a cemetery seen by neighbors would bring a group of enraged citizens to the scene." The body snatchers might escape into the night but would lose all their equipment or be caught and punished. For example, as described in an 1828 newspaper report, three resurrectionists were "apprehended at Chateaugay," New York. "They had disinterred the body of Mr. Andrew Foster but being pursued, they threw the body naked into the river, with a rope round the neck." The "three" were apprehended and made to take the body of the deceased back and reinter it. Afterward they were turned over to the "civil authorities."[3]

However, if all went well, two strong men could "complete a disinterment in an hour from the time they entered the cemetery and be on their way. The return would be uneventful "unless [as noted above] discovery had been made and pursuit followed."[4]

Early Laws Regarding Grave Robbing

The phrase "grave robbing" was the common term for the stealing of the effects of dead bodies from their graves. According to common law, a "dead human body" itself "is not property."[5] The principle had been upheld in both English and American court decisions, and even today courts have ruled that "there can be no property rights in a dead body.... The next of kin does not have a property right in a relative's dead body but does hold some limited right to possess the body for purposes of burial."[6] However, the statutory law of England that governed the American colonies provided no penalty for the exhumation of a human body; however, if one took property such as a shroud, this was considered a felony under common law. The law determined that the property "remains ... [with] ... the executor, or that of the person in charge of the funeral." Also, whoever owned the soil could bring trespassing charges against those who dug up or "disturb[ed] it."[7]

English law that governed the American colonies contained no statutes for penalizing the digging up of dead bodies. However, it should be noted that the application of laws in the early colonies was contested due to the various jurisdictions in the colonies. Some believed that English law should always apply, while others believed that colonial law should take precedence and English general regulations should take precedence if there was no colonial law for the specific case.[8] Nevertheless, the early laws passed in the New England colonies, the *Body of Liberties* (1641) and the *Connecticut Code* (1650), make no mention of grave robbing. The witchcraft law that passed in England in 1604 under James I followed the repeal of the Elizabethan witchcraft act of 1563, which was more severe than the latter. A "new offence was added: dead bodies were not to be taken out of their graves" and used for the purposes of charm, witchcraft, sorcery, or enchantment.[9] The punishment was death and entailed intent for using the bodies "in any manner of witchcraft."[10] The law was applied in Massachusetts in 1692. The 1604 witchcraft law was later repealed in 1735; at that time many people believed that those who claimed to have extraordinary powers were con men and vagrants.[11]

The first laws on grave robbing in New England were passed in New Hampshire in 1796, Vermont in 1804, Connecticut in 1810, and Massachusetts in 1815. The Massachusetts law was titled "An Act to Protect the Sepulchers of the Dead." This act would be applied in the grave-robbing episode that took place in Massachusetts in 1818.[12]

A Grave-Robbing Incident in the Parish of Chebacco in Ipswich, Massachusetts

In April 1818 a year before the parish of Chebacco was incorporated into the town of Essex, the people of the parish were "startled and excited to an unparalleled degree" when it was discovered that "eight human bodies had been surreptitiously taken from their resting place in the village burying-ground." The occurrence, as related by a resident of the village, had a powerful and lasting effect on the people of what later became the town of Essex. He wrote that he had come to the town twenty-two years after the incident; "there was still a pungency and acerbity in every occasional allusion to it by the majority of the adult population, who freshly remembered all the circumstances."[13]

At the time of the incident there were approximately 1,107 inhabitants in the parish.[14] On the night of January 10, 1818, the townspeople saw light coming from the "graveyard of Chebacco Parish," a telltale sign that something was amiss.[15] This aroused the suspicions of the townspeople, especially the family of Sally Andrews, age twenty-six, who had died from consumption (tuberculosis) on Christmas day and was soon after buried in the parish cemetery. Although the weather was especially mild that winter, six inches of snow had fallen that night, providing cover for the body snatcher's activities.[16]

The townspeople were concerned that the body of Sally Andrews might have been taken out of her grave for anatomical purposes. This suspicion made such an impression on several in the town, particularly her parents and neighbors, that it was determined to make an examination in the spring.[17]

On the morning of April 17, 1818, "Sally Andrews' parents Jacob and Sarah (Tyler) Andrews and other family members went to the burying ground armed with picks and shovels...."[18] The grave was opened, and the "painful discovery ... made ... their suspicions were too well founded. Her body was gone!"[19] Their misgivings that more than one grave might have been disturbed led to an examination of other graves, leading to such a "shock ... never felt before" in that community. In going forward to examine other graves, the townspeople thought they would be examining "the extent of the evil"; instead, they found themselves having to quiet "the troubled minds of those who had recently buried friends...."

Apart from Sally Andrews's empty grave, there were seven other bodies missing. Among them were Cesar Conway, a former slave and servant of the highly esteemed Choate family, who had died of consumption years earlier, and two youths both age ten, William Allen (not listed in Robert Crowell's necrology but in his sermon), and Philip Harlow (son of John Harlow), who died on October 11, 1817, from a "nervous fever." Others included Elisha Story, age sixty-four, who died of "lethargy on October 21, 1817, William Burnham 79 who died of consumption on December 23, 1817, Mrs. Mary Millet 35 who died of consumption March 4, 1818, and Samuel Burnham 26 who died from consumption the following day."[20]

Reverend Robert Crowell wrote that the townspeople suspected that the reason for the body snatching was because the corpses were to be used for "anatomical purposes" or medical dissection. At the time, the dissection of the dead body was acceptable only for criminals who were executed and considered to have died outside Christian society. Reverend Crowell would preach in his sermon (to be discussed later) that the dissection of the bodies was both a sacrilege to Christian teachings and morally reprehensible.

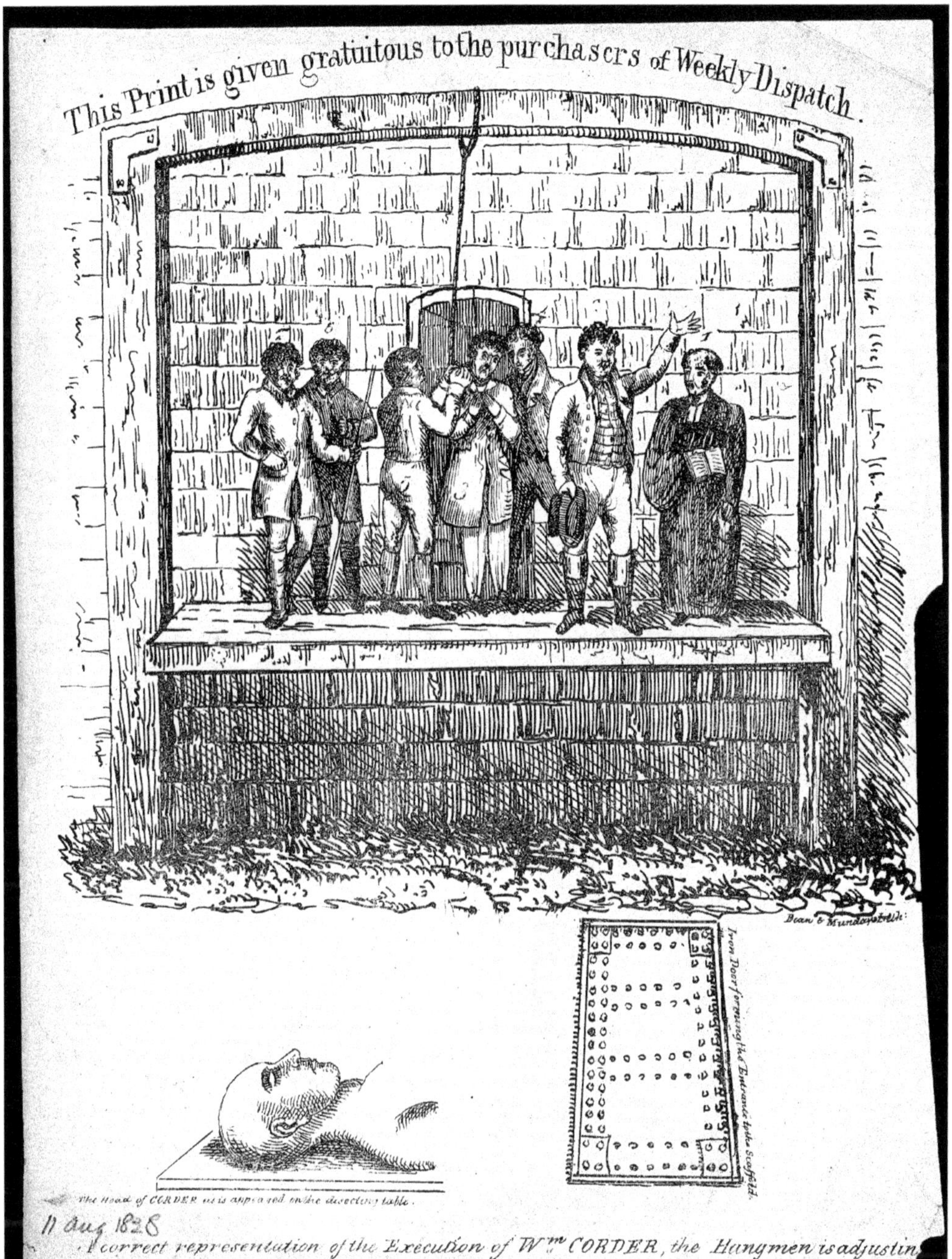
This Print is given gratuitous to the purchasers of Weekly Dispatch.
Iron Door forming the Entrance to the Scaffold.
11 Aug 1828
A correct representation of the Execution of Wm CORDER, the Hangmen is adjustin
the rope round the Prisoners neck, while an Assistant is supporting the wretched ma
Mr Orridge is announcing CORDER's acknowledgement of the justness of his sentenc

William Corder was convicted of murder and hanged on August 10, 1828. A dissection of his body was carried out the next day at Cambridge University. Note that his head is shown on the dissecting table. Lithograph by Bean and Mundays (courtesy Wellcome Library, London).

Here it was especially troubling because it caused "unusual distress through a very extensive and respectable circle of relations and friends."[21]

At a parish meeting held the evening of April 17, 1818, a committee was appointed to raise money to offer a reward "for discovering the authors of the late horrid deed." On April 21, 1818, the *Salem Gazette* reported,

> A great excitement has been produced in Chebacco by the recent discovery of the removal of a number of dead bodies from their graves. No less than eight empty coffins have been found in the grave-yard of that parish, and one in the neighboring precinct parish of Gloucester. A parish meeting has been called in consequence of this outrage and a large reward has been subscribed by individuals for the discovery of the perpetrators, which we hope will be effectual, and that hereafter the bones of the dead will remain undisturbed in the place where the affection of their friends has placed them.[22]

Interestingly, on April 24 a Boston newspaper reported the same story, adding more information on the size of the reward and saying it had "seen a letter which mentions the names ... four of the persons had borne, whose bodies have been taken.... And a suspected individual thought it necessary to have a guard round his house."[23]

Two days before the Boston newspaper's report, a meeting was held in which the families of the victims pledged to do more than just offer a reward. Viewing "the empty coffins now lying exposed to public view," they were determined to appoint "a day for solemn reintering [*sic*] of said coffins in one grave in some conspicuous part of the burying ground" and, in addition, have a "monument erected over them by subscription with the names of the deceased whose bodies were stolen inscribed thereon to perpetuate the memory of the horrid deed." It seems likely that suspicions may have surfaced that the culprit was the town doctor, Thomas Sewall, and he was the person mentioned placing the guard around his house.[24]

On April 28, the townspeople followed through with their first proposal to offer a reward. A "sensational advertisement" appeared in the *Salem Gazette* as well as other newspapers throughout New England and New York. Three prominent members of the parish signed the following advertisement:

> 500 Dollars Reward.
> *Most daring and sacrilegious Robbery.*
> STOLEN, from the grave yard in Chebacco Parish in Ipswich, the bodies of eight persons, seven of whom were interred since the 13th of October last; the other, a coloured man, about six years ago. As without doubt they have all, ere this time, passed under the dissecting knife of the anatomist, either of the rude novice in the art or of the skilful [*sic*] professor, little hope is entertained of recovering any relict of them for the consolation of the deeply afflicted friends. But whoever will give any information of this atrocious villainy, so as to detect and bring to justice, either the traders in this abominable traffic, or their inhuman employers, shall receive the above reward, and the thanks of an afflicted and distressed people.
>
> WILLIAM ANDREWS jun.
> THOMAS CHOATE
> NATHAN BURNHAM
> *Ipswich, Chebacco Parish, Committee. April 25th 1818.*[25]

The three were either "a parent, a brother or son" of each of the bodies taken.[26] The advertisement captured "the powerful reaction produced by the terrible discovery at Chebacco." The body snatching was described as a "daring and sacrilegious robbery." A reward of $500 was offered to "anyone who could give any information of this atrocious villainy, so as detect and bring to justice, either the traders in this abominable traffic, or their inhumane employers."[27]

The Salem newspaper *Essex Register* published an editorial on May 2, 1818, attempting to "thread the needle" over the outrage of the Chebacco townspeople and the needs of the medical community. However, what is important in understanding the editorial is what is not mentioned, the notion that stealing bodies from burying grounds was not wrong and was necessary. The argument was debated in the salons of New England, a debate the editors of the newspapers would be fully aware of. It was argued that the end justified the means to improve medicine for the living, and there were even those who argued the dead were "articles" and were "wasted on the bottom of the grave." The editorial suppressed these callous views and couched their argument in more ambiguous language. Later Reverend Robert Crowell at the interment service for the missing dead would preach against this view, as would a host of others, sparing no group or idea in the process.[28]

The editorial began with "the great alarm at Chebacco has made the subject of disturbing the dead a very serious concern." Next, "something must be done to render the public mind quiet on the subject." The editorial introduced the idea that the business of dissection (not using the term) is important to physicians as a method to learn from and help their patients. "Few who regard the living will be disposed to deny the human system should be understood." The editorial then cautions that it is the responsibility of the government to "put … the safety of common graves" beyond the "temptations to violate them" by providing "proper subjects for the Anatomist and Physician." Those proper subjects are criminals, "those who have forfeited their lives and liberties to the public."[29]

The editorial, perhaps to mollify the public, addressed the history of memorializing the dead by noting that it is "no peculiar sentiment of our own time." In the past and even today, "other enlightened nations have erected the most costly monuments and have spent the greatest wealth upon the graves of their friends." The editorial referenced Jesus, who accepted the tomb of his wealthy friend Joseph of Arimathea "without any reproof of sentiment." As a result, "Christians had been honoring it ever since." The editorial stated that even before Christianity, in ancient Rome violation of the dead was punishable by death.

The biblical and other references to past practice and traditions were to indicate to readers (and those who argued for exploiting the graveyards for subjects) that the writer was not recommending that bodies in the burying grounds be turned over to physicians. The editorial concluded with the following: "It is the wish of sober citizens that no temptations exist to actions which violate the best affections and the memory of the dead. Let the Medical faculty make known their wants to the government, and let them obtain the knowledge of life, without violating all the best hopes of it."[30]

There was a provision in the law for the purpose of turning over the cadavers of executed criminals for dissection; however, there were not sufficient executions of criminals to meet the demand. Of those executed, there were other limitations to prevent the cadavers from being delivered to the dissection table, such as family and friends who requested the bodies for a proper burial.

Reinterring the Coffins, July 23, 1818

Following the disclosure of the Chebacco incident that the body snatchers had not limited themselves to Chebacco but had also stolen a body from Gloucester, one observer in Salem wrote that "many towns have been alarmed." This also seems to have lifted the veil on what was known to take place but not discussed openly in public. As William Bentley, pastor of the Second Congregational (East) Church in Salem, wrote in his diary, "It has been disclosed that the wife of Micah Saunders, in our New Ground, was taken from her Grave, but for a long time the alarm has been prevented till this great excitement brought it out."[31] In another case of hysteria flowing from this incident, people had come to believe that the "grave of a Suicide had been violated in Salem but to relieve the public mind a search was made and the body found where left."[32]

During this time, in New England there was a lack of cadavers for the established and newly opened medical schools of anatomy. Stealing bodies was an open secret, especially in Boston. Body snatching had become more dangerous, and the cost of the dead bodies for the anatomy programs had continued to escalate.[33]

John Collins Warren, MD, wrote that after he opened a "dissecting room" in 1806 in Boston as more medical schools began opening in New England, cadavers had become more expensive. He turned to "procuring them from New York. The cost $25.00 per subject." Even this was considered a "great expense," and there was a "great hazard of being

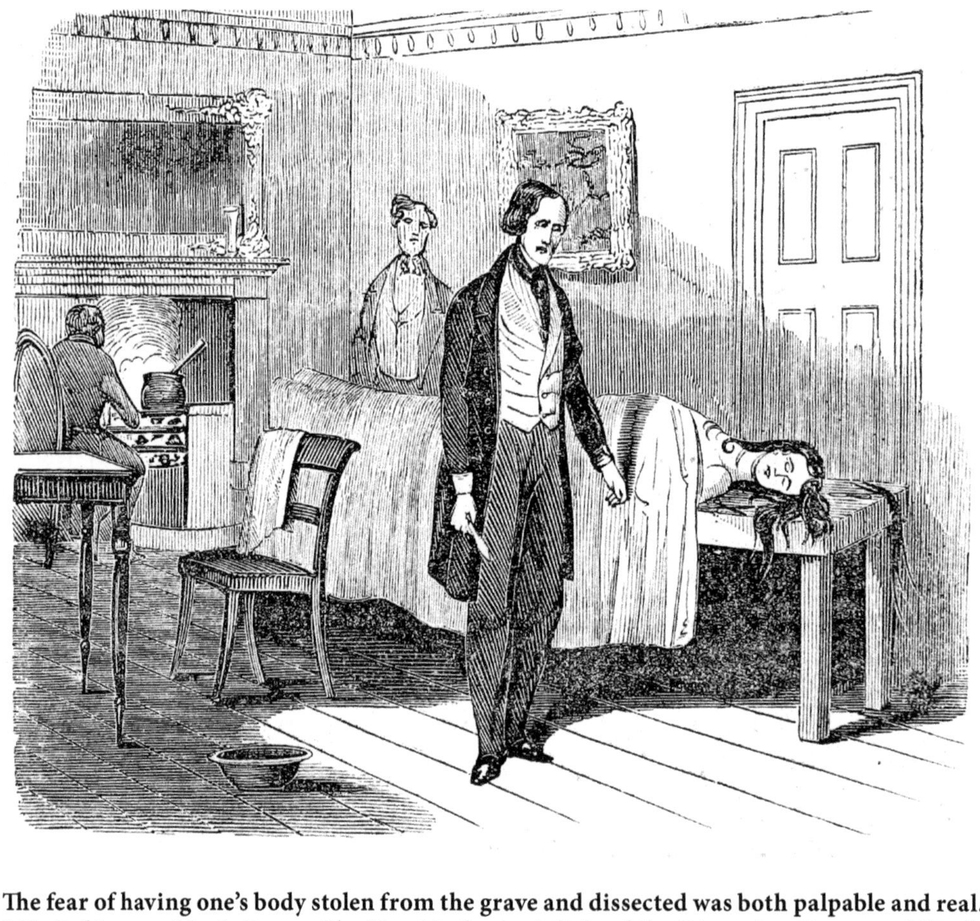

The fear of having one's body stolen from the grave and dissected was both palpable and real. J.H. Robinson, *Marietta, or, The Two Students: A Tale of the Dissecting Room and "Body Snatchers"* (Boston: Jordan & Wiley, 1846), 7 (courtesy Wellcome Library, London).

discovered."[34] Clearly, the price of dead bodies had continued to increase, at least for locally obtained bodies (obviously fresher and more useful to the anatomists), because later when the Chebacco culprit was discovered, Bentley wrote that he boasted "he could get 50 dollars for every body he had disturbed."[35]

The fear of one's body being stolen from the grave and dissected was real. Robert Crowell told the story of the near hysteria and fear of dying of a consumptive young woman who believed she might become the victim of body snatchers, be dissected, and perhaps more. She was the daughter of a clergyman, "a pious young lady ... in this vicinity." She feared "such a use of her body (an exposure from which her modest and refined sensibility shrunk with horror), and heard her repeated and dying request" of her parents to protect her from "suffering in anticipation" of this fate. Her parents "set a watch" after her burial ensuring that those who sought her body "were disappointed of their prey."[36]

Based on the words used to describe the young lady's anticipated horror, she likely feared necrophilia from the grave robbers themselves, in death lying naked in front of an assortment of young men, undreamt of while alive, possibly brutally handled and then dissected. It is no wonder that she asked her parents to do everything to help her avoid this horrible fate. Her fear was not unfounded, as later critics noted. "Body snatching, and dissecting-room jokes, and narratives often had a sexual" component. The violence of "body snatching figured as a rape of the grave, while dissection was a public undressing, a rape of the dead body."[37]

At the time, handbills with "startling headlines, and printed verses" were scattered about the village of Chebacco following the discovery of the missing bodies. An example of the depth of the feelings at the time can be found in the title of one flyer and an accompanying poem:

Recent Inhuman, Barbarous and Atrocious Affair
Perpetrated at Chebacco in Ipswich

Hark! The sad tidings from the bell now sounding,
To warn the people of some wretched monster,
Who, for the sake of gain and filthy lucre,
Robbed the grave-yard!
O! what is this my eyes are now beholding?
See the graves open and spectators mourning,
Friends and relations stand amaz'd to see this Sad profanation![38]

Eight empty coffins had been standing in full view of the inhabitants for four months and were presently scheduled to be interred in a common grave in the Chebacco burying ground on July 23, 1818. They were to be buried, and a monument was to be erected. Unfortunately, adequate funds were never raised for the monument.[39] A "solemn religious service was held in the Congregational Meeting-house," and a sermon was preached by the parish minister, Robert Crowell. "He later published his sermon as a forty-page pamphlet entitled *Interment of the Dead*." His printed sermon provides more information on this incident and its effect on the families and other inhabitants who were horrified by what happened in their town.[40]

This was an extraordinary sermon and served as a touchstone of criticism for the entire body-snatching enterprise of the anatomists. Crowell highlighted many arguments that served the opposition to grave robbing in the service of medicine well into the nineteenth century.

Frederick C. Waite in his article "An Episode in Massachusetts in 1818 Related to the Teaching of Anatomy" wrote that Crowell said that "dissection in itself was not unchristian"; he suggested by inference that if there was a law that allowed dissection of all criminals and not just "duelists and murderers," this would protect private graves. Crowell presented arguments "of those who defend private resurrection for anatomical study and examined each." He further suggested that these ideas were probably "derived from a physician."[41]

On closer examination of the sermon, Crowell offered no supportive arguments for dissection except one, and he hardly needed to consult with a physician, as these ideas were likely known and discussed among the New England educated elites.[42]

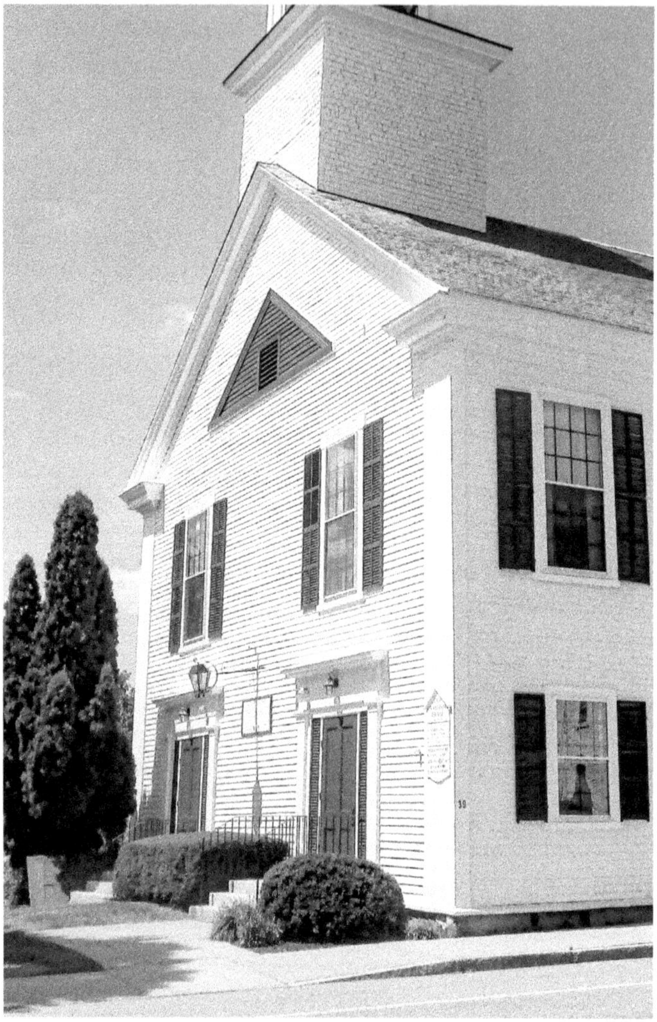

The meetinghouse today of the First Congregational Church in Essex Massachusetts, built in 1793, where Reverend Robert Crowell gave his sermon on "Interment of the dead.... A sermon delivered in Ipswich, Second Parish, [Chebacco, was called the second parish], July 23, 1818, on the occasion of reinterring the coffins which had been robbed of their contents" (photograph by the author).

The Sermon

Although much of Crowell's sermon deals with religious justifications for the proper burial of the dead, my primary interest is in his arguments against the justification of stealing bodies for dissection and its effect on the families.

Crowell began the sermon with a brief introduction concerning who had their bodies stolen from their graves and some general background already discussed. He then began both a secular and religious justification for treating the dead and burying them with "affection," piety, and respect, all three "sanctioned by the word of God...."[43]

Crowell's first illustration was the risen body of Jesus from his tomb and the despair of Mary and the disciples when this first occurred. They did not know where the body was and believed it had been stolen until Jesus appeared to them resurrected. Crowell believed that this example and other instances found in the Old and New Testaments justified proper burial.[44] He also gave examples of other societies in which the veneration of the dead was paramount.[45] He wrote that those who saw the pious and reverential treatment of the dead body as a mere "superstition" would have "their dead tumbled into a ditch, or thrown to the dogs, or, still better, in having them dissected, and exposed, for the inspection of the curious, and the promotion of useful knowledge, than in having them decently buried, and rest in their graves."[46]

Crowell had no sympathy for either the body snatchers or their employers. The "anguish" of the family and friends of the "dead stolen" is incalculable. They disturb the dead for "filthy lucre's sake," and he condemned their employers engaged in this "unholy traffic" because for whatever "purpose the latter appropriate these stolen bodies," they are guilty. If the saying is true that the "receiver is as bad as the thief," they should not be hidden from any of the "odium, which is attached to a stealth and merchandize of the dead; since if it were not for their patronage and suggestion none would be guilty of this outrage upon decency and humanity."[47]

For those who volunteer their bodies to science and "forgo the rites of burial; and the resting in their graves until the resurrection," they are putting themselves on the same level as the "notoriously wicked" and making a sacrifice that any good that can come from doing so in the "advancement of a particular science will more than counterbalance the evils of weakening the principles of nature, of impairing the salutary influence of a distinction between … those, who have forfeited their persons to civil justice, and of those, who have demeaned themselves in a manner to be entitled to its protection."[48] Dissection was reserved as a specific punishment for felons following their execution but had to be specifically ordered by a judge as part of the punishment. This was not done on a regular basis, contributing to the shortage of criminal bodies available for dissection at this time.

Crowell argued further that "we do not believe that any Christian has a right to dispose of his body, which is the temple of the Holy Ghost, in a manner which God has thought fit only for the vilest criminals." Whatever we think "of willing our bodies to be used for the advancement of an important science, it is very certain that we cannot use the bodies of our friends, or suffer them to be used, in this manner, unless … they may and do thus bequeath them, without a destitution of all-natural affection, and a violation of every principle of justice."

As for the simple act of dissection of a human body, there must be "Christian tenderness in the dissector." The body should have been obtained legally, and the dissector must approach the body with "proper views and feelings" and should leave with "exalted views of the wisdom, power and goodness of their Creator." Here, I believe that Crowell means the body should be that of a "vile criminal" outside the boundaries of the Christian community, as he has just argued that only these bodies are proper for dissection.

Further, "if there be guilt in obtaining the body, and they be knowingly partakers of this guilt, it is very certain that they cannot come to the examination of it, with any proper or religious feelings; but the contrary. And if they dissect, and examine, the human system with levity, and infidelity, and impiety, instead of receiving any good their wickedness and guilt will be greatly increased by it." Whatever the "guilt or innocence of the dissector, we still maintain that the body is thereby subjected to an evil; an evil which ought to be inflicted on none, but those who by their crimes, deserve it by the hand of man."[49]

Crowell rebuked the body snatchers who played a critical part in this "merchandizing of the dead" and condemned them and their foul methods used in obtaining cadavers, writing that after we "solemnly, and affectionately, … inter our dead, and … desire that they may rest undisturbed, then it must be unnatural, and inhuman, and impious; to violate their graves, and forcibly to remove them." They are thieves who "break open the houses of the dead, and, with a halter about the neck, violently pull the dead from their coffins."

He contrasted the body snatchers and their medical confederates with the worthiness of those who piously honor the dead and asked if we should send our "dead to the anatomist to be dissected for the promotion of medical knowledge, or if we are poor, … sell their bodies for the maintenance of ourselves and surviving family?"

If this is "unnatural and brutal," is it not the same for those who "violate the graves of our dead, and drag them out, almost as soon as they are in?" It cannot be right to bury our dead "merely to give others the trouble of going in the night and stealing them away." What of the poor man who goes through the expense of a solemn funeral for his wife and children, only to have others obtaining the "profits of the selling of their bodies."[50]

Crowell then turned to ideas that likely circulated among physicians and their elite supporters concerning a justification for obtaining these bodies even if the act is illegal. They agree that stealing dead bodies for "filthy lucre" is an insult to the dead and a "vile and inhuman act." But if the bodies are taken to acquire better knowledge of the "human system" and improve the "healing art," then one should "do away with the imputation of guilt to the person thus taking and using them." Crowell noted that there are many who are partially "inclined to justify the practice." They do not fully agree but believe there is "something not quite regular," but in the end "absolutely necessary" for the advancement of anatomical science.[51]

Then it is argued there is no harm done to others, "especially if it is never known to them, is so trifling, that they conclude, it is one of those evils, which must be winked at, and which can bring no great guilt upon the authors of it." Crowell concluded that there is no stronger refutation of this "fallacious reasoning than the fact, that none wish to have it applied to themselves, in regard to the dissection of the bodies of their own relatives, whom they tenderly love, and sacredly venerate."[52]

Third, Crowell noted that if it is argued by those who support grave robbing and dissection of bodies obtained through this method, "the motive of the actor determines the moral quality of the action[;] … if this object be a bad one, it makes the action put forth to obtain it, bad[;] … if it be good in itself, the action of seeking it cannot be wrong." He also stated that this is "specious" reasoning, and "it is radically defective, and has brought more sin, and mischief, upon society, than any other of the deceitful workings of the depraved heart."

Crowell argued that if the removal of the dead is for the "benefit of the living, [it] is and must be, a harmless thing, provided it be done with such caution, and prudence, and that the friends never know it"; therefore, it is "right and harmless to take these bodies, in a clandestine manner, and appropriate them to some useful purpose." According to this line of reasoning, "all our graveyards may be lawfully emptied of all their dead." Crowell makes an analogy regarding the sin of body snatching (or stealing) and adultery. "The man, who can commit adultery with his neighbor's wife without being detected in it, is no adulterer; nor is his neighbor at all injured by him, so long as he is ignorant of the fact. He is not at all the less happy for this crime, any more than he would be, if his neighbor were to take the body of his dead, and he knew it not." Unfortunately, the body snatching was not a secret in Chebacco, and the dead had been "torn from their coffins for monied and scientific speculation and exposed to the rude gaze of unbearded youth."[53]

Fourth, Crowell raised the question of the treatment of strangers who had no one to claim their bodies and had led an "upright life." Why should their bodies be "treated no better than the worst of felons?" The dead are "insensible" to the treatment of their bodies. "If it become [*sic*] a general practice to take the bodies of strangers without regard to age or sex, the suffering in anticipation of such an evil ... of such an exposure of their bodies upon anatomical theatres, must be no small punishment for the innocent to undergo, merely because they are strangers."[54]

On this topic Crowell concluded that there is no justification for stealing the dead from their graves for any purpose and added that this practice is "built on the most corrupt and pernicious principles."[55]

Crowell offered a solution dripping with sarcasm and pointed out the hypocrisy of those who support this "imperious necessity" of grave robbing for the "maintenance of the very important science of anatomy." If the "necessity is so great, that with the knowledge of anatomy already possessed by the world and the legal means of promoting it, and especially the dissection of the bodies of all who are executed by the hand of justice, the science must essentially suffer and be eventually lost, without an extensive, and indiscriminate dissection of the dead?" Therefore,

> And why then do we not see these liberal and zealous patrons of the science, and especially those, who are professionally interested in its advancement, taking their own dead, as well as the dead of others, for this benevolent purpose? If charity should begin at home ... in making those sacrifices, which are necessary to enable her to do good? That charity is of a very suspicious kind, which sparing her own, is very liberal with the property of others. May we not expect then, that all medical gentlemen, and others, who advocate an indiscriminate dissection of the dead, and who mean to act consistently with their principles, will first volunteer their own bodies, and if these are not sufficient, proceed to take the bodies of their deceased wives, and children, and parents, and other relatives, to be dissected, and exposed, both in private and public seminaries? If they should conclude thus to act, in consistency with their own principles, we might reasonably expect, that such a numerous corps of volunteers, as they would make, would be amply sufficient for the well-being of anatomy, and that the rest of the public might, for the present at least, safely dismiss their fears, and the painful anxiety, and trouble, of watching, night after night, for the security of their dead.[56]

For some, Crowell's recommendation was a commonsense solution to the ongoing demand for cadavers for the dissecting table. Throughout the nineteenth century when many of the arguments concerning proposed anatomy laws were debated, opponents would ask why these anatomists and their students did not will their bodies for dissection after death or have family members undergo the procedure. Their opponents answered the "dissection of physician's bodies would distress family and friends...."[57]

However, as the following shows, even a renowned physician might have second thoughts about having his body dissected. Thomas de Haviland of Philadelphia recounted that on the evening after the burial of Dr. Benjamin Rush on April 19, 1813, in

Philadelphia, another famous physician, Dr. Philip Syng Physick, who had attended the burial of Dr. Rush, received a troubling visit from a "large black man" who asked him, "Would you like Dr. Rush?" Physick replied, "What do you mean? Dr. Rush is dead." The visitor said, "I can take to the college tomorrow morning at 9:00 am for $20 dollars." Dr. Physick did not see his visitor again and did not hear any more of Dr. Rush's body. "He long wondered if the great man of American medicine and signer of the Declaration of Independence ... had not gone through a dissection room."[58]

Clearly, this early episode must have haunted Dr. Physick up until his death, because he left strict instructions on the disposition of his own body. "A dissection was absolutely prohibited, no one was to touch him but two females who had been his domestics for the last twenty years." His body was to be "warmly wrapped" and not to be moved from his bed for some time. The room was to be kept warm until "putrefaction commenced." He was then to be covered in flannel and placed in a wooden coffin, with the coffin placed in a leaden one and "soldered up closely."

He requested that a "public notice be given of the period of his interment, but no invitation issued."

On December 21, 1837, Dr. Physick was sepulchered in the burying ground of Christ Church in Philadelphia. The procession included individuals from the university, students from Jefferson College, and representatives from several medical societies as well as politicians and the public. Among the arrangements attending his death was a "rigid watch being kept for six weeks during the night over the place of his interment and which it was said to be according to his directions, to prevent his body from being disturbed."

Dr. de Haviland wrote that Dr. Physick's peculiar instructions may be "very properly regretted by ... admirers of his reputation, as it was calculated to create obloquy and unjust suspicion against individuals, if not against his profession by leading the public to infer that no place nor person was too sacred for the anatomist."

However, Dr. Physick's greatest error, because he was a famous surgeon, was his "prohibition against the examination of his body after death, [which] may be considered as among the sentiments incompatible with his career of surgery and anatomy." This restriction and the severe instructions gave credibility to those who opposed the stealing of cadavers for anatomy research in two ways. First, no one was safe from these odious thieves of the dead no matter their position, because this famous surgeon gave instructions to protect his body. Who would know better the tactics of grave robbers than one who was or had colleagues that were their customers? Second, he did not want his body dissected, although he spent his professional life in the field of anatomy and surgery. This gave some credence to their opponents, who argued that those who engaged in dissection should be the first to volunteer themselves and their families as subjects rather than using the victims of grave robbers.

Unfortunately for de Haviland, he could offer no better excuse than that Physick had deviated from sound thinking on this matter, likely "produced by long continued retirement and indisposition."[59]

There was never a groundswell of physicians willing their bodies for dissection. According to one historian, there was a "medical tradition of private autopsies on the bodies of practitioners, often performed by friendly colleagues."[60] Nevertheless, it appears that these dissections were not the spectacles imagined when stolen bodies were used. One example was that of John Collins Warren, MD, the first dean of Harvard

Medical School. Prior to his death on May 4, 1856, he left a letter that was not to be opened until his death and before the funeral. In the letter he gave instructions that his body was to be injected with arsenic after his death. He was to be given a full funeral service at St. Paul's Church, and after the service his body was to be brought to the medical school and "examined or dissected according to circumstances." His bones were to be "carefully preserved, whitened, articulated, and placed in the lecture-room of the Medical College near my bust…." He asked that his family forgo "any natural feeling of opposition" to his final request because he was doing it in the "interest of humanity." In addition, he concluded that he hoped to "enjoy the society of our blessed friends who have gone before."[61]

It should be noted that his desire to have a full funeral service and his expectation of a life hereafter run contrary (even though he was not buried) to much of Crowell's earlier argument based on biblical authority. Perhaps it was Warren's way of demonstrating that not all physicians who engaged in dissection believed that burial of the body was a precondition for an afterlife and that even those engaged in this practice could still be believing Christians.[62]

Nevertheless, returning to Crowell's sermon, he does not give any quarter to the physicians who want to use the poor, strangers, or even volunteers for dissection. Crowell concludes that it is unchristian. Examples from the Old Testament and God's wrath toward those Jews who angered him include imagery in which the bodies and bones of "their kindred and friends" are "cast forth from the earth," not to be gathered up and buried. Crowell concluded that "from these maledictions we learn that not only is the want of a decent burial a great evil, but also to be taken out of the grave after we are buried."

Using the example of the punishment that God inflicted on those who disobeyed him, Crowell wrote that "in no case whatever, except that of criminals, is it proper, and right to omit sepulchering the dead?" As noted above, the dissection of "murderers and duelists" was legal in Massachusetts.

Crowell added that if any good can come from what is being done to the dead for society, "it must not be sought in the violation of the rights of the dead to a decent interment and repose unmolested." If a "particular good which yet cannot be obtained, by ordinary means, without sin, He [God] can easily work a miracle to effect it."[63]

In closing, Crowell spoke to his congregation and the assembled townspeople that they should "make every lawful effort" to bring the perpetrators of this "sacrilegious robbery of the dead" to justice and, if possible, "to repentance and reformation." To not take every "prudent and lawful measure, in such a case, to bring to justice the guilty authors of the deed, is to partake of their guilt." He praised them for "keeping their counsels with prudence and justice." He said that "suitable measures" had been taken "to expose the authors of it, and to restore, if possible, our wonted confidence in the security [of] the dead."[64]

Crowell finally turned to the task at hand, to "inter again those coffins which once contained the bodies of beloved friends, but which are now all that sacrilegious hands have left us, as memorials of them. As precious, though but poor relicts of the stolen dead, we will again inter them, and erect a monument upon their grave which shall declare to children's children the melancholy scene we have witnessed, and which may bid the hand of avarice beware of making merchandize of the dead."[65]

It is not without irony and is perhaps a pointed reference to Crowell's most famous sermon that at his funeral in 1855 a fellow minister wrote that "we bore his mortal remains to the neighboring cemetery, committing them earth to earth, ashes to ashes, dust to dust, there to rest with his sleeping congregation and arise with them in triumphant, glorious resurrection."[66]

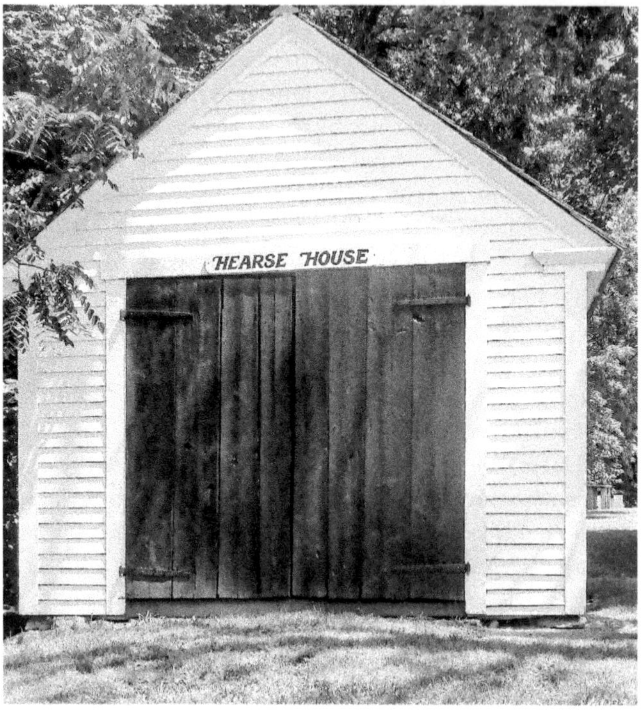

Present-day view of the Hearse House built in the mid-1800s in the "Old Burying Ground" in Essex, Massachusetts. The empty coffins of the stolen dead are believed to be buried under this building (photograph by the author).

The dogged and persistent resistance to body snatching was not simply possession of the relic of the departed for its own sake or to prevent the shame of dissection. There was a religious motivation against body snatching and dissection because it went against the most basic tenet of Christianity. This was articulated in April 1854 by Henry Raymond, editor of *Harper's New Monthly Magazine*, who wrote an editorial on the "sacredness of the human body." A good portion of the article discusses religion and dissection. There are also echoes of the arguments that Robert Crowell made in his sermon in 1818.

Raymond identified the core problem with the stealing of the dead and their dissection as an "increasing indifference to the grave and its sacred contents." There was an inherent disdain of the most basic tenet of the Christian religion, the resurrection of the body, as shown in the death and resurrection of Christ. Like Crowell, he saw the body as a shrine to the "human spirit." He concluded there are illnesses that are beyond discovery and should remain a mystery because trying to discover the cause is too high a price for the "best feelings of the soul."[67]

On the question of dissection, he saw the cutting up of the body as a dishonorable, humiliating, unwarranted abuse of the body itself.[68]

Other problems included the attitude of disrespect shown to the body itself in the laboratory by the physicians and their dissolute students and the focus on the poor as raw material for the dissection tables.[69]

The mainstream Protestant belief at this time in the actual resurrection of the physical body as fundamental to the founding of Christianity no doubt was one important motivating factor in the general opposition to body snatching, dissection, and reforms in the anatomy laws in antebellum America.

2

Dr. Thomas Sewall of Chebacco

The members of the Chebacco parish and the town of Ipswich were justifiably shocked to learn that they had been betrayed by their town physician, Thomas Sewall. Not only was he the town doctor, but he had also married into one of the most prominent families in Ipswich if not New England, the Choate family.

Thomas Sewall was born on April 16, 1786, in Hallowell, Maine. As a young boy he met Reuben D. Mussey, who was "courting his older sister Mary Sewall."[1] Reuben Mussey received his medical degree from Dartmouth College in 1803. Dr. Mussey became the town doctor in Ipswich. He married Mary Sewall on August 1, 1806, thus becoming Sewall's brother-in-law.[2] The two were not only brothers-in-law but were also later suspected of involvement in the selling of bodies. As noted, in Henry Bowditch's memoir of Amos Twitchell, while Mussey was attending Dartmouth, "deeds were to be done, either by myself, or by someone else, with my knowledge and full consent, but abhorrent to my inmost nature[;] … it was the absolute and fixed fate of every medical student to do this."[3]

Thomas Sewall first traveled to Ipswich to stay with his sister and brother-in-law. Likely, Sewall was planning on attending medical school. He studied medicine under a preceptor and began his practice in Chebacco in 1808, succeeding Dr. Mussey as town physician.[4] In 1810–1811 Sewall attended the Medical Department at the University of Pennsylvania, where Dr. Mussey had recently taken his second medical degree. In 1811–1812, Sewall attended Harvard Medical School and completed his MD in 1812.[5] (This was only the second year this degree was awarded. Only the bachelor of medicine was previously awarded.)[6] In 1812 he joined the Massachusetts Medical Society.[7]

While at Harvard, Sewall studied anatomy, and we learn from the eminent Dr. John C. Warren the atmosphere surrounding Sewall and perhaps expectations of a medical student while studying for his degree. Warren wrote that nothing gave him more "anxiety" than obtaining "subjects for dissection in his medical lecture." His father, John Warren, had himself resorted to body snatching as a student at Harvard. According to Edward M. Hartwell, the Anatomical Society and the Spunker club at Harvard were formed by John Warren. The club was a student organization whose purpose was to obtain subjects for anatomical instruction. According to a letter sent to John Warren prior to 1775 from another student, "as soon as the body of Levi Ames was pronounced dead by Dr. Jeffries, it was delivered by the sheriff to a person who carried it in a cart to the waterside, where it was received into a boat" on its way to Dorchester Point. "When we saw the boat at Dorchester Point, … Norwood, David, one Allen and myself took chaise [*sic*] and rode round to the Point, Spunker's like, but the many obstacles we had to encounter made it eleven o'clock before we reached the Point, where we searched ... in vain!... There was no corpse to be found.... [W]e have since heard that Stillman's gang rowed him back from the Point up to the town, and ... buried him—God knows where!"[8] Later as a physician during the American Revolutionary War, John Warren obtained numerous cadavers for dissection because of the many soldiers who died "without relations." However, when the war was over it became increasingly difficult to obtain subjects for his lectures at Harvard College. "Bodies of executed criminals were occasionally procured; and sometimes a pauper subject was obtained averaging not more than two a year."

While the younger John C. Warren was at Harvard College in 1796, he devised a plan to obtain more bodies for his father's lectures. He knew of a man who was to be buried in North Burying-Ground in Boston who had no relations. He and a Boston physician, Dr. William Ingersoll, went to the fresh grave at ten o'clock that evening but "were led to suspect a mistake and went to another place." They realized their mistake and returned to the original site. They "proceeded rapidly, uncovering the coffin by breaking it open. They took out the body of a stout young man, put it in a bag and carried the body to the graveyard wall. They saw a stranger approaching. Two other members of the group distracted the stranger and led him away. When they returned the body was loaded on a carriage between two of the grave robbers who drove off to Cambridge with their booty."

Warren and another member remained behind to fill in the grave. Warren's partner became "alarmed" and quickly fled the cemetery. He noted that "the importance of covering up the grave and effacing the vestiges of our labor, remained, with no very agreeable sensations, to finish the work." He finished up and drove off with the tools and arrived in Cambridge before daylight. When his father found out just before his morning lecture that his son had been involved in this "scrape, he was much alarmed." When he saw the uncovered body and "what a fine healthy subject it was, he seemed to be as much pleased." The body lasted for the entire course.[9] Warren wrote that things went along this way (body snatching?) until 1806, when he opened a dissecting room in Boston, a private facility not under the scrutiny of the public. "Here, with the aid of students a large supply of bodies was obtained for some years, affording abundant means of dissection to physicians and students."[10]

Even so, conditions were changing as more medical schools were opening in New England. Students were being sent to Boston to obtain bodies, and body snatchers became careless. The police became suspicious. Watchers were sent to the burial grounds. Obtaining bodies locally became dangerous, and their number quickly "diminished." The schools resorted to acquiring bodies from New York. This was a "great expense," and there was a "great hazard of being discovered." Two or three times their agents were arrested by the police and had to appear in court. The punishment for a finding of guilty was a fine. Warren remarked that law officers were more liberal than the city officials, and the former tried to "make the penalty as small as possible." Nevertheless, it was a constant effort "to carry on this business, and every species of danger was involved in its prosecution."[11]

Warren related two incidents that occurred during this time demonstrating the danger in body snatching. He asked two students to obtain a subject for dissection. The two students observed a body being taken from the "Alms-house to the burial ground on the Neck, which was appropriated exclusively for the interment of paupers." They marked the grave by placing "a piece of stick on it." After midnight, they waited for the watch to appear and leave. They opened the grave, removed the body, and filled in the grave. One of the students went into town to procure a pre-engaged wagon. The other student remained behind awaiting the wagon. As they tried to remove the body "a group of watchmen" came after them. One student was seized, and the other hopped on the wagon, "laid a lash upon his horse, and went off at full speed, dragging with him two or three watchmen some distance."

The student managed to lose the watchmen and headed for the countryside. His partner escaped his captors by bolting into Boston's Back Bay (then a marsh). The watchmen raised the alarm; "their rattles filled the town with their cries, set all bells a-ringing." The student "to his great enjoyment … heard all the riot, of which he was the object." Eventually he approached a toll house, and as he tried to pay the toll he was recognized and recaptured. He escaped again and hid in a "mass of shavings" where a house was being constructed. He finally made his way home. The other student had a "quiet time in the country and the next morning returned … unsuspected to the town." The student who drove the carriage he called F did not continue in the medical profession and instead turned to business and was still "living, in good health and prosperity." The other student he called T in trying to escape the watchmen "brought on a hemorrhage from his lungs." He appeared to be a "stout and well-formed young man," but later "the complaint, followed by a cough, … terminated in consumption and carried him to a premature grave."[12]

At times "popular excitement was got up," and the medical college was threatened. Warren feared attacks on his home as well. When the dissection lectures approached "a state of incessant anxiety came with them." The pressure became so great that the medical men decided to resolve it through legislation, although at the time Warren felt that "there would be little hope of success."[13]

It was during this time that Thomas Sewall attended Harvard and took his course in anatomy. He likely participated in grave robbing while at Harvard, and it was even more likely that he and Dr. Mussey carried on a trade in stolen bodies until Dr. Sewall was caught stealing eight bodies from the Chebacco burying ground in 1818.[14] As Bentley wrote, "As to Sewall in his profession he was a partner of Mussey of Dartmouth College & could boast he could get 50 dollars for every body he disturbed. He was the grave digger of the Club."[15]

Oddly enough, in a court case in Manchester, Massachusetts (see Chapter 3), Dr. Grosvenor of Manchester was accused of not paying a note of $50 to Dr. Mussey. Dr. Mussey was questioned. "Did you ever put into the hands of Dr. Thomas Sewall, of Ipswich, any demand you had against Dr. David Grosvenor of Manchester, for collection?" Dr. Mussey answered somewhat cryptically, "I did; a note for fifty dollars signed to me by said Grosvenor. And further saith not."

Dr. Mussey did not volunteer any information on what the note was for, but the questioner said he asked it for another purpose, so the question itself was "irrelevant to the deposition," and he did not follow up any further. Given what William Bentley has written regarding the value of a body at that time and the involvement of Sewall and Mussey and that all three doctors were involved, it seems likely that this could have been a note for the sale of a cadaver for dissection.[16]

Thomas Sewall managed to ingratiate himself with one of the most prominent families in Ipswich. He became a boarder at the home of Miriam Choate, whose husband David had died in 1808. Sewall followed Dr. Rueben Mussey, who had been a member of the Choate household for several years previously. Like Dr. Mussey, Sewall tutored Miriam Choate's two sons, David Jr. and Rufus Choate, especially in Latin as well as other subjects. Sewall developed a close relationship with Rufus Choate and courted his sister Mary Choate, whom he married on November 13, 1813.[17]

As befits one of the town elites, Dr. Sewall began playing an important role in town governance. "In October 1816, Sewall was appointed treasurer of the parish."[18] In January 1818, oddly enough when the grave robbing incident first appeared, he served on an important committee that eventually succeeded in "separating Chebacco from Ipswich and incorporating it as the town of Essex." Yet, while on the committee Dr. Sewall served alongside men with familiar names who were likely relatives of the people he had been digging up. The graves that were robbed were those of William Burnham, Samuel Burnham, Elisha Story, and Sally Andrews. Nathaniel Burnham, Captain Francis Burnham, Jacob Burnham, Jonathan Story, Jacob Story, Joseph Story, and Elias Andrews served on the committee. By his marriage to Mary Choate, Sewall's actions would be especially embarrassing to three other members of the committee: George Choate, Nathan Choate, and Colonel John P. Choate.[19]

Dr. Sewall, a prominent member of the community, had a secret life. It is difficult to know who was aware of his grave-robbing activities. It is not clear how long he had been digging up the local dead, but one of the empty graves was that of Cesar Conway, a former slave freed in 1775 who was buried in 1811.[20]

Christopher Benedetto raised the question of why Sewall would have removed seven bodies during a six-month period from October 1817 to March 1818. Benedetto wrote that the weather was unusually mild during this time and that conditions were appropriate for grave robbing.[21] I wrote earlier that it was known that Sewall claimed he could get $50 per body (adjusted for inflation, over $1,000 in 2022). It was certainly a lucrative side business for the doctor and must have been worth the risk. Sewall may have dissected some of the bodies, but at this time there was a market for fresh bodies.[22]

Grave robbing for the use of private instructors teaching their students and for "physicians occurred at all seasons of the year except the hot months of the summer." However, the acquisition of bodies for the medical colleges in New England was dependent on their sessions. New England colleges held their sessions primarily from early November until February. Some schools gave spring sessions that lasted from early March to late May. Sewall and any partners, if he had any, might have seen the mild weather as opportune, allowing them to acquire more bodies than through a normal winter and benefit from both the demands of independent

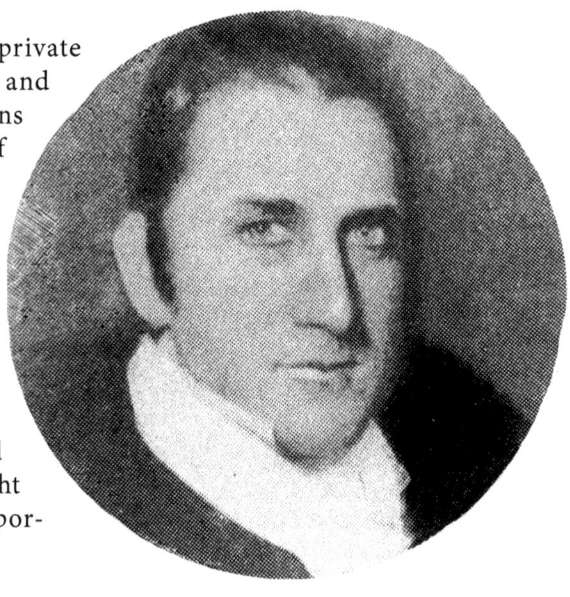

Portrait of Dr. Thomas Sewall (National Library of Medicine).

physicians and the competition from the medical schools at the precise time they needed fresh bodies during their anatomy sessions.[23]

Surely Sewall would have justified his actions of robbing the Chebacco burying ground and perhaps disinterring his own patients for himself. In the words of John C. Warren, "the surgeon and the teacher have a high moral duty to perform to their patients and the community; and, in the eye of reason and religion, they will be less culpable for preserving articles [cadavers] so very important and useful, than if, through fear or neglect, they allowed them to be wasted in the bottom of a grave."[24]

An Act to Protect the Sepulchers of the Dead

Unfortunately for Dr. Sewall, the Massachusetts legislature had passed a law titled "Act to Protect the Sepulchers of the Dead" in 1815, only a few years before he was accused. The act was a result of the activities described earlier by John C. Warren regarding the increased boldness of medical students and others in grave robbing. In addition, the people expected that body snatching would only get worse with the increase in the number of medical schools in New England and more "private dissecting rooms" opening in Boston. There was also "a bitter public discussion over the petition to establish a medical school in Boston" and over a legislative grant request by Harvard to build a "new building for the Medical School." The public demanded that something be done "to prevent the robbery of graves."[25]

The latter had led to an earlier legislative act passed on February 13, 1812, that obligated the sheriffs of jails to either give the dead bodies to relatives or friends of the deceased or ensure that they received a proper burial. If not, the penalty was either fines or imprisonment.[26]

The Act to Protect the Sepulchers of the Dead quickly followed on March 2, 1815. There were basically three parts to the act. The first was "that if any person not being authorized by the Board of Health or selectmen of any town in the Commonwealth shall knowingly and willfully dig up, remove or carry away, or did assist in digging up, removing or carrying away any human body, or the remains ... shall on conviction of such an offense ... be imprisoned not more than one year, or fined, not more than one thousand dollars according to the nature of the offense." The second part criminalized any "person or persons who knowingly and willfully receive, conceal, or dispose of any human body or the remains thereof, which shall have been dug up or carried away as described in the first section of this Act, he or they shall be subject to the forfeitures and penalties as in said section as provided on conviction in the court aforesaid." The final section notes that all fines collected were to be distributed "one-half to the informer, one-half to the town in which the offense was committed."[27]

What had previously fallen under the purview of common law had now been codified into statute. The conflict with this new law was that the Massachusetts legislature had given the Massachusetts medical community the power to require that all on entry into the practice of medicine had to have "an adequate knowledge of anatomy," a knowledge that could only be acquired by dissection.[28]

The act did not constitute a complete legal barrier to dissection, although one physician summarized it thus: "A man who is found with a human body for dissection shall be considered guilty of a felony."[29] Because of this new law, medical men in Boston turned to other means of obtaining dead bodies both legally and illegally. Legally, cadavers could still be obtained through the courts upon the execution of convicted criminals. For example, when Dr. John C. Warren and Nathaniel Niles requested the bodies of four criminals, the court ordered that the four bodies be turned over to Warren but required that he accommodate Niles "with one of said bodies." Illegally, one procurer explained, "the place where I generally obtain them [dead bodies] is the Charlestown Hospital—where through the kindness of Dr. T. it is wholly unattended with the unpleasant circumstances & risks usually connected with such business." As noted previously, another option was to obtain bodies from New York or even Philadelphia, thus avoiding the danger of being caught in a local cemetery.[30]

Nevertheless, there were simply not enough bodies to meet the demand, and cadavers continued to be obtained both locally and illegally. This explains why Dr. Sewall was involved in this practice, but it does not explain why he thought the wholesale removal of the local townspeople in the town burying ground would go unnoticed (see below).

The Trial of Dr. Thomas Sewall

According to the newspaper accounts carried in Salem (about twelve miles away) and later accounts based on these reports on April 17, 1818, a newspaper article appeared officially (although rumors abounded) alerting the public to what had happened in Chebacco titled "Exhumation of the Dead. Great excitement prevails in Chebacco because it was discovered that no less than eight bodies have been taken from the graveyard. They adopt methods for detecting the person or persons concerned in the act."[31]

There are no records detailing what occurred in Sewall's trial or of his defense by Daniel Webster. We have some limited documentation and commentary by outsiders who appear to express accounts they learned in the courtroom proceedings. The proceedings were extended over a two-year period. The Supreme Judicial Court of the Commonwealth of Massachusetts first met on this case on April 28, 1818. The case was delayed to November 3, 1818, and the justices postponed the case again until April 1819. The court levied its decision in November 1819.

First Session, April 28, 1818

The Supreme Judicial Court of the Commonwealth of Massachusetts convened in Ipswich on April 28, 1818. A grand jury produced one bill against Sewall for receiving a human body:

> On the first day of September now last past, with force and arms at Ipswich aforesaid in the County aforesaid did knowingly and willfully receive, conceal, and dispose of a certain human body and the remains thereof which human body had been there and there recently dug up removed and carried away by some evil minded person or persons to the Jurors aforesaid unknown, the said person or persons not being authorized by the board of Health or the Selectmen of any town in this Commonwealth to dig up or remove or carry away the same, against the peace of said Commonwealth and against ... [the] statute in such case made and provided.[32]

On April 29, "the Justices summoned" Miriam Choate, Sewall's mother-in-law, and his two brothers-in-law David and Washington Choate "who lived with Dr. Sewall and ten other individuals from Chebacco to testify." Although there is no record of these proceedings, it appears "it was ... sufficient to indict Dr. Sewall...." On May 2, he was "notified by the sheriff, Michael Brown, to appear before the Supreme Court in November to answer charges against him."[33]

Bentley wrote in his diary in May 1818 that the "disturbing of the Dead has given great alarm at Chebacco. Eight graves have been found without the bodies. A Dr. Sewall has been charged with it [and] a bill has been found by the Grand Jury. The case is to come on at the next November term. Many towns have been alarmed." Bentley specifically mentions "Dr. Sewall is Brother-in-Law [*sic*] to Mussey."[34]

Second Session November 1818

Dr. Sewall hired Daniel Webster to defend him. The fee for his defense was $100, noted on November 13, 1818, in Webster's private correspondence.[35] The period following Sewall's accusation must have been a difficult time for him and the Choate family, especially after Crowell's sermon on July 23, 1818, and the burying of the eight empty coffins. Dr. Reuben Mussey wrote to Miriam Choate that she and the family had been "called ... to severe trials ... as of late" and that "even though 'some of your neighbors reproach you and your family, you have a thousand friends ... as attached to you ever.'"[36]

On November 3, 1818, Thomas Sewall and his attorneys, Daniel Webster and Asa Andrews of Ipswich, appeared at the Supreme Judicial Court in Salem, Massachusetts, for the second session. The first indictment read "Thomas Sewall, Ipswich Physician," on the "twelfth day of January A.D. 1818 with force and arms ... [did] ... conceal and dispose of the human body and remains ... of Sally Andrews ... [who] had been recently dug up removed and carried away by some evil disposed person or persons." The jurors could not identify these persons, so as noted above Sewall was not charged with grave robbing itself but rather receiving and concealing the body of Sally Andrews.[37] The second indictment read the same for the "human body" of William Burnham, except the charges noted above occurred on January 10, 1818.[38]

As for the other bodies, there were no further indictments probably because there were no remains identifiable or the cadavers had been sold to other doctors (perhaps in Boston). Daniel Days, the solicitor general, decided not to prosecute a third indictment; the court noted that the indictment was "inaccurately drawn and there being two other indictments found at this term against the defendant for the same offence, the Solicitor General says he will no further prosecute this indictment."[39]

The community was shocked by the testimony heard during the trial. On November 7, 1818, Bentley wrote, "The affair of Sewall the Grave hunter at Chebacco has his hearing in this term. The graves were robbed without decency & bodies dragged from their deposits by ropes." He noted there was possibly a trade in bodies. "It was supposed it was a matter of traffic as may be seen at the report today."[40] On November 10, 1818, he wrote, "We learn that Dr. Sewall of Chebacco pleaded guilty of violating the graves of that place. It was believed that the grave of a suicide had been violated in Salem but to relieve the public mind a search was made, and the body found where left. The fact discovers into what agitation the indiscretion of this man has thrown the public mind." He concluded that now the public would be suspicious of all doctors.[41]

On November 12, 1818, Bentley recorded that "Sewall the grave searcher has been pursued with great indignation. The Court has delayed the trial till April Term which will give him the opportunity to abscond, but at Ipswich not to be more patiently heard." Bentley suggests that he would probably have to leave Ipswich due to his nefarious activities that created such bitterness toward him. "The truth seems to be that the practice had become so common of opening graves that the common cautions were neglected or forgotten. Sewall took a row of graves without missing one & left appearance on the surface which obliged suspicion." Bentley concluded that "to the study of Anatomy in our Colleges, the frequent use of dissection, and the reputation of the study abroad must be imputed both the suspicion & the practice."[42] Finally, on November 19, 1818, he wrote, "Sewall's matter of the Graves has passed out of all conversation, since his Case is put off. We are told the Court has adjourned till after Thanksgiving."[43]

The trial was continued to April 1819 and again to the November 1819 term. Daniel Webster and Asa Andrews defended Sewall and argued that the commonwealth "ought not further impeach or molest him" because the matter was "insufficient in law to put him, the said Sewall to answer to said Indictment … and that he may be discharged from the Court here." The solicitor general of the commonwealth argued that the indictment "is good and sufficient in law" to have Sewall "answer to the same."[44]

The November 1819 Session

The indictment was continued from April 1819 to the November term 1819. On November 12, 1819, Bentley reported that the "Essex Sewall grave affair [Chebacco had since been incorporated as the town of Essex, Massachusetts] is not settled by the sentence of the judge. The friends of Sewall plead his health that he might not be present at the sentence, but the Judge excused no absence. We shall soon have the event."[45] On November 29 the court met, and Bentley wrote, "Dr. Sewall … was fined 4 Hundred Dollars for each offense in removing bodies from their graves which he did in a most shameful manner."[46]

Interestingly, throughout his commentary on the Sewall trial, Bentley was focused on body snatching as a more serious issue, probably because to him, as a minister, body snatching was seen as sacrilegious and a higher crime.

However, the record shows that Sewall was convicted on the charge of "possession rather than disinterment" of Sally Andrews and William Burnham.[47] Sewall's punishment according to the court was that "and now all and singular the premises [legal action, complaint] being seen, and by the Court have fully understood and mature advisement being thereon had, the Court are of the opinion that the indictment is good and sufficient in law. It is therefore considered by the Court … [that] Thomas Sewall [is to] pay a fine to be appropriated according to the law of four hundred dollars, [for each case] that he pays costs of prosecution and stand committed till sentence be performed."[48]

The fine of eight hundred dollars was a significant sum and the maximum amount according to law. Sewall was lucky he was not imprisoned. The fine was likely a signal to discourage others who would trade in the dead. With these convictions, there was little doubt that Sewall would have to leave his medical practice in Essex.[49]

Although Daniel Webster had lost the case, perhaps his arguments had kept Sewall out of prison and had the charge of body snatching dropped to "possession of a body." As one physician later wrote, "Only Mr. Websters ingenious eloquence, sympathy, devotion averted prison ! [*sic*] but not exile beyond the circle of distressed, harrowed, friends of the violated dead, and of public sentiment" and object of curses. "Dr. Thomas Sewall was driven, in his household's apprehension and dismay from his native Ipswich, Massachusetts, to Washington, D.C." Daniel Webster at the time was a member of Congress and invited the disgraced physician to Washington, D.C. The former was grateful for "Daniel Webster's, good will and furtherance, which our profession gratefully acknowledges."[50]

Sewall moved to Washington, D.C., during the winter of 1819–1820.[51] He paid his fine of $250 to William Andrews, Jr., and the rest of his fines to the treasurer of the County of Essex for the Commonwealth of Massachusetts. "It appears all the fines assessed by the Court were paid" and his "accounts settled on February 20, 1820."[52] Sewall did not remain quiet. Between March 1820 and June 1822, he sued some of his former patients and his victims' families including Ebenezer Andrews, the older brother of Sally Andrews. When "eight other defendants failed to appear in court ... the justices awarded Dr. Sewall over $200 in damages. It appears that no one paid Sewall."[53]

Unfortunately for the Choates and especially Dr. Sewall, they had to live among their neighbors. Obviously, Sewell's medical practice in Essex was ruined. As to the elites such as the Choate family, Bentley summed it up nicely: "The evils in our County from the pretended great in it are blots on our escutcheon."[54]

When Sewall first arrived in Washington, we learn of his state of mind. Although his wife and son were still in Essex, he wrote to Rufus Choate on March 18, 1820, inviting him to Washington. "We shall here be surrounded by the best of friends and acquaintances, while the family at Essex will be forsaken and surrounded by wolves and tigers on every side!"[55]

We should not be surprised by the local reaction to Sewall's crime. Religion still played an important role in the lives of these people. Only recently, in Ipswich there had been a religious revival (this was going on throughout the country). In June 1817 the members of the Second Congregational Church in Ipswich numbered nineteen; six new members were admitted, including Captain Samuel Burnham and Captain Frank Burnham.[56] There was religious ferment by other sects and denominations beginning to openly question the privileges of the Congregational Church as the only officially established church in Massachusetts (it was not disestablished until 1833).[57] Nevertheless, there is little doubt that the "moral and social" views of the people remained unchanged even for those not in the Congregational Church. One minister writing of an earlier period, which I believe is relevant to this situation, stated that the "transgressor was made to feel himself odious to the whole community, a blot upon its fair name and a disgrace to himself and his friends." Public opinion "drew the line sharply between good and evil and no one was left in doubt as to which he would be expected to choose."[58] Clearly as we have seen, the good doctor had to leave Exeter and pursue his medical career elsewhere.

It was fortunate that Sewall, under the auspices of Daniel Webster, relocated to Washington, D.C. Unlike many of the cities and towns of New England, with their rigid society and social mores, Washington was a more welcoming city in 1820. One traveler described Washington thusly: "This skeleton city affords few of the amusements of a metropolis. It seems however to possess the advantage of very choice society; the resident families are of course few, but the unceasing influx and reflux of strangers from all parts of the country affords an ample supply of new faces to the evening drawing rooms. To this continual intermixture with strangers and foreigners is perhaps to be ascribed the peculiar courtesy and easy politeness which characterize the manners of the city."[59] As we will see in a later chapter on Washington, D.C., it was a perfect environment in which to start over for Dr. Thomas Sewall, convicted receiver of stolen bodies.

3

"Witnessing angels sorrowfully turned their faces aside"

Coincident with the uproar over the body snatching in Ipswich, the neighboring town of Manchester, Massachusetts (its official name today is Manchester by the Sea), found itself in turmoil over accusations that the town minister, Reverend James Thurston, had attempted to attract a young doctor to the town by promising him bodies for dissection.[1]

The betrayal by local elites of their community, as was the case with Dr. Sewall, does not compare to that of James Thurston, minister of the Congregational Church in Manchester. He was the spiritual leader of his community, and his actions seemed more damning to his flock than the actions of a physician such as Thomas Sewall.

To understand why and how this was significant, some background on town and church relations in Manchester is necessary. The area that became Manchester was originally populated at the time of John Winthrop's settlement in 1629. It was called Jeffrey's Creek and was part of Salem, Massachusetts. In 1645 the inhabitants petitioned the Massachusetts General Court to separate from Salem. They called the new town Manchester, as many of the inhabitants had come from Manchester, England.[2] Manchester borders the Atlantic Ocean and the Massachusetts towns of Beverly, Gloucester, and Ipswich, which included Chebacco.[3]

There was no separation between church and state in Massachusetts until 1833. The town "called the minister, voted his salary, built the meeting house, and set apart ministerial lands, planned his ordination, in short transacted all business involved in ecclesiastical relations ... that would later be transferred to the parish. The town was the parish. The ministerial tax was levied on the taxable property irrespective of creed or religious preference."[4]

Manchester clergy had a history of strict Calvinism and congregationalism. It was not until 1792 that church members voted that the minister "Baptize all children who Shall be offered upon what is called the Half Covenant."[5] This controversy was settled in most congregations in the last third of the seventeenth century, although in its time it led to much dissension in the Congregational Churches of New England.[6]

Following the death of the long-serving minister Ebenezer Tappan in 1790, Manchester entered a period of difficulty retaining ministers. Following Tappan's death, the town saw the premature death of the next minister in 1794, an interregnum (1794–1801) with at least forty ministers, and a new minister installed in 1801 and his dismissal in August of 1808. Yet, the town soldiered on and built a new meetinghouse. In 1809 the town hired Reverend James Thurston.[7]

The sermon given on the day of Thurston's installation augured well for him. He was told that he possessed the "appropriate talents and are receiving the charge of the people." The advice by the Reverend Dr. Manasseh Cutler to Thurston was "keep thyself pure, supporting the expectation of the office and give no offence in anything, that the ministry be not blamed." He continued, "Church and Christian society ... with ... unanimity, invited you to and be their minister."[8]

If only Thurston had taken the advice of his fellow clergyman. As the town historian, Reverend Darius F. Lamson, later wrote, cryptically and without explanation, a series of events tore the town and church apart and forced Thurston's dismissal on July 9, 1819. "Thurston's pastorate seemed bright with promise.... But the day that dawned so bright, was soon clouded, and Mr. Thurston's pastorate was on the whole a stormy one. An unfortunate cause of misunderstanding arose, criminations and recriminations followed, and witnessing angels sorrowfully turned their faces aside."[9]

The parishioners made eight charges against the minister. The most serious was that he wished to entice another physician to Manchester and attempted to persuade the physician to settle there by promising that "he might have a fine opportunity for private dissection in Manchester, as there would not be the least difficulty in obtaining subjects there."

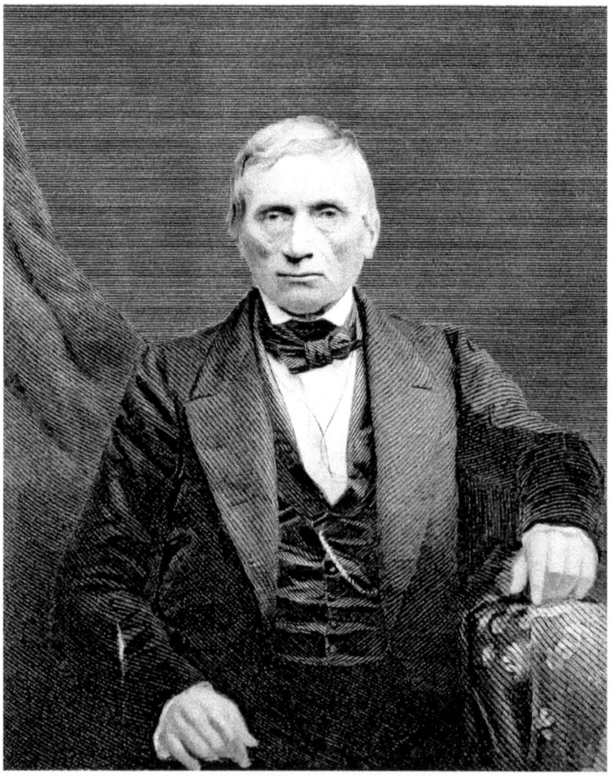

"Doct. Dewey he might have a fine opportunity for private dissections in Manchester, as there would not be the least difficulty in obtaining subjects there." Dr. Mussey's letter to Dr. Sewall set off a great commotion in Manchester, Massachusetts. Portrait of Dr. Reuben D. Mussey (National Library of Medicine).

Other related charges included that Thurston had pretended to go on a journey to see the doctor he was alleged to have invited to town to obtain a letter "to exonerate him" and that he had "forged a false letter" from the doctor, "which he sent to his home and circulated among his friends to show that he had not invited" this doctor "or offered him the inducement of an opportunity for private dissection in Manchester."[10] Additionally, reports circulated of "such a nature as tended to bring the members of the church as a Christian society, into disrepute."[11]

The charges concerning the business of dissection originated in a letter written by Dr. Reuben D. Mussey, chair of anatomy and surgery at Dartmouth College and former brother-in-law to the now notorious Dr. Thomas Sewall.[12] Somehow the information in the letter was leaked. Tyler

Parsons, a church committee member investigating charges against Thurston, called on Dr. Sewall to examine the letter and to make a copy:

Hanover, October 26, 1818

To Doct. Thomas Sewall

Doct. Dewey was in town the other day, and on reference to your difficulties, [accused of grave robbing] he repeated his surprise that the Rev. Mr. Thurston has interested himself so ardently against you; inasmuch as he urged him to tarry at Manchester in the capacity of a physician, by a motive which seems to be in opposition to the course he is now taking. He told Doct. Dewey he might have a fine opportunity for private dissections in Manchester, as there would not be the least difficulty in obtaining subjects there.

Yours, &c.
Reuben D. Massey[13]

Parsons wrote to Dr. Mussey on November 18, 1818, stating that Dr. Sewall's letter had been made known to Mr. Thurston. "He has denied the conversation between him and Dr. Dewey." Parsons was told that Thurston expected to get an affidavit from him. Parsons wrote, "Dr. Dewey's testimony ... will be of the first importance to the inhabitants of Manchester. I shall not be disappointed if Mr. Thurston is found guilty of the conversation with Dr. Dewey, and also of denying the same."[14]

Parsons was out to get Thurston, as shown in the last sentence. Parsons also wanted Dewey's testimony because he believed it would show that Thurston was immoral, unchristian, and a liar. It would be crucial in helping him force Thurston from his position. There were some in town who did not think a minister of God would promise such an unchristian and immoral act to attract a doctor; however, there were plenty among the church members and parishioners who had been induced "to believe that Thurston was a bad citizen, a bad minister, and a bad man."[15]

Dr. Mussey's reply to Thurston on November 28, 1818, is of interest because he does not understand why Dr. Dewey's remarks in his letter to Sewall were "made known to Mr. Thurston." However, he does not doubt that the doctor's statement is true even if Mr. Thurston now denies it. Mussey wrote that perhaps Thurston "has forgotten the conversation" that it struck him "that a gentleman should offer to one physician the facility of obtaining and dissecting dead bodies, as an inducement for him to settle in his parish and persecute another physician [Sewall] with unremitted zeal for the same thing, even before any adequate evidence was obtained of the fact. But men, even good men, often act inconsistently, and it may be argued in Mr. Thurston's favor, that he has had time to change his views upon the subject."

Dr. Mussey's latter assessment of Thurston is hardly something church members and parishioners would find acceptable in a minister and is thinly veiled sarcasm on his part. Mussey does not want to become involved in this dispute. He rightly says that Thurston wants to "put the most favorable construction upon the whole of his conduct. Whether Dewey may think it worthwhile to give an affidavit in confirmation of his statement, I do not know—nor does it particularly interest me to know; but I presume he will never deny any thing I have stated." Further, "I am of opinion, that no one who is acquainted with me, will charge me with falsehood or misrepresentation in this thing; should this, however, be the case, I shall be ready, when legally called upon, to make oath; the statement which I mentioned in my letter to Dr. Sewall, as coming from Dr. Dewey."

However, if Parsons wanted an affidavit, Dr. Mussey suggested that "your best way is to write to Dr. Dewey for it." He concluded that "about the time I wrote Dr. Sewall, he [Dewey] passed through this town, on his return homeward from a long journey; he will probably not be again in Hanover for many months."[16]

According to Parsons the enmity between Thurston and the current town physician, Dr. Grosvenor, began shortly after Thurston arrived and began interfering with Dr. Grosvenor's "medicine and practice." The two were frequently "at odds with each other." Thurston was "peculiarly ungrateful" and "vengeful" and began "speaking in a sarcastic manner from the desk [lectern]."[17]

Dr. Grosvenor was well liked in Manchester and was a member of the church. He had begun his medical practice in 1810 shortly after Thurston's installation. We are never told exactly what Dr. Grosvenor in his medical practice had done to earn Thurston's animosity.

An affidavit by Captain John Girdler provides some background about Thurston's invitation to Dr. Dewey, the affront to the town, and Thurston's attempt at damage control. Girdler related how Thurston had called on his sick sister knowing that Dr. Grosvenor was attending her. Thurston told her that she would soon be "relieved from the imposition of Dr. Grosvenor's medicine and practice, for there was a physician on his way to town." It was believed that it was Dr. Dewey that "Mr. Thurston alluded to."

A second source, Major Burely Smith, said that when he moved back to town in 1815, he found Thurston and Dr. Grosvenor feuding as usual. When Dewey came to Manchester, Thurston brought him to his house and told him that Dr. Dewey came to Manchester to establish himself "in the line of his profession as a doctor." Thurston left the two men, and Dewey confided that he understood that Dr. Grosvenor had "but little practice in town." He wanted to know if he should be encouraged "to settle in Manchester, as a physician." Smith, having only recently returned to town, said he could offer no opinion. Dewey replied that after speaking with other leading citizens of the town, no one "would give me an opinion on this.... I should not like to settle in any place, where I could not be useful to myself and society generally." Smith said that he would make further inquiries and a few days later reported that "Dr. Grosvenor had no intention of leaving town; and that Mr. Thurston and Doct. Grosvenor were at variance."[18]

Smith was concerned that this feud would harm the town and tried to determine the cause and resolve the issues between the two men. As there was much talk about Dr. Dewey coming to Manchester, Smith asked Thurston if he had invited the doctor there. Thurston said that "he had no agency in it whatever."

Nevertheless, Smith reasoned that if the dispute was not settled, "Doct. Dewey would not tarry, and Grosvenor perhaps would remove to get rid of the noise."[19] Smith spoke to both men. Thurston would not meet with Dr. Grosvenor, so Smith asked him if a letter pointing out "the way and manner this thing shall be settled" was amenable to him. He agreed. Then Thurston told him that "you must not let Grosvenor know that I have any desire to have difficulties settled." After hearing this, Smith said that it "confirmed in his mind" that "Thurston ... was a bad man, and a dangerous man in the community."

Dr. Grosvenor wrote a letter to Thurston, who refused him a reply and "appeared indifferent about the business." Smith decided to drop the matter. When Dr. Dewey returned to ask him what he had found out about his settling in town, Smith told him that "the inhabitants of Manchester are determined to support Doct. Grosvenor." Dewey thanked him for his "candor."[20]

The following day after church, Thurston invited Smith to his house in the evening. Soon after arriving at Thurston's home, Thurston began talking about Dr. Grosvenor in a "reproachful manner." Thurston said that Dr. Dewey was from a good family and was a "man of the first medical talents for his age." Thurston then asked Smith if he had told Dr. Dewey "that if he settled here his encouragement was small or nothing." Thurston said that Dr. Dewey had informed him of this the prior evening and that "he was going to leave the town in the morning for that reason."[21]

It appears that Thurston was set on the young doctor, a modern doctor and one trained with dissecting experience.[22] Perhaps Thurston thought he could entice Dr. Dewey by emphasizing the possibility of private dissection and implying he would not give the young doctor any trouble if his acquisition of bodies was discreet. Unfortunately, we do not know how successful Grosvenor's medical methods were (although he did seem to have the support of the town), but it appears that Thurston thought an improvement was needed and perhaps that he was criticizing Grosvenor's practice when he was quoted as saying "there would not be the least difficulty in obtaining subjects there," implying he lost many patients.[23]

Thurston informed Smith that because Dr. Dewey was leaving town he had "ruined" him and his family. Smith said to Thurston that he had tried to end the feud between him and Dr. Grosvenor and even told people that Thurston had no "agency" in bringing the doctor to town, telling them "neither did you know of his coming here, as you said before he came here."

Smith told him many people believed Thurston had knowingly lied when he said that he did not know of Dr. Dewey's impending visit and that he had advised Dr. Dewey to leave town. Thurston then accused Dr. Grosvenor of being a cheat and claimed he had bilked Dr. Mussey out of fifty dollars (this was a lie, as Dr. Grosvenor had an affidavit from Dr. Sewall certifying he received the payment from Grosvenor to Mussey). Smith replied that "if Dr. Grosvenor is such a man as you represent him to be, then you have got the devil in your church."

Smith advised Thurston to "settle his difficulties" with Dr. Grosvenor "or I believed he would have to leave the town himself." Thurston retorted that "before I will muckle to Doct. Grosvenor, or any of this people, I will lose the last drop of my heart's blood, for you are a covetous, malicious, and Indian set of people." Smith concluded his testimony: "being treated by Mr. Thurston in such a manner, and his disposition that he shewed me at his house, such malicious, wicked, and impious language astonished me, coming from a priest."[24]

Thurston Attempts Damage Control

The fact that Thurston attempted to bring another doctor to Manchester was an affront to many people in the town. However, when news of the "dissection business" began circulating about the same time as gossip and reports in the newspapers of Dr. Sewall's grave robbing and trial, Thurston found himself on the defensive.[25]

As for his invitation to Dr. Dewey, Captain John Girdler had earlier told Thurston he was not employed by the town "to invite physicians here into town nor turn them out of town." He also reported on the circumstances of Mussey's letter to Sewall dated October 26, 1818, on "Thurston's being charged with this conversation with Dewey about the dissection business, that it was the letter from Mussey that created serious difficulties." Girdler and others spoke to Thurston on this matter, and "he denied ever having any conversation on the subject of dissections with Doct. Dewey … and insinuated … this letter from Mussey was got up by some one probably in Manchester, for to ruin him and his family."[26]

Thurston raised an interesting question. Why would Dr. Mussey commit to paper such a damaging accusation when he knew Dr. Sewall's trial had been moved to November 1818 (a verdict was not rendered until the following November). Is it possible that Dr. Sewall showed someone the letter to get back at Thurston. As Dr. Mussey later said in his affidavit on March 15, 1820, in a conversation with Dr. Dewey, "I stated to him Dr. Sewall's difficulties at Ipswich, and the strong part the Rev. Mr. Crowell of that place and the Rev. Mr. Thurston, of Manchester had taken against Doctor Sewall."

Thurston offered Dewey "among other inducements for him to remain in Manchester, the facility of procuring subjects, [from the cemetery?], and of prosecuting private dissections there."[27] The truth concerning the procuring of bodies for dissection hinged on Dr. Dewey's testimony.

After Thurston told Girdler that the dissection charge was made to ruin his family, Girdler went to Chebacco to obtain the original letter from Dr. Sewall for the purpose of showing it to Thurston so that he could have an opportunity to "acquit himself."

Thurston said he would visit with Dr. Dewey and obtain proof that would "exhonerate [*sic*] him." The records indicate that Thurston and his wife went on a pretended journey; he was gone for less than a week. On his return he was asked if the trip had been successful. He replied that "some future time would explain the enquiry more perfectly."

Girdler never received any "satisfaction" from Thurston, including his "pretended journey in the country notwithstanding." Soon after, Thurston sent for Girdler and asked if he had the "original letter written by Doct. Mussey to Doct. Sewall, in [his] possession." When Girdler replied in the affirmative, Thurston wanted to know if he planned to return it to Dr. Sewall. Thurston became upset, letting Girdler know that the letter would be his undoing. Thurston informed Girdler he had "engaged … a lawyer in New-Hampshire." Thurston asked him what the people thought of him "respecting these charges." Girdler refused to answer. Thurston then asked him "to hold that letter and keep it. I am determined to see the matter closed … [and] … make use of such means as God shall give me." Girdler told him he would seek the advice of a friend as to what to do with the letter and left.

Shortly after in December, Thurston came to Girdler's house with his wife and Miss Abigail Hooper. After pleasantries, Thurston asked Girdler if he still had the letter. Girdler informed him that a friend had advised him to return it, but he had not done so yet. Thurston asked to see the letter, and Girdler showed it to him. Thurston said "it was a false letter, got up for to ruin him and family." After a short conversation about Parsons (derogatory and "unchristian" on Thurston's part), Thurston said, "I wish you to keep that letter for as long as you keep that letter, I am safe."[28]

Here is a mistake on Thurston's part. If the letter were hidden, he could not disprove its contents. Girdler does an odd thing. Thurston asks him to give the original to a female friend of his. Girdler does so. When he asks for it back, the woman tells him it is in the hands of a Mr. Norwood. After multiple threats, Norwood returns it to Girdler with two "copies of the original." As we will see, when Thurston cannot dispose of the letter, he will have a letter from Dr. Dewey forged that purports to exonerate him.

Insulted by the way he was treated by Thurston about Dr. Mussey's letter to Dr. Sewall, Girdler wrote to Thurston for an apology but received no reply. When Girdler next saw Thurston, he confronted him. The minister acknowledged receiving Girdler's letter and threatened him to "beware of what you do; I am a gentleman, and a minister; and you have vilified my character." Girdler told him he was the cause of his own difficulties and that "you may now expect to meet me and some of my brethren in the church. Said Thurston, I care not what you do."[29]

Discord in the Church

Although Thurston proclaimed that he would be "proven innocent," Girdler told him the "church and town was much excited about the matter" and said that he needed a better explanation "to satisfy the church members and others, respecting his innocence." Thurston replied, "Don't be worried, be easy, I am an innocent man; this was in the month of December 1818."[30]

Thurston should also have been concerned about his actions in the church. Although the accusation of facilitating the acquisition of dead bodies for Dr. Dewey was bad, his actions in the church "were deplorable" and enough to remove him without this charge. It started in November 1816 when a committee of church members, including Tyler Parsons, had written up rules for church discipline. The articles were presented to Thurston. He tried to substitute other articles, but they were disallowed, and the church accepted the committee's rules. Thurston was unhappy and blamed Mr. Parsons for the committee's actions. Thurston spoke of Parsons as a dangerous man "especially in the church" and began to circulate rumors against Parsons, claiming that he "eventually would overthrow the present system of faith and belief in Manchester." These rumors were considered "injurious to the character of the church."[31]

Church members tried to negotiate with him, but in the end it was agreed that he had to be dismissed. Due to his antics, "two thirds of the male members of the church had withdrawn their fellowship" because of his "pointed allusions frequently from the desk, and the history of prevarications out of the desk by Thurston, ... [this] ... parted the cords of affection, and sowed discord and confusion all around us." In addition, "communion was suspended."[32]

A town meeting was held on January 20, 1819, to inquire about reports circulating concerning Thurston's character. Thurston claimed he was not prepared to answer any charges but at the end of the meeting said if agreed upon he would be "sifted; like wheat" and that everyone "should know the character of your minister."

A second meeting was held on February 15, 1819, to hear charges against Thurston. He strangely came forward with the following charges. He accused himself of fornication, "of getting one girl with child ... [and] getting a bundle of shingles from the schoolhouse in a fraudulent manner" and of advising Dr. Dewey "to settle in Manchester for the purpose of carrying on private dissection; or in other words, to barter away the dead bodies of his people ..." and of "slandering the inhabitants of Manchester indiscriminately."

In answer, the opposing party led by Tyler Parsons observed that the first two charges had "never been a subject of litigation either in church or town," and claimed that he had raised them to prove they were false charges in hopes people would see the others as false as well. As for the charge of obtaining the shingles, he said, "We ... presume it can be proven," and as for advising the doctor, "it is believed by many, and probably will prove true eventually." To prove the last charge, Parsons introduced the testimony of Major Burley Smith, which concluded with Thurston's own words that the people in the town of Manchester were a "covetous, malicious, and Indian sett [*sic*] of people." Smith's testimony also shed light on the charge related to the dissection business.[33]

In the end Thurston was only charged with slander, the question of his involvement with Dr. Dewey having been raised in the testimony; no doubt the town committee (which claimed it would make a report never did) decided to wait for a resolution on the "questionable letter" supposedly received from Dr. Dewey (see below).

Evidence of the unresolved tensions in town due to the inaction of the February 15 committee meeting can be inferred from the town meeting held on March 8, 1819. One of the agenda items was to raise money for Thurston's salary. The opposition argued that Thurston's slandering the town and giving advice to Dr. Dewey per Mussey's letter to Sewall was evidence he had not met the conditions for his salary. They argued that "he had agreed to be a teacher of piety, morality, and virtue ... and had ceased to perform these duties." Those arguing in his favor said he only had to perform "parochial duties." Thurston's opponents countered that "if slandering the inhabitants and other unchristian like conduct, was considered parochial duties, then Thurston had amply fulfilled them and ought to have his salary." The disaffected lost the vote on his salary by a slim majority. There were "some hard sayings on both sides, alienated the affections, and produced ill blood."[34]

Thurston had done himself no favor within the church and town. "Mr. Thurston screening himself from examination, at the meeting of the 15th of February, led us, a majority of the church, and a respectable part of the town, to inspect the situation of Thurston closer than ever. At length we who seceded came to the conclusion that Thurston was guilty of sundry base charges, such as rendered him, unfit for holding the office of minister."

The Dissection Controversy

The dissection controversy led to several issues that lay behind the accusation on Thurston's character and played an underlying role in the fractiousness of the town committee meetings, hearings, the church councils, and the ecclesiastical council that would later settle Thurston's fate in the town. At this time, it is appropriate to discuss exactly how Thurston responded to his "dissection" accusers and why those who opposed him were so militant in their opposition to him.

Thurston was caught in a bind of his own making. At the same time, he was under assault by an opposition to his ministry in the town. He had been a prominent critic of Dr. Sewall along with Robert Crowell, the minister in Ipswich. Sewall had been remanded for trial for "body snatching" in 1818, a trial that would not conclude until November 1819. When the Salem minister Bentley wrote that "Sewall's matter of the Graves has passed out of all conversation, since the Case is put off ... , the implication being it had been at the forefront of much speculation prior to its continuance."[35] Obviously, the matter weighed heavily on Thurston's mind as he saw rightly that the accusations contained in the Sewall letter would ruin him and his family.

Thurston's character and trustworthiness were tied up in references to how he reacted to the accusations of his involvement in the Dr. Grosvenor fiasco and the dissection business. What had Thurston been doing to mitigate these accusations? At first, he had written to Dr. Dewey on December 4, 1818, asking him to clear his name. Thurston had received no reply. He knew he was going up before the town committee in January. Desperate for an answer, he wrote a second time to Dr. Dewey on January 14, 1819. Thurston asked Dewey to repudiate the accusation that he was guilty of "bartering away the dead bodies of his people." For the second time Thurston asked for an "honorable letter." He threatened Dr. Dewey and wrote that if he did not receive such a letter, "painful consequences must ensue both to you and myself." Undoubtedly, Thurston was threatening Dr. Dewey with a lawsuit.[36]

A Spurious Letter

Initially, Thurston may have thought he would receive the reply he wanted. He proclaimed his innocence whenever he was questioned about any accusations. In a deposition taken in March 1823, Daniel Annable testified that Thurston had gone into the country in December 1818 to obtain a statement from Dr. Dewey "to clear himself from the dissection business." When Thurston returned "he gave me to understand … he had accomplished his object.… I then asked him how he made out with Doct. Dewey, and how the report of the dissecting business was. He said it was without foundation."[37]

In January, Thurston received a letter he claimed was from Dr. Dewey. The "famous letter, so long predicted by Thurston, made its appearance—it came by mail." To many, it looked suspicious. "It was dated about the latter part of January 1819." The letter was sent from Vermont, about thirty to forty miles from where Dr. Dewey lived. Thurston stated that the letter would "acquit him" of the "gross charge of the dissection business." He was "elated when the letter got here … and congratulated by his friends and some.… Thurston considered his enemies."[38]

The letter was immediately distributed to Thurston's friends "with astonishing rapidity" and even read out in "Mr. Ebenezer Tappan's store." Parsons and others were suspicious of the letter; it was too "agreeable to Thurston's predictions … , especially its contradicting the testimony of Smith of his agency of getting Dr. Dewey to Manchester." They believed it was a "downright false letter got up for the express purpose of exonerating Thurston from the base charge of the dissecting business … as stated" in the Sewall letter.[39]

Parsons and other members of the church asked to examine the letter. Thurston at first resisted but finally gave it to them. Parsons recognized the handwriting as resembling that of a young woman. The signature was also questioned. Later Captain Abiel Burgess testified that he knew Dr. Dewey's handwriting and the way he expressed himself. The letter was not written by him, and "notwithstanding it was signed John Dewey, the body of the letter and the signature was two hands writing, as appeared to me."[40]

Dr. John Dewey's Deposition, March 13, 1820

Dr. John Dewey's deposition made on March 13, 1820, showed that he was careful in his answers and appeared to fear legal action. "I have never in any conversation, at any time been disposed to injure the said Mr. Thurston." Dewey then discussed his correspondence with Thurston and claimed never to have written any letter to Thurston, stating that he had been "in this part of the country since the close of 1817" and did "know that there was some probability of his going to Manchester[;] … he had some agency in relation to my going there, although he has by letter requested me to give … a statement to the contrary, or … to what I think he must have known to be false."

Following the deposition, Dr. Dewey was asked if he had written to Thurston "on the subject of dissection, since you was at Manchester, by way of denying or confessing what you said to…. Mussey, at Hanover, or anywhere else on the subject." Dewey answered carefully and said "he had not written any letters to Thurston since the end of 1817." Regarding the "famous letter," Dewey was asked, "Then you say if Mr. Thurston has got a letter by mail or otherwise purporting to come from you and directed to him" since 1817… "then it is false," and if your name is on the letter "it was written by some-one else, and is a forgery." Dewey replied that he had written no letters to Thurston since 1817, and "neither have I signed such a letter."[41]

Dr. Dewey would not admit that Thurston promised him dissection opportunities in Manchester as described in Sewall's letter. In a second deposition on April 20, 1820, Dewey was asked more detailed questions on the dissection business.

> **Quest.…** [D]id Thurston state to you, or intimate to you that said town would be a convenient place to practice dissections, and that subjects for dissection might be easily obtained there?
>
> **Ans.** I do not now recollect conversation of … dissections. It is not improbable that I might say something to him upon the subject. His answer if he made any, or his conversation, I do not recollect.

Other questions related to the previous deposition were asked again, then the questioning returned to the business of dissection. "Did you relate what said Thurston had said to you on the subject of dissection to … Mussey of Hanover, … when the same was fresh in your memory?" Dr. Dewey answered that he could not recall any "conversation with Dr. Mussey when Mr. Thurston was present." Dewey was also asked if he had a conversation about the same when "Mr. Thurston was not present." Dewey answered that he did not. He was asked if he remembered a "conversation with Dr. Mussey on the subject of said Thurston's conduct towards Dr. Sewall, or with regard to Dr. Sewall's difficulties?" Dewey answered, "Not any in which Mr. Thurston took a part."[42]

On the issue of dissection, it makes sense that Dewey was not forthcoming. In 1815 Massachusetts had just passed the Sepulcher Act (the statute Sewall was tried on), and New Hampshire had passed a law against grave robbing in 1796 (a year before Dartmouth College founded its medical school). Penalties in New Hampshire for grave robbing included a fine of not more than one thousand dollars, imprisonment for not more than one year, and a public whipping not to exceed thirty lashes, the penalties to be imposed at the "discretion of the court." The whipping penalty was abolished in 1810.[43]

A secondary consideration was the possible punishment that could be inflicted on a doctor who engaged in grave robbing or illegal dissection. "To steal a body, cut it open, and take it apart is a transgression against the dead and the living. Grave robbery …

could result in imprisonment, ostracism, a tar-and-feathering, or beating."[44] For example, Dr. Thomas Sewall was hated and shunned in his own community, while Dr. Charles Knowlton, a self-confessed grave robber, was sent to a Massachusetts prison in 1824 for "illegal dissection" and taking a cadaver and cutting it up.[45]

Town Meeting, March 29, 1819

On March 29, 1819, members of the Congregational Church of Christ in Manchester called a meeting with the intent of asking for a "mutual ecclesiastical council" provided the town approved the measure. The church's true intent was "to ask the town's advice" and take "reasonable measure," in hopes that Thurston would see his own situation and make "dispatch in setting his discharge from his people."[46]

Once the proposal was submitted, Thurston and the disaffected church members argued over the way the charges should be presented to the ecclesiastical council. The opposition wanted the charges presented on the day of the council; Thurston demanded that individuals who wanted to make accusations should do so twelve to fourteen days in advance of the council meeting so he could refute them.[47] The disaffected argued that Thurston was a proven forger; he would likely forge other papers to disprove individual charges. Besides, he had been accused of dissection, one of the "grossest of charges that it is possible to conceive of—especially a man who pretends to preach the gospel."[48]

Thurston claimed that he was unaware the church had made charges against him. He thought they were only made by individuals and wrote, "But that the church, as a body, were at war with their pastor, is what I had no reason to believe, nor do I now believe it."[49] Parsons gave numerous examples of how the church was at war with him and made the following sarcastic remark: "Look at the time Doct. Dewey was at Manchester, when counseling Dewey, as Mussey says in his letter to Sewall. That is what I call being at war with our bodies after the soul has departed."[50]

Thurston replied with a threat: speaking "as your pastor ... do not make the charges of others your own, and thus expose yourselves to the displeasure of God."[51]

Town Meeting April 15, 1819

At the town meeting on April 15, the disaffected believed they had sufficient charges against Thurston, especially on dissection and the forged letter. The town selectmen argued that Thurston had a right to know all the accusations against him so he could prepare a defense. The opposition agreed for the sake of peace that "we have once and again proposed to Thurston, and now to the town, to try James Thurston before an ecclesiastical tribunal, such as one he last proposed, the 15th of February."

A vote was taken to request an ecclesiastical council to settle matters in the town concerning their pastor. The disaffected lost the vote. The majority decided it was not a good idea to proceed "to choose an ecclesiastical council, as it would probably have been attended with much confusion." Prior to the vote, the opposition threatened to secede from the church and town affairs. In addition, they said "you can have James Thurston till you are sick of him."[52]

That evening the disaffected made good on their promise; they assembled and agreed "to secede from society, as the best way for peace in this society and the church." A committee was organized, and an appeal was made to the First Baptist Society in Beverly (Massachusetts). Altogether, forty-three men and three women left the Manchester church. Because the minister's salary and church upkeep depended on taxes paid to the town, there was great concern as to whether those who remained in the church would have to bear a higher tax burden.[53]

Those who remained in the church thought that the disaffected "intended to impose a burthen [*sic*] of taxes on them, to support Thurston." This caused a great deal of hostility in them "and for a season divided families in affection." Thurston told them that "it should not make any difference in their taxes."[54] Having gotten the disaffected to leave the church, Thurston likely felt that without their interference and the fact they had joined a Baptist society, he could settle the conflict in the town and retain his position by calling for the ecclesiastical council.

On May 6, Thurston wrote a letter to the remaining brethren of the church "to unite with me in calling for a mutual ecclesiastical council for advice, and … if the council judge it expedient that our connexion be dissolved." He also called on the brethren to join with him and asked the town to call an ecclesiastical council to settle this conflict.[55] At the May 15 town meeting, it was agreed to call the ecclesiastical council as requested by Thurston, the church brethren, and the town moderator.[56]

The Ecclesiastical Council

The ecclesiastical council met on June 2, 1819, "in concurrence with the town … for advice, also to decide on the subject of their difficulties and the dissolution of Rev. Mr. Thurston's pastoral and ministerial relation among them." The council received information from Thurston, the church committees, and the town "in relation to the unhappy difficulties subsisting among them."[57]

Members of the council were appointed to communicate with the disaffected, now members of the Baptist Society of Beverly. This was allowed because "the council are disposed to give them opportunity to make communications to the council that they may deem proper." Their representatives "appeared, and exhibited their papers, which were read." After dinner the council met and heard "statements in explanation of their written communications."[58]

Tyler Parsons and Captain Smith wanted Thurston to be put under oath. Reverend Robert Crowell of Essex replied "that Ministers of Christ were always considered under oath." Someone in the room countered "that we wished they would conduct as such."[59] It was proposed "to go into the investigation of Thurston's having slandered the inhabitants. (Some considerable clamor.)" Crowell said that "all that they have produced is nothing but a bubble." Dr. Worcester, of Salem, replied that "what had been said by the disaffected had great weight and would have weight always.… The council forbore going into the merits of any of the causes on any investigation whatever." The council "after deliberating on all that had been laid before them, the council proceeded to consider the expediency of dissolving the connexion [*sic*] between the Reverend Mr. Thurston and his church and people."[60]

The council determined that all concerned return in two weeks and subscribe "to an explicit declaration of their intention to adhere to the congregational order and discipline agreeably to the established usages of our churches, provided the Rev. Mr. Thurston be dismissed; and to seek the regular settlement of a congregational minister as his successor, shall be recognized by this council as constituting the congregation church of Christ in Manchester." A committee was appointed to investigate compensation and equity for Mr. Thurston in the event he was dismissed. The meeting was adjourned until June 17, 1819.[61]

On June 17, 1819, the disaffected agreed to accept the recent "covenant and articles adopted by the tabernacle church in Salem[;] ... we do consider these to contain ... the necessary discipline and government in the church of Christ, Manchester." On the same day the opposition said they would adhere to the congregational order and that they did not want to remain separated from the church and would be willing to return if Thurston was dismissed. Also, their opinion was that if Thurston was not removed, the church would lose "seven eighths" of his parishioners "in the next twelve months." Finally, when the disaffected were asked to adhere to the congregational order, this suggested to them that Thurston had been at work behind the scenes trying to convince the council members that his opponents were "heretics." This showed why they had been right not trusting Thurston and was evidence of his propensity to lie and dissemble. They told the council members, "if there have been any insinuations, by any one presented to you ... introducing a new system of belief, faith or practice, the insinuation is ungentlemanlike, unchristian like, and false."[62]

The council's decision was that Thurston "should be regularly dismissed" and determined that there was no possibility of "a restoration of union and harmony, nor ... any prospect of his ministerial usefulness, or his receiving a competent support, so long as he remains in this place."

Other recommendations were more controversial. The council suggested that "the pastor should ask a dismission of the church, and that the church should grant his request, with fair testimonials of his Christian and ministerial character." That the "council would forebear entering into the causes and merits of the controversy which has involved them in so much distress and peril, any further than to state, they do explicitly, and with heartfelt satisfaction, that after opportunity afforded a full hearing of all parties, nothing prejudicial to the moral Christian, or ministerial character has been sustained." This finding and a recommendation of four hundred dollars compensation was later roundly criticized.[63]

However, in the end the disaffected felt that the only charge they could make against Thurston to the council was that he had slandered the people in the town. The council declined to investigate any charges, deciding instead to recognize the longtime dissension in the community. From the view of the council members, there was no good outcome. Thurston had devasted the comity of the church in Manchester, and there was no getting it back. The best solution was to get him out, have the church reunited, and replace him with a new minister. Likely this was explained to Thurston, which is why he agreed to leave but with the condition he would receive a good review and compensation. Undoubtedly, he gave the council the amount he was owed, to be forwarded to the town for payment.

Parsons was bitterly disappointed that an investigation of the slander charge was not undertaken: "If the council on Thurston had gone into the merits of the case, of Thurston's slandering the inhabitants of Manchester, that would have led them to the dissection business; and that false letter that Thurston circulated in Manchester; in order, as we believe, to acquit him of the charge as in Doct. Mussey's letter to Sewall."[64]

Parsons said that "at the time of the meeting of the council at Manchester" the disaffected did not have Dr. Dewey's deposition, admitting he had not written Thurston any letter since 1817; "the circumstances," however, "warranted us to believe that the letter was false." Parsons argued that by not following through on the charges, the council could do much damage in the future, essentially covering up the "bad character" of Thurston and moving him along to another position where he could do additional damage (which seems to be a problem with clergy even today).

One important question to be answered is why the council did not go through with the full investigation. Why was Robert Crowell immediately willing to dismiss the evidence that the disaffected had produced? Likely Crowell saw firsthand the dissension and turmoil that grave robbing and dissection produced in his own community. As Reverend Bentley in Salem observed regarding Sewall's activities, the public lost trust in doctors and were in a great agitation over this. Perhaps Crowell and others feared the same uproar if a minister of God was implicated in the heinous crime of countenancing body snatching and dissection as described in the Sewall letter.[65] For believers this flew in the face of the basic tenet of Christian doctrine: the redemption and resurrection of the physical body.[66]

In addition, prior to the meeting of the council, the Sewall trial had been continued from April 1819 to November 1819, with no decision rendered while the council was in session. Two of the charges—dissection and the supply of bodies promised by Thurston and his having forged a letter related to these accusations—would have suggested to many people that he was guilty by lying to cover up the charges in the Sewall letter. The latter would have been a great embarrassment to the church if it were to go on record. Also, two elite groups would have been under attack. Although physicians had not achieved a high social position at this time, Sewall's elite standing can be attributed to his marriage to Mary Choate, whose family enjoyed high social status in the town. Clergy held higher social status than doctors at this time by virtue of their position as leaders of the church and the community.[67]

The matter of dissection and the suggestion of the ease of obtaining bodies was sinful and would have been a huge embarrassment to the congregational churches and fellow clergy. Crowell and likely others were willing to ignore the evidence, because at the time the council did not have a letter from Dr. Dewey stating he had never communicated with Thurston concerning the dissection and related charges, as the forged letter stated. In addition, according to Mussey's letter, Thurston had been a great supporter of Crowell inveighing against the body snatcher, Sewall. Perhaps Crowell also believed that it was Sewall who made Mussey's letter public about Thurston's dissection offer to embarrass him. Likely Crowell could not believe that a fellow minister who supported him so vigorously would have made such a damning proposal to attract a physician to his town. Crowell seemed to think as noted above and likely convinced others there was enough gray area not to go forward with the charges. However, the congregation had been irrevocably ruptured enough that Thurston had to go but in such a way as to avoid needless embarrassment to the church and the town.

In addition, if they had pursued the matter, an honorable dismissal for Thurston would have been out of the question and would have made it impossible for him to obtain another position. It appears that this was the result the council wanted. The council worked diligently with the town leaders and the church to ensure he received one.

Before the council adjourned, the church members who previously "seceded were invited to join them" in giving Thurston a dismissal and a recommendation. To a man, they refused to give him a recommendation, saying to the council's committee that "Thurston was a bad man and ought not be imposed on any society whatever, as a minister of the gospel." The committee informed them that they had to vote for his dismission even if they could not vote to recommend him for another position. Ten opposing brethren left for further discussion, and eight returned to participate in the vote. They were informed that the vote for dismission and recommendation were blended and that this was how they had to vote on the issue. They refused to vote. There were four church members present who had never seceded. The council called the vote, and the measure passed with the votes of the four church members. The council declared that the measure was passed unanimously. The disaffected had been tricked, and the church members who had never left the church sided with the council's decision.[68]

The church followed with a separate dismissal in concurrence with the town: "we dismiss and recommend him as a member in regular standing, to any regular church, where, in providence he may be called to reside."[69]

As for Thurston's remuneration, the town council was not as cooperative, writing to him that "the town does not consider the council to have authority to act upon concerns which do not belong to such bodies.... This recommendation the town ... do[es] not feel it to be their duty, under existing circumstances, to comply with it."[70]

Parsons Sued by Thurston

According to Parsons, since Thurston did not get the money he felt was owed him from the town, he decided to get his money "by the law." Thurston accused Parsons of slander, saying he had stolen a bundle of shingles from the schoolhouse in Manchester. The charge relied on in court was "stealing," and Thurston claimed special damages as the minister of Manchester.[71]

In February 1820 the sheriff attached Parsons's real estate, which he estimated to be worth $3,000. The case was to be held in the Ipswich court in March 1820. The case was moved to April. There is little doubt that Parsons planned to introduce into the proceedings much of the evidence used in the town meetings and the ecclesiastical council to discredit Thurston, especially the charges related to the "dissection business." Parsons acquired the two depositions from Dr. Dwight previously discussed on March 13, 1820, and April 20, 1820, and Dr. Mussey's deposition on March 7, 1820.

The case was moved to the Salem court in June 1820, where it was turned over to a court of reference. The court of reference consisted of a three distinguished Massachusetts men: Artemis Ward, Lemuel Shaw, and Samuel Hoar. Daniel Webster and Leverett Saltonstall argued for Thurston. William Prescott, Benjamin R. Nichols, and Davis Cummins argued for Parsons.[72]

The writ was read by Saltonstall. Thurston was accused of "lying and stealing." Both sides presented witnesses with their evidence.[73] The newspaper report on the verdict stated that "the award of the referees, in the case of the Rev. James Thurston vs. Tyler Parsons of Manchester, for slander ... [Salem] May last, was opened, and read in this

Court [Supreme Judicial Court of Massachusetts]. The award is in favour of the plaintiff—damages fifteen hundred dollars."[74] Besides the initial fine reported by the newspaper, Parsons was also required to pay $400 for court costs.[75]

The matter of supplying dead bodies for dissection or the forged letter does not appear to have come up in the proceedings. According to Parsons, "the only evidence they had was he was a bad man[,] … not being a man of truth, and that we had no confidence in him as a member of the gospel—and that he had created much disturbance in the town." The other business of dissection was not considered pertinent to the case at hand, and Parsons believed that the reason he lost was because "on the part of the defense, we are not allowed to state anything but what has a bearing to the action pending, *of course here is where the failure took place.*"[76]

Even if Parsons had produced the three depositions in court, Dewey claimed that he could not recollect any such conversation about the dissection business, thus making Mussey's letter to Sewall hearsay and inadmissible.

Thurston moved to Exeter, New Hampshire, and died there on December 12, 1835. According to the town history of Exeter, he is not listed as having served as a minister in the town.[77]

4

"A prodigious bustle" at Dartmouth

Dr. Nathan Smith, physician and anatomist, founded the medical school at Dartmouth in Hanover, New Hampshire, in 1797. He later became a distinguished member of the Yale faculty in New Haven, Connecticut, from 1813 to 1829. Smith organized the medical department at Bowdoin College in Brunswick, Maine, in 1820, and cofounded the University of Vermont Medical Department in 1822.[1]

When Dr. Smith first came to Dartmouth College, he found himself in more difficult circumstances than his colleagues in larger cities. For Dr. Smith, "teaching always meant performing dissections and having students do them as well.... [D]issections were crucial to the teaching of surgery; this, he believed, was how a doctor learned enough anatomy to do effective surgical work."[2]

An early event in New Hampshire involving Dr. Smith showed the hardship of acquiring cadavers, the lengths he was willing to go to to procure a body, and his somewhat callous approach to obtaining one from the state.

Concerning the latter, Dr. Smith's involvement began with a letter addressed to the governor of New Hampshire, John Langdon, on June 19, 1806. The letter concerned a convicted murderer named Josiah Burnham. Originally Burnham was to be executed on July 15, 1806. Dr. Smith had heard that Burnham "was about to apply to your Excellency and the Council for a reprieve that his execution may be put off until a better time than that preferred by the court that had sentenced him." Dr. Smith continued:

> If your Excellency would think it proper to grant him his request, it would be of a great advantage to the medical school established at Dartmouth College to have his execution on or about the last week in October next that his remains might be usefully employed in teaching a large class of medical students.

Interestingly, in a postscript he wrote, "If the execution above alluded to should be deferred to the time or about the time, I have suggested I can obtain the body without any breach of law, a very desirable thing & I believe no person will be dissatisfied with the measure."

Dr. Smith may have been in contact with Burnham about securing the reprieve for the purpose of having a freshly executed corpse for his classes, although there is no direct evidence of this. However, what is more interesting is a somewhat veiled threat in the postscript that he would like to obtain the body "without any breach of law, a desirable thing."[3]

Dr. Smith was denied his requested time for Burnham's execution. Burnham was hanged on August 12, 1806, in Haverhill, in Grafton County, New Hampshire, about forty miles distant from Dartmouth.[4] One newspaper reported that "when the body was hung 30 minutes, it was taken down and buried, but afterwards dug up by the Doctors who took it into possession, having previously purchased it, and conveyed away."[5]

It is possible that Dr. Smith obtained his cadaver, although no doctors' names are mentioned in the newspaper report. Dartmouth was the only medical school in the vicinity in 1806. The fact that the body was purchased may suggest a prior agreement with Burnham to pay off his family's debts, as he was in debtors' prison when he committed the murders, sending him to the gallows.[6]

That Dr. Smith appeared overeager to obtain a fresh cadaver in Grafton County makes sense when it is realized how rare executions were in that county. The first execution in Grafton occurred ten years earlier on July 28, 1796; a "mulatto," Thomas Palmer, was convicted of rape. After Burnham's execution there would not be another until 1849 when the Methodist minister Enos G. Dudley was hanged for murdering his wife.[7]

Unfortunately, subjects "were more easily obtained in larger cities, where the unclaimed remains of paupers were available and where the large and numerous cemeteries made it relatively easy to find corpses that would not be missed. In contrast, Hanover was rural, isolated, and thinly populated; if a body were dug up anywhere in the vicinity, everybody would soon know. Consequently, … Smith at times hired people to find bodies for him or attempted to get subjects sent to him from Boston."[8] One method to avoid detection was to have bodies shipped in from out of state in whiskey barrels or, if caught, simply to claim that the body was from out of state.[9]

Nathan Smith was never open about his procurements. "He tried to keep as much out of the messy business as he could. Among those he relied on to help him were students[;] … one who became especially adept" was a former student, Amos Twitchell.[10] "Dr. Smith depended almost wholly … upon his young and ardent friend [Twitchell] for the procurement of subjects for dissection.… He did this for many years for Dr. Smith."[11]

Dr. Smith's concern about finding cadavers for dissection in New Hampshire haunted him from the beginning of his time at Dartmouth. In the letter written in 1806 to Governor John Langdon he also wrote, "Nothing is more important to medical science & no part of medical education in this part of the country is obtained with so much difficulty" as acquiring cadavers.[12] This anxiety remained with him his entire time in New Hampshire. Public attitudes toward the "cutting up of dead bodies" and concerns about what harsh laws might be enacted for the "digding (?) or dissection" that "the New Hampshire legislature might enact" would eventually help prompt Dr. Smith to remove himself from Hanover.[13]

The Body Snatching "Bustle" at Dartmouth

In 1807 Dr. Smith assigned his anatomy lectures to the famous professor Dr. Alexander Ramsay of Edinburgh, whom Dr. Smith hired as a visiting professor. The lectures were a success. "So many students attended the Course given … that subjects [cadavers] became rare in spite of those that Dr. Spalding had brought from Portsmouth."[14] When Dr. Ramsay left in 1809, Dr. Smith returned to teaching the anatomy course. That fall while teaching the course, the Dartmouth body-snatching uproar occurred. Details about the event are provided in a series of letters written by his student, Ezekiel Dodge Cushing, son of "a wealthy… [Pembroke, Massachusetts] shipping family."[15]

Cushing's letter to his father gives not only a graphic description of the uproar but also an interesting account of Dr. Smith's role in the episode. In a letter dated December 2, 1809, Cushing wrote, "In this part of the country the people are so enraged, to the distance of 50 miles round that it is as much as ones [*sic*] life is worth to attempt getting a subject for dissection." He continued,

> Under these circumstances and considering that the law was much more severe here than in Massachusetts, the penalty being 2000$ [*sic*] fine, two years imprisonment, setting on the gallows, 50 lashes, from what I considered prudence, but what some called cowardice, rather declined being engaged in any undertaking of the kind. And to get clear honourably. I proposed to the medical class for each one to contribute so much as would be sufficient to induce some one to undertake the business, this was accordingly done, and a subject procured about a week ago.

Ezekiel Cushing continued to describe how the body of a ten-year-old child was discovered missing in the graveyard:

> The very night that it was procured they were by the suspicion of a woman at a toll gate so far put out of their gard [*sic*], by her close questions that they lost their senses almost and the one that paid the toll in making change took out his pocket book and left at the toll house, it contained a letter without a signature, addressed to the student [Cushing originally wrote "students," but the "s: is crossed out in his letter] who left the pocket book. They instantly began searching the grave yard pointed out in the letter, and yesterday found that a boy of 10 years of age was gone.
>
> At six o'clock that morning the authorities arrived at the college with the sheriff. He "demanded leave to search for the body, they had in the night set a guard to every window and door leading to the lecture room." Dr. Smith's reaction was repeated many times throughout his career of not wanting to be involved or questioned when it came to obtaining "subjects." Cushing wrote Dr. Smith wished me to attend the sheriff in the search and saying that to my prudence he committed the conducting of [the] whole affair, he was scared almost to death. The body was thrown into a closet which was rather concealed a little in the wall as we could not remove it.... Sylvester [Ruggles] and I attended the sheriff in his search[;] ... there was two men with him ... [and] they after a long search found it.

When they found the body, one of the men "threatened to destroy the Anatomical Museum and to open the door and let in their companions for that purpose." When Cushing refused to let the others in, "one of them took up an ax and threatened to knock him over." Cushing told him that "if he valued his own life to be quiet" because otherwise the students outside "would tear them limb from limb," and he "deliberately unbuttoned" his "coat to let them see the Drs. Pistols in my jacket pockets, that stilled them."

Here, I suspect he may have exaggerated his response to the men who threatened to destroy the anatomical museum. However, it is curious that he claimed to have the "doctor's" pistols to defend the anatomical museum. Where was Dr. Smith while his student was being threatened, and why did he give his pistols to Cushing?[16]

Once the body was found, Cushing took a no harm, no foul approach and wrote, "I then told them it was to no purpose to make a noise about it[;] if they would be quiet, I would help them sew up the belly and sew on the leg and arm that had been cut off." The men agreed, and Cushing "went to work and put all the parts together as neat as possible." He reported that the men seemed to grow "good natured and perhaps it was over." Cushing then had to "persuade the father of the child not to see it. They got a coffin and have gone home." He added somewhat incredulously, as if this was unexpected, that "not without stopping and telling the whole story at the town, ... they threatened to expose the body to public view as soon as they got home. If they do it is possible that a mob will be raised."

There was no mob raised, but the episode had repercussions for the college and the medical school (noted below). Cushing informed his father that Dr. Smith told him he had "acted nobly."[17] A few days later, Cushing wrote to his mother informing her that Dr. Smith asked him at the end of term to board with him. Cushing wrote, "I have so behaved myself as to gain his good will, and confidence as he made me the offer without any solicitation on my part."[18]

In the following letter from Dr. Smith to Dr. Lyman Spalding dated February 13, 1810, Dr. Smith references some bad luck keeping him busy, but he "obtained a Truce for a time." He continued: "Toward the close of our last course of Lectures I contracted with a certain person to go to Boston to procure, if possible, a Cadaver.[19] But instead of going to Boston, he went to Enfield, [New Hampshire, about ten miles from Hanover], as it appears, & procured a subject, which was taken by an Officer when about half dissected. The circumstances made a prodigious bustle for a time & gave me great inquietude, but I believe we shall survive the accident without material injury either personal or to the Institution."[20]

Dr. Smith asked a person (he does not say a student) to procure a subject, but according to Dr. Smith, he asked him to obtain the body in Boston. Smith gave the person a letter. There was a letter found, but it was unsigned, and as Cushing noted, it was "a letter without a signature addressed to the student who left the pocketbook." One question not answered was whether Cushing had written the name of the local graveyard on the unsigned letter and that was how the authorities knew where to look for the empty grave.

It would have made sense if Cushing had written the unsigned letter to the students to help them obtain a body closer to Hanover, saving them a trip to Boston. However, in a letter to his sister Mehetabel dated February 11, 1810, he wrote, "I have been very much engaged in anatomical studies and

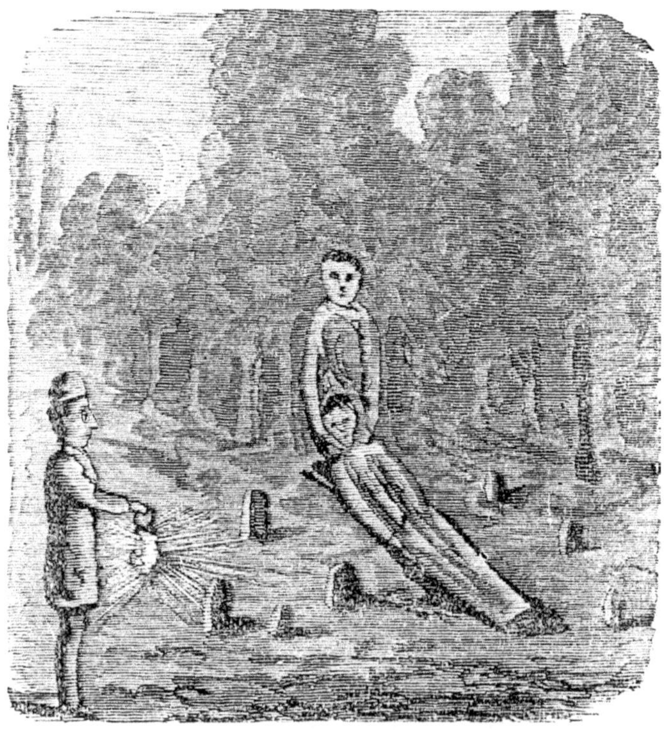

Since the founding of the school, it had always lived under the suspicion of grave robbing. "Grave Robbing, Dartmouth Medical College, 1877–1878" (courtesy Rauner Special Collections Library, Dartmouth College).

believe that I have proved that I was not concerned in vain in digging up the body of Daniel Doyle."[21]

Based on Cushing's letter to his sister, it appears that he did not want to get involved in this body-snatching episode, and his concern appeared well founded. However, he certainly had foreknowledge concerning the enterprise. If Cushing did not write the letter, then who did and named the graveyard in Enfield? Was it possible that Cushing was somehow implicated in this episode anyway in place of Dr. Smith? However, in the end the records only show that Sylvester Ruggles was charged for this body-snatching event. For a medical student, a body-snatching episode would not have the same effect on his future as it would on a professor such as Dr. Smith.[22] This would have endangered Smith's professional reputation, the reputation of the college, and ongoing sensitive negotiations with the legislature of New Hampshire concerning its support for the Dartmouth College Medical School.

Dr. Smith's letter to Dr. Spalding does not mention his part in refusing to become involved in the assault on the medical building. Smith had hired a person to obtain a body from Boston, not the body being sought by the authorities, but perhaps to ensure complete "deniability," he expected his student, Cushing, to handle the entire affair "once the sheriff arrived on the scene" to search for the body of the boy.[23]

A member of the Dartmouth College faculty, Ebenezer Adams, provides some clarity on the situation concerning the college's faith in Dr. Smith's innocence. Adams wrote to Dr. George Shattuck on December 6, 1809, about the effect of the incident on the school. Adams was not sanguine on the business of body snatching in his remarks. "But for the present the medical department occupies all our attention." The local population was highly distressed, with good reason "with regard to a subject taken up for dissection." He noted that Dr. Smith was not being blamed for the latter. "He had contracted with one of his pupils and given him a letter to you upon the subject [recall that Smith told Spalding he intended the person to get a 'subject' in Boston; apparently he was counting on Shattuck to help]. The pupil to save expense, took [one] up in a nearby town, kept it 3 or 4 days, [based on Cushing's December 2 letter I estimate that the body snatching took place on November 25, 1809] and then brought it forward for dissection." When the body was discovered missing "from the grave, search was made, and [it was] the body of a lad 9 years of age, of a very reputable family. Some abuse and insult offered by the students to those who came in search of the body, irritated to a high degree the public resentment already justly very great." Adams did not know what the consequences would be but concluded, "I think it must either overset the institution, or at any rate work as an effectual cure for the evil."[24]

According to Adams, Dr. Smith had the excuse of a letter written to Dr. Shattuck and even at this early time believed in Dr. Smith's innocence. However, it is curious that Adams blames the "abuse and insult offered by the students" for further inflaming public opinion. Perhaps if Dr. Smith had taken some responsibility initially during the search, the latter could have been avoided.

Following Adams's letter, we have more information on the situation. Cushing wrote to his mother on December 15, 1809, that things had quieted down and that most of the faculty had left. "We find it easy to pacify the enraged people [for the half dissection of the Enfield boy]." He added more information on the situation. "One of the Medical Students [Ruggles Sylvester] has had a trial and is bound over to the Supreme Court in May in bonds of 1000$ and there are nine men gone different routs [*sic*] to apprehend another who has fled for his life."[25]

Sylvester Ruggles was "responsible for digging up the body of the boy in Enfield" and "Cushing's companion in the search instigated by the sheriff." Curiously, a $10 charge against Dr. Smith appears in his lawyer Mills Olcott's personal ledger on December 5, 1809, in regard "to attending at the examination of Ruggles Sylvester for digging up a dead body at your request at Ralston [possibly a tavern in Claremont, New Hampshire, said to have a large meeting room] and arguing the same." The notation in Olcott's ledger strikes me as ambiguously written; likely he is referring to the examination, not to the fact that Dr. Smith requested that Ruggles Sylvester dig up a dead body.[26]

Dr. Smith was always anxious about repercussions from any corpse-snatching rumors and how it would affect his own reputation and the impact on his ability to obtain financial support from the New Hampshire legislature for the medical school.

Since the founding of the medical school, it had always lived under the suspicion of grave robbing. Before New York, the states of Massachusetts, Virginia, and Pennsylvania had anatomy laws, the New Hampshire Legislature "passed a stringent act against grave robbery in 1796, a year before the Dartmouth Medical School was organized."[27]

The relationship between the Dartmouth College administration and the medical school was limited. The college awarded the medical school degrees and hired the appointed faculty. Otherwise, the medical department was an independent entity, including its financial operations. However, in December 1809 President John Wheelock induced the board of trustees to accept new rules concerning student discipline because of the "notoriety" resulting from the body-snatching episode.[28]

When the Enfield, New Hampshire, body-snatching episode was first discovered, President Wheelock moved swiftly to salvage the situation and tried to protect Dr. Smith's reputation. The following is Wheelock's response to this incident given on December 9, 1809, only a few days after its occurrence:

> You have doubtless been informed of the great disturbance lately excited at this Institution by the base and unjustifiable conduct of some individuals also in secret and clandestine manner opened a recess of the dead and taking there from a body, exposed the same (instead of a subject regularly and lawfully procured without wounding the feelings of humanity) in the medical department for anatomical dissection.[29]

President Wheelock told Benjamin Gilbert, a Hanover attorney and justice of the peace, that his administration would do everything in the future to "prevent this criminal act" and told Gilbert he could depend on the "full cooperation of the faculty and governors in any investigation of any members of the college participating in body snatching or illegal dissection."[30] To quiet the excitement, officials from the surrounding towns were selected to form a "visiting committee with the right to examine the medical department labs and lecture rooms and the rooms of the medical or science students to pursue any rumors or reports of grave robbing." A committee of five students was elected who "made a formal admission and apology to President Wheelock," and the faculty said that their actions were "nothing short of sacrilege" and had "unfairly damaged Professor Smith's reputation."

President Wheelock had many reasons to take this approach to quiet the situation. The college was under threat by the community. By involving the public with a committee to investigate the activities of the students at the medical school, he likely calmed some members of the public with the belief that there would be an investigation and that the body snatching would stop. Wheelock no doubt disapproved of this activity and couched the actions in almost mellifluous terms—"in secret and clandestine manner opened the recess of the dead"—and later had five medical students apologize to him and the faculty. (Was there an apology to the boy's family and the community?) The problem with all the apologizing was that there were not enough cadavers legally available for the needs of the medical school. Although the medical students and faculty might apologize, it was known at many medical schools that these apologies were not sincere and were "made with a wink."[31]

Nathan Smith's correspondence with his student Ezekiel Cushing (and Cushing's correspondence with his family and others) suggests that Smith was more involved in the incident than anyone admitted.[32] As for the great concern of legally obtaining cadavers for dissection, note how cavalier Dr. Smith is in the following quote about involving a student in obtaining "subjects" in his letter to Dr. Shattuck on January 7, 1821, requesting cadavers for the new Bowdoin College medical school that he had recently helped found: "Can you find some young man in Boston who would agree to furnish us two or three subjects. They could be sent to Portland by water. The College expects to pay the expense and be willing to give a reasonable compensation."[33]

Another consideration by the college was Nathan Smith's involvement with the New Hampshire legislature. Between 1809 and 1811, Smith had been negotiating to obtain building funds for a new medical building at Dartmouth. Funds had been approved in June 1809, but groundbreaking was not scheduled to begin until 1811.[34] The grave-robbing incident was on Dr. Smith's mind and possibly Wheelock's as well when it came to the public and the legislature. On February 13, 1810, the *Concord Gazette* published a letter from Grafton County, New Hampshire, accusing the governor and "several members last June [who] met in Caucus and agreed to give Dr. Smith the sum of money mentioned in the Grant, and that this measure was carried in opposition to their representatives in the Legislature. What say they, are we to be taxed for the purpose of giving Dr. Smith 3 or 4000 dollars to build a slaughter house?"[35]

In view of the controversy in Hanover, Cushing seemed unconcerned in the weeks following the "riot." Perhaps he knew he would not be prosecuted. On December 27, 1809, he wrote to his father rather jokingly about the sensitive topic of digging up the dead and the lack of bodies. "I received yours of the tenth instant, and am happy to inform you that at present we are tolerably quiet, about digging up people. The anatomical lectures have been rather dry, from our misfortune with regard to subjects."[36]

On May 23, 1810, in a letter to his father, Smith made a joke that his colleagues in the dissecting business might have found humorous (probably his father would have found it simply morbid, as he was in the shipping business). "If I should die, I should make an excellent subject for I have fed so much on salt meat that I should be sufficiently preserved."[37]

An Ominous Turn of Events

On Oct 7, 1810, Cushing wrote to his father that "all things go on well[;] ... it is probable that we shall have no difficulty from the lectures this year. Dr. Smith intends by the middle of December to go to Boston and see how he can make out there."[38]

Just as Nathan Smith feared regarding body snatching, he and Ezekiel Cushing were charged by a grand jury with "raising the dead" in Massachusetts, although the charge against Dr. Smith was later dropped. On November 18, 1810, Cushing gave the following sworn deposition before Benjamin Gilbert, justice of the peace, in Grafton County, New Hampshire. Cushing swore that he did not at "any time ... procure ... a subject or subjects for dissection" and that no one else including Dr. Nathan Smith asked him to obtain "a subject or subjects for dissection either from Boston or any other place ... [and] that no one has ever given me money, or in any way engaged to give me money to obtain any subject."[39]

In "his deposition [Cushing] utterly failed to discuss what happened in the anatomical museum or the role he admitted to his father that he had played in proposing how the medical students should obtain a 'subject' at the end of the previous autumn's course of lectures."[40] There is "considerable room to question the veracity of what he did say to the Justice of the Peace."[41] Conversely, perhaps on the advice of his lawyer, he was told to make the deposition relate only to the specific act he was being accused of in Boston.

On November 28, 1810, Cushing appeared worried about the case but at the same time resistant. He wrote to his father that "the lectures have been peaceable entirely so here, and the rumbling of distant thunder is all we have had to disturb us, whether it will burst on our heads I cannot tell, and only inform you that armed with conscious innocence, we feel ready to meet its vengeance, ... directed by two [of] the most skillful Doctors in Boston."[42]

On December 4, 1810, Dr. Shattuck wrote to Cushing that "despite of all my efforts to prevent it you are indicted by the Grand Jury for an attempt to raise the dead. I have consulted Mr. Blake about what you ought to do in relation to appearing in Boston for trial. He thinks it advisable that you come into town: otherwise, a warrant will be issued from the Governor of this Commonwealth to the Governor of New Hampshire for your being apprehended and brought to Boston. It is true you may avoid being taken by concealment at Hanover or going into Vermont. But it will make more noise, and the rumors will be the most unpleasant part of the business. Mr. Blake says the probable extent of punishment will not exceed a fine of twenty dollars. The testimony adduced against you was furnished by your confidential friend Mr. Whitman. Both the Board of Health and the Grand Jury believe Dr. Smith entirely now free from implication in the late attacks on the rights [rites] of sepulture." Dr. Shattuck closed the letter by telling Cushing he was contacting the Massachusetts attorney general to let him know "you would come to town as soon as possible" to conclude this "unsavory subject."[43]

The last we hear on this subject is a reference to the matter in a letter to his father dated January 22, 1811: "how does my lawsuit come?"[44]

It does not seem possible that Cushing's indictment for "raising the dead" was related to the episode in New Hampshire, as has been suggested by Dr. Smith's biographers Hayward and Putnam.[45] The incident most likely occurred in the early fall of 1810. Dr. Smith used professionals, friends, and even students to obtain cadavers in Boston. As we saw earlier, Boston was a hotbed of body snatching in the early 1800s.

Why would there be a trial in Boston if the body-snatching episode had occurred in Enfield, New Hampshire? According to Dr. Shattuck, the incident in Boston was serious enough to involve the governors of two states if necessary. Cushing was advised to return to Boston to face a trial. Trying to evade arrest in New Hampshire or Vermont would have caused more trouble than it was worth to him, and "the rumors would be the most unpleasant part of the business." The fine was estimated by Dr. Shattuck at twenty dollars. The key to this event is in the statement from the Board of Health in Boston and the grand jury relayed by Shattuck that they did not believe Dr. Smith was implicated in the "late attacks on the rights of sepulture." Cushing's body-snatching charge was recent; his close confidant was likely Isaac W. Whitman (also from Pembroke and a fellow classmate at Harvard) who bore witness against Cushing. It is likely this charge was not linked to the New Hampshire episode.

One historian, although he did not give his source, wrote, "Cushing was subsequently indicted by a Grand Jury for 'raising the dead' and seems to have been fined twenty-five dollars for the offense. Such incidents, often involving students, were not rare, and as a result the school acquired an unsavory reputation in the region."[46]

The strain of obtaining cadavers by dangerous and illegal methods weighed heavily on Dr. Smith.[47] As early as May 14, 1810, he wrote to his friend Dr. Shattuck that he wanted to leave Hanover. Smith feared that the New Hampshire legislature might enact more laws against dissecting and obtaining cadavers for his teaching. "If the thing should take its course, it will afford me a good pretext for leaving the College and State—a thing which will not be disagreeable to me.... The conduct of people and parties here has cooled my ardor ... and determined me to sell my talents to the highest bidder in physic and surgery."[48] Nevertheless, even after escaping the charge of body snatching in Massachusetts, Smith was back to obtaining bodies for his classes at Dartmouth in the fall of 1811. He wrote to his friend Dr. Shattuck on December 20, 1811, that "we were very fortunate in obtaining subjects and have dissected three who were all pretty good; the one brought by T. [Dr. Twitchell] was excellent."[49]

In summary, it is hard to believe that Dr. Smith did not have some involvement in his students' body-snatching activities. His most recent biographers also suspected that he might have been more involved with the Hanover-based body-snatching event and saw the fact that (at least for historians) this was a lost opportunity. "If Smith himself had been indicted in 1809, it is possible that he would have been in sufficient trouble with both college and law-enforcement authorities to destroy his effectiveness as a teacher [even if not as a physician]." This may explain why the college made every effort to blame the students for this "disturbance," even going so far as to have selected medical students to apologize to the faculty and Dr. Smith. If Dr. Smith had been blamed, this would have affected the negotiations with the state legislature for the funding of the medical building and also tainted the overall reputation of the college and the faculty. He was simply too important to be involved in this embarrassment.

On the positive side for historians, Smith's biographers argue that "an indictment might also have left us with information that would have helped us understand better how he managed to accomplish so much as a teacher of anatomy [while in Hanover] despite the stumbling blocks." Smith may have avoided more incidents in Hanover due to "his contacts in Boston and elsewhere," or his students avoided "collecting bodies to close to home" and avoided his own involvement by getting others, his students or colleagues, "to handle ... [the] resurrectionist activities found in every anatomy department of the day."[50]

Fortunately for Dr. Nathan Smith, he was not ultimately charged in New Hampshire or Massachusetts with body snatching or "raising the dead," though two of his students were charged and convicted of the crime of body snatching. Smith was free to seek employment elsewhere. He set his sights on Yale College, where in 1824 he would have to confront a full-blown riot over accusations of body snatching by Yale medical students.

As for the two students tried and convicted for body snatching, Ruggles Sylvester and Ezekiel D. Cushing, both received their bachelor of medicine degrees from Dartmouth College in 1811.[51] Dr. Ruggles Sylvester migrated to Allegheny County, Pennsylvania, and was "probably the first medical doctor in the area." He died in 1834.[52] Dr. Ezekiel Dodge Cushing had a short but distinguished career. He practiced in Boston and then moved his practice to Hanover, Massachusetts. He died in 1828.[53]

Looking for New Opportunities

Dr. Smith saw opportunities elsewhere to continue with his work unfettered by the threats he foresaw in the anatomy laboratory in Hanover. For him to leave Dartmouth, he would have had to remove himself from financial and personnel obligations. Dr. Smith's former student, Timothy J. Gridley, who knew Jonathan Knight, a tutor at Yale, wrote to him about Dr. Smith's interest in relocating to teach at Yale College. If Dr. Smith was to teach surgery, he would need cadavers for his research. Gridley wrote, "The difficulty and danger of procuring subjects for dissection is another consideration which induces Dr. Smith to remove from this place. Without these, you may know, the study of anatomy is but trifling with time and expense, to say nothing of the danger to [which] the patient of the merely descriptive anatomist is subject."

Gridley described the hostile environment in Hanover. "But the inhabitants within forty or fifty miles of this place are constantly on the watch, lest the silent repose of their departed friends be disturbed by the nocturnal visitations of medical students." He noted the difficulty and distance required to obtain cadavers and thought that because New Haven is on the water, obtaining bodies would be much easier. "Boston is the nearest port from which subjects can be obtained without great hazard and difficulty. At New Haven the water communication with New York, and even with Philadelphia would completely obviate this difficulty, as subjects might be procured as frequently and as expeditiously as occasion might require."[54]

Dr. Smith did move on to Yale College in 1813, but it was not the "promised land" he imagined it might be. It did not meet the expectations for easily procuring subjects, as suggested in Gridley's letter. As one historian later wrote, "During the long history of Harvard and Yale they were allowed one body a year. After dissection the body had to be restored."[55] When Dr. Smith arrived at Yale, "procurement and the attendant problems should have been the concern of Dr. Jonathan Knight [now professor of anatomy and physiology], to whom Smith had turned over the teaching of anatomy. But Smith himself, as professor of surgery, was of course also very much concerned with the problem and could not altogether escape responsibility for finding bodies."[56]

Rumors of body snatching and the discovery of empty graves in the towns surrounding New Haven fueled suspicions that there was wholesale robbing of graves under way by Yale medical students. As we will see, these suspicions would be confirmed with the discovery of the empty coffin of a young woman buried in a West Haven, Connecticut, cemetery in January 1824 that led to an attack on the medical college, a weeklong riot in New Haven, and later that year the passage of an anatomy act by the Connecticut legislature.

5

The Yale Medical School Riot

Hannibal Hamlin's "The Dissection Riot of 1824 and the Connecticut Anatomical Law" is generally seen as the seminal article explaining the Yale medical school riot of 1824 and its consequences leading to the passage of the Anatomical Act by the legislature in Connecticut in 1824, an act "relative to the disinterment of the dead."[1] Hamlin wrote about two of the three professors responsible for the Yale Medical School at the time, Dr. Jonathan Knight, who served as professor of anatomy and physiology, and, tangentially in a digressive note, the famous Dr. Nathan Smith, professor of theory and practice of physic, surgery, and obstetrics.[2]

Dr. Knight was responsible for procuring subjects for dissection. However, because of Dr. Smith's interest in surgery and, as we saw previously, his experience in procuring subjects in the past, Smith was also involved in this activity.

The Yale Medical School Under Suspicion of Body Snatching

From the founding of a medical school at Yale, suspicions over body snatching had surfaced in neighboring towns. Before Jonathan Knight was appointed a professor at the college, in 1810–1811 he was commissioned by Professor Benjamin Silliman, the "prime organizer" of the medical school, to obtain specimens for the new school while taking lectures in Philadelphia. "None of the businesses in the City of Brotherly Love trafficked in human anatomy, he, like the medical students, was left to his own devices." Knight dutifully collected and prepared the specimens himself. After landing in Norwalk, Connecticut, he put the specimens in temporary storage. The locals became aware of this and "worked themselves up into something of a frenzy, suspecting he had dead bodies in his boxes." Under cover of night, he loaded his "gruesome packages onto a wagon" and "stole quietly out of town toward New Haven." There he "received a cordial reception."[3]

Dr. Smith wrote to a fellow physician, Dr. George C. Shattuck, on May 14, 1810, that there was "strong feeling against cutting up of dead bodies."[4] In New Hampshire and doubtless where schools of medicine were founded, rumors of grave robbing flourished. Early on when the Yale Medical School was established in Sheffield Hall (where the medical school operated until 1859), rumors were rife that its location was "attributed to proximity of the Grove Street Cemetery[,] … the belief being current that resurrectionists found it all too easy to introduce subjects for dissection disinterred from … the cemetery across the street."[5]

This may be a reference to what a traveler from Scotland reported when he visited New Haven in 1818 and 1819. He wrote that the "Medical School connected to Yale

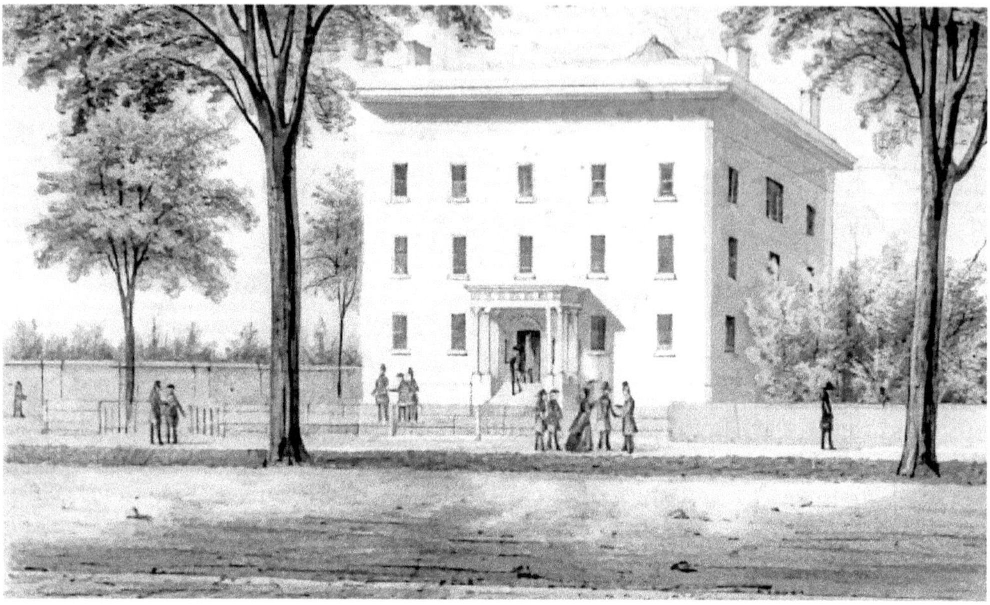

"View of the original building housing the first School of Medicine at Yale College, New Haven, Connecticut. Contemporary engraving (image from later postcard). Circa 1814." The building was built as a hotel; Yale rented it until 1814 when through "the efforts of Dr. Nathan Smith" the school received a grant from the Connecticut legislature for $20,000 and purchased the building for $12,500. The building contained "lecture rooms, sleeping accommodations, study rooms" and a "commons" in the basement. Thirty-seven students were admitted to the medical school in the fall of 1812. In 1814 "the first class of three members was graduated with the degree of doctor of medicine." Yale Medical School, *Memorial of the Centennial of the Yale Medical School*(New Haven: Yale University, School of Medicine, 1915), 25–26 (courtesy Harvey Cushing/John Hay Whitney Medical Library, Yale School of Medicine, Yale University, New Haven, Connecticut).

College, is under a bond by the State Legislature that no bodies shall be taken from the New Haven burying ground [the recently established Grove Street Cemetery, also called Westminster at Yale] for anatomical purposes."[6]

At Yale in March 1818, there had been some trouble in obtaining cadavers. Dr. Smith wrote to Dr. Lyman Spalding that "of late, owing to some headstrong and unforesighted young men in procuring subjects, we have been brought into much trouble, and perplexity, which I trust, will however pass over."[7]

There was no doubt that grave robbing was going on, and the public was becoming increasingly suspicious. Dr. Smith was circumspect in his correspondence and generally did not provide details on this matter. His former student Cushing basically admitted this approach, having written to his father these cautionary words: "for fear my letter should be opened at the Post Office here."[8] This was no doubt good advice provided by Dr. Smith or his lawyer, Mills Olcott.

The lack of "subjects" and perhaps a complaint or two by Dr. Smith in class or an aside may have motivated several students to attempt a "resurrection" from a local graveyard. It appears that Dr. Smith must have known something; otherwise, why write that the perpetrators were "headstrong and unforesighted." Perhaps they, like Dr. John Warren's son, suspected that if they delivered a fresh cadaver undiscovered, all would be forgiven. We know that Dr. Smith inspired almost unwavering loyalty in his students. For example, Ezekiel Cushing refused to say that Dr. Smith was involved in the Dartmouth body-snatching incident detailed above.

Dr. Lyman Spalding, whom Dr. Smith mentored in his youth, and Lyman's son, Dr. James Spalding, called Dr. Smith his teacher. After graduating from Harvard, James Spalding helped Dr. Smith found the Dartmouth medical school in 1797. He wrote that my father "left his practice at Portsmouth [New Hampshire] for two or three months at this time, dissected and made beautiful preparations under [Dr.] Ramsay's instructions and gave various lectures at intervals at Dr. Smith's request."

James Spalding added, "We can imagine him [Lyman Spalding] setting out for Hanover on the stage coach [*sic*] with these rum-preserved subjects toiling on behind over 100 miles of rugged road between Portsmouth and Hanover" envisioning a "hearty welcome… [and] … thanksgivings[,] … for, on this material depended the success of the great lecture course now under way."[9] Dr. Smith's student Timothy J. Gridley, who earned his MD at Dartmouth in 1812, wrote to Jonathan Knight[10] the following about his professor: "I was conversing with Dr. Smith [and] … I observed that a medical institution was contemplated at New Haven and asked his opinion of the probability of its success. He answered … in … a few years it would excel any medical school this side of Philadelphia.… *I also expressed a wish that in case of a medical establishment at New Haven he could be one of the professors.* He said if there was a vacancy, and the faculty of Yale College should request him to fill it, *he would accept without the least hesitation*, although by dissolving his relation to this college he might hazard considerable pecuniary loss."[11]

Gridley's letter was extraordinary for a student writing a letter feeling out the situation, recommending his teacher for the position in New Haven, and saying he told him if offered he would accept! As Smith's biographers, Hayward and Putnam noted, various "points in Gridley's communication to Knight … suggest Smith helped compose the letter."[12]

There is little doubt that Dr. Nathan Smith seemed to have an uncommon effect on his students and friends, who seemed inordinately loyal and willing to go to extra lengths to work for him and protect his reputation.

Outrage over the Body-Snatching Episode of Major Tiff in January 1819

The following year on January 16, 1819, a body-snatching episode occurred in Southbury, Connecticut, a town about nineteen miles northwest of New Haven. The body of Mr. Tiff, a revolutionary war soldier, a man who had been impressed into the British Royal Navy for seventeen years, had returned home a broken man and since lived off the charity of his neighbors. Upon his death he was buried in the Southbury north burying ground. A few days later, mourners at another funeral noticed that his grave had been disturbed. On checking further, they found an empty coffin. On February 16, 1819, the *Connecticut Courant* reported that "the circumstances have produced on the town a feeling of general indignation at so atrocious a crime as that of disturbing the ashes of the dead."[13]

On February 15, 1819, the town of Southbury held a special meeting to take "measures to detect and bring to condign punishment such wretches as are in the habit of resorting to our grave-yards and stealing from graves the remains of deceased friends and relatives." Their suspicions fell on the medical school in New Haven. The notice continued: "People of New Haven and adjacent Communities, Take Notice!! That north burying ground in this town was entered on or about the night of the 16th of January last, by some of these felons of the tomb, and the body of Major Tiff (recently interred) was dug up and taken from the grave!" The article also reported that the body of a Mr. Towner was stolen from his grave from a churchyard in nearby Oxford, Connecticut.

The people of Southbury were so outraged that they passed resolutions to make every effort to capture the "miscreants, who perpetrated the above outrage"; not to employ or support any physician or surgeon who may have been involved or whose student was "directly or indirectly, … [involved] … in so nefarious a transaction"; and to offer a $100 reward for information about anyone "hereafter, within the limits of the town, [who commits] a similar outrage upon the peace of society." Finally, to show there was no doubt who they thought was responsible for the outrage, it was ordered that the results of the meeting be published in the papers of New Haven "for the information of the public" so they "may be on their guard."[14]

The people of Southbury were right to suspect a Yale connection. On February 24, 1819, Alanson Beecher, a grand juror of the town of Southbury, made a complaint "in writing to William Hinman Esq., justice of the peace," that charged Joseph T. Waldo (a medical student at Yale) "with having opened a grave in Southbury, and with having taken therefrom, and carried away, the body of Major Tiff, deceased for the purpose of dissection." Waldo was arrested and brought before Shadrach Osborn, a justice of the peace. Osborn judged the testimony and evidence credible. Waldo pleaded not guilty. Osborn ordered Waldo to appear before the superior court in New Haven on the second Tuesday in August and set bail at $200. Waldo did not appear after three notices and forfeited the surety. Later, the state treasurer sued Waldo for the surety, and the case dragged on until July 21, 1821. (The defendant argued on several objections to the court's procedures, including that the court had his name wrong, and that this explained why he did not appear. Waldo lost the case on his claim of the superior court's error and had to pay the surety. The original charge of body snatching does not appear in the resolution of the proceedings. Joseph T. Waldo received his medical degree from Yale on September 8, 1819.)[15]

In reference to the above episode in May 1819, Dr. Nathan Smith wrote to Dr. George Shattuck that "we have had a little of the old Hanover spirit [i.e., 'resurrections'] here this winter." He noted he was not involved "and so was not immediately concerned."

We learn more of this episode from a letter Dr. Nathan Smith wrote to his lawyer Olcott Mills in Hanover, New Hampshire, in May 1819. Dr. Smith and Dr. Jonathan Knight "were both summoned to give in evidence" of what they "knew on the subject" of the body-snatching incident in Southbury. Dr. Smith again tried not to get involved and told Dr. Knight he "had patients, on the way, I would be there soon, but he had so much reliance on my former experience in such cases that I could not prevail on him to go an inch without me. So, I had to go on & meet the mob in the [Southbury] town meeting who treated us with great civility and as it so happened, that I knew nothing of the matter & having bowed very respectfully to those we hate they let me depart & appeared very well satisfied. The subject, Major Tiff who was named Major and it was said that he was a drum major, but notwithstanding his title he died a pauper unlamented but after it was discovered he had descended from (?) he became of great consequence, especially as a certain man in your profession [lawyer] wished to ride his bones into Hartford as deputy at the next election. The business … has terminated without any serious injury." He "had to meet with another Committy [*sic*] on the subject," and it was not unpleasant.[16]

It is important here to understand the context of this letter. The Connecticut legislature was meeting in May 1819 and was considering a bill "relating to digging up dead bodies for dissection."[17] In his letter to Shattuck, Dr. Smith seems to be making a little joke about what has happened at Yale, writing that "we have had a little of the old Hanover spirit here." Shattuck would know exactly what he meant by those words: students at the college had been robbing graves for dissection. Since both doctors used dissection in their classes, they had been called upon to give evidence. In the letter, Dr. Smith once again claimed that he was not involved and so was not "immediately concerned." He used the excuse that he had patients and so could not attend an inquiry. Dr. Knight, who was relatively inexperienced in these matters and was a young doctor (he had only been licensed to practice in Connecticut in August 1811), expected more support from Dr. Smith.[18]

We only have Dr. Smith's interpretation but can imagine Dr. Knight pleading for his support. Dr. Smith tells us that Dr. Knight convinced him to go and "meet the mob in the town meeting" at Southbury, who nevertheless treated them "with civility."[19] However, Dr. Smith could not contain his contempt for those who questioned the two of them. He added that he met with a "mob" but acted "respectfully to those we hate." This was no doubt a carryover from his contempt for the activities of the New Hampshire legislature that had helped him decide to leave Hanover.

Although Dr. Smith was not involved in the stealing of Major Tiff's body, he does demonstrate a callous attitude toward the action. He has no sympathy for those upset by what happened and seems to suggest because Major Tiff was poor and unlamented, his stolen body should not be a cause for alarm and that he only saw "Tiff's bones" being used for an advantageous political purpose by the anatomists' enemies.

Finally, Smith had to meet with a committee on the subject, which may have been a separate committee from the town of Southbury. Unfortunately, Dr. Smith does not give any more information concerning this meeting except that it was not an unpleasant meeting.

At the same time as Dr. Smith's letter to Mills Olcott in May 1819, a Connecticut legislative committee was meeting about preventing the digging up of the dead for the purposes of dissection. The newspapers reported that a bill was introduced by representative Curtis Hinman of New Haven, perhaps the politician Smith referred to as "riding the bones" in his letter "to prevent the disinterment of the dead."

After much debate, the bill was passed by committee to the Connecticut House on May 20, 1819. The punishment "directed by this act to be inflicted on such as remove bodies of deceased persons, for the purpose of dissection, is a fine, imprisonment, sitting in the stocks, and disenfranchisement."[20] If the students and teachers did not know where their "subjects had been obtained," they would have been "ineligible to hold civilian or military office in the State" and also "lose the privilege of being an elector, and on conviction could not collect debts for professional services."[21] The bill does seem to be an expansion of some of the ordinances passed earlier at the Southbury town meeting on February 15, 1819.

The bill was tabled twice and read a third time and passed in the Connecticut House on June 1, 1819.[22] Nevertheless, when it went to the Connecticut Senate it was "negatived by the Senate" and never became law.[23]

The bill only punished those who stole bodies and those physicians who received illegal bodies but offered no solution to the overriding issue that Connecticut physicians were required by law to have dissection experience with human bodies. There were simply not enough legal bodies available to meet this requirement. As the English physician and sanitary reformer Thomas Southwood Smith summarized, he did not blame Americans for attempting to "abolish exhumation" but maintained that "it is both absurd and criminal, to make this practice a felony, without providing in some other method for the cultivation of anatomy."[24]

As we saw previously, there were elites who did not oppose the use of criminals and stolen pauper bodies in the dissecting laboratories. Besides the religious opposition, Americans were also becoming more democratic in their "anti-aristocratic beliefs about the individual value and equality of human beings, unalienable dignities that supposedly continued into death."[25] Public opinion made it difficult to not only pass but even introduce legislation that expanded access to and increased the number of legally acquired cadavers for the medical schools. For example, in Massachusetts in 1830 the committee on the judiciary tasked to reform the 1815 Sepulcher law, when asked about the status of its proceedings, replied, "The Committee Are aware that the subject is as delicate as it is important, and they do not think it expedient to propose any alteration of the law at the present time; because in a community like ours, it is necessary the laws should proceed from and be supported by public opinion."[26]

Even though public opinion supported harsh penalties, the law was one-sided and offered no solution to the need for additional cadavers for the medical community. It could be argued that if passed it would have virtually ended the teaching of anatomy with human subjects in Connecticut because of the harsh punishments in the law. In this case, the Connecticut senators were likely influenced by the Yale faculty, the medical societies, physicians, and those who had originally approved the medical school to defeat the bill with the hope for another opportunity to pass anatomical reform legislation for Connecticut.

The Yale/New Haven Body-Snatching Riot of 1824

According to Dr. Smith, the instances of grave robbing in and around New Haven led to suspicions that the medical school was responsible. The measures passed by the town of Southbury (including the order to publish them in the New Haven papers) were a direct warning to the students and faculty of the medical school that their actions would not be tolerated. But the failure to pass a law to prevent body snatching by punishing the participants failed in the legislature and led to frustration and a smoldering resentment by the public.

In the fall of 1823, the following body-snatching incident occurred in Vernon, Connecticut. The "grave of a Mrs. Hammond of Vernon, wife of a respectable gentlemen, of that place, was robbed of its tenant, and although a large reward was offered for his detection, the villain has not been discovered."[27] Vernon, being quite a distance from New Haven and its surrounding towns, probably did not excite the people but continued to add to their resentment as evidence that nothing was being done to prevent and punish those who "perpetrated ... [this] ... outrage upon the feelings of the living and the rights of the dead."[28]

The public in New Haven and the surrounding towns had reached their breaking point; seething with frustration, they were ready to take matters into their own hands. They finally got their opportunity when the body of nineteen-year-old Bathsheba Smith of Orange was stolen from her grave. (The parish of West Haven since 1822 was part of the new town of Orange.)

Bathsheba Smith was the daughter of Laban Smith, a farmer. She died on December 30, 1823. Her body was brought to the old burying ground in West Haven, Connecticut, and interred on New Year's Day.[29] The funeral and subsequent events are described by Henry Peck, a New Haven historian writing in 1889 who interviewed eyewitnesses, family members, and others.[30]

> At the funeral of Miss Smith, which was largely attended, there happened to be present a student from the medical college, on the corner of Grove and Prospect streets, since occupied by some of the departments of the Sheffield Scientific School, of Yale. The young lady died from consumption and dropsy, and her complexion and features after life had departed were very beautiful. The body was buried in the old cemetery, near the Episcopal Church, West Haven. A few nights after the burial, Mrs. Smith, the young lady's mother, was visited in her dreams by an Intelligence which will perhaps forever be a mystery. She was made certain that the grave would be despoiled. For succeeding nights, the bereaved mother dreamed that the body of her child was being molested in the grave. So deep an impression was made upon her mind that she communicated the dream to her husband, and for nine consecutive nights he watched by the grave, gun in hand, to prevent desecration.[31]

Peck in his introduction refers to Laban Smith as a sea captain rather than a farmer, as he is currently referenced. It is likely that in his earlier days Smith was a seafarer, as it was a common vocation for young men in New Haven. The reference to the "student from the medical college" at the funeral is interesting because if it is accurate, it would explain why her parents became especially anxious that their daughter's grave might be despoiled, leading to Mrs. Smith's disturbing dreams and the girl's father watching over her grave for nine consecutive nights. In addition, how common was it for medical students to show up at funerals? It is possible that someone at the school was informed that Bathsheba was an excellent candidate for dissection and would be of interest because she had a combination of consumption and dropsy, her body was in good condition, and the cold weather would help to preserve it. The earliest obituary published seems to have been on January 10, 1824, simply reading "Died-In Orange, on the 30th ult. [last month] Miss Bathsheba Smith, aged 19, daughter of Mr. Laban Smith."[32] It is possible that the students were waiting for an opportune time and, on the night of Saturday, January 10, read the obituary, visited the grave, saw no one watching over it, and took her body. Sunday morning after attending church services, Laban Smith returned to his daughter's burial site. Having previously marked the grave, he

> saw evidences that there had been a disturbance of the ground. Some stalks of straw which had been laid upon the top of the coffin to muffle the dread sound of the falling earth while the grave was being filled, were scattered about. Mr. Smith immediately communicated with his neighbors[;] ... they decided to re-open the grave. A few feet below the surface of the ground was found a tortoise-shell comb which had been placed in the hair of the deceased. When the coffin was reached, it was seen to have been split open and a log of wood had been substituted for the body.[33]

To avoid discovery, it was necessary that the grave be filled in and arranged so there was no evidence it had been disturbed. Placing straw on the coffin may have muffled the sound of the dirt landing on the coffin but also served a second purpose; if any of the straw was discovered on the surface of the grave, it would be telltale evidence that there had been a disturbance. Leaving the tortoise comb in the grave just below the surface was also inept, because when it was found it only motivated the father to dig down to the coffin.

No doubt the students were careless; however, placing the log in the coffin suggests that they may have gotten advice from someone more experienced. Although I have found no reference this was standard procedure, it makes sense if the coffin was "split open." Perhaps the advice of placing a log in the coffin was recommended in case the coffin did break (substituting for the body) to prevent the ground from settling after the culprits left, thus giving away the crime.[34]

> Among those who were present was Simeon Filch, brother of Mrs. Lewis Fitch and cousin of the young woman, William Kimberly, and Sidney Painter. It was reported at the time, that the body had been taken to New Haven in a chaise, by two young men [some reports said there was but one] and was held in an upright position by the person driving.

Moving the body disguised as a passenger, usually sleeping or drunk, is a common description in the body-snatching literature. The chaise would likely have been "an open, horse-drawn carriage for one or two people, usually with one horse and two wheels." Most likely there would have been no way of finding out whose chaise was used for this purpose.[35]

In contrast to Peck's description as reported to him by family members and friends of the family who claimed to have witnessed the event, there is a letter dated January 12, 1824, written by Erastus Osborn, a constable, to his father Shadrach Osborn, postmaster in Southbury, Connecticut, describing the events.[36] He wrote that "this morning I was called to the Medical College with a search Warrant to look for the Body of young woman 19 years old which was taken from the Grave in West Haven burying ground Night before last, rather yesterday morning [or Sunday morning]. a Waggon [*sic*] was heard to pass a House near the grave yard between Midnight & 2 O-Clock. this [*sic*] excited suspicion and yesterday the appearance of the grave confirmed it. it [*sic*] was open and a flat stone found broken on the head part of the lid the stone was removed & the lid found broken in & the Body missing."[37]

The description of how the grave was found by family and friends, as told to the historian Henry Peck, long after the event and Erastus' account recorded at the time, are distinctly different. There is no mention of the constable being at the burial site when Laban and friends dug up the grave. He likely observed the grave after the fact. He noted that it was opened. Perhaps Laban placed the stone over the open grave to deter curiosity seekers and to prevent anyone from falling in. Naturally, when the stone was moved, the grave would have been empty. It seems to me unlikely that the grave robbers would have left the grave in such an obvious condition because suspicion would have immediately fallen on the medical school. At least if the grave was returned to a look of normality, by the time it was discovered, Bathsheba Smith would have been dissected and disposed of without an identifying trace.

Both accounts agree with the estimated time of the grave robbery. As we will see, many of the other incidents are described by both accurately.

According to Peck's account, the "young men of West Haven were in a great state of excitement. They left the village about midnight, in a large body and accompanied Laban Smith to the city, where they arrived at the dawn of day. General Dennis Kimberly, a New Haven lawyer, but whose home was in West Haven, was called upon. He advised them to obtain a warrant to search the medical college."[38] Erastus Osborn wrote that they wanted the search warrant prepared "without giving the alarm." He left to meet General Kimberly at the home of Dr. Knight. The three men went to the medical college "without it being generally known." They searched the medical college and "found just as I suppose usually to be found at such institutions and concluded further searching would be unavailing." Then Osborn quickly changed his mind; he "determined to be thorough & I took 5 or 6 West Haven and New Haven Men with me."[39]

According to various accounts the following likely occurred, causing Osborn's abrupt change of mind. "Mr. [Laban] Smith was not satisfied. Nor—were hundreds of young men of West Haven, New Haven, Fair Haven, and from the outlying districts, who had heard the story of the crime and who met on the Green, where they were addressed by different persons who urged an attack upon the medical college and the razing of the building. The people appeared to be generally determined that the college building must be pulled down."[40]

The "excited crowd ... having obtained possession of one of the town cannons, advanced upon the medical building." The militia was called out by the high sheriff of New Haven County. The commander, Major Granniss, raised a detachment of twenty men "to assist in suppressing a riot at the medical college and save the college from being destroyed."[41] The "late Dr. Jonathan Knight and Dr. [Nathan] Smith were officers at the college. After a speech from Dr. Knight and some parleying, it was agreed that Mr. [Nathan] Smith and a committee should further search the building."[42] The "militia ... held the crowd at bay while the building was searched" by this committee.[43]

The members of the committee searched all the rooms and finally descended into the subcellar. Osborn wrote that in a "low Cellar, we came to a place in the pavement (the Cellar being paved with large flat stones) which looked generally like the bottom of the Cellar throughout but appeared to have a trifle of fresh dirt lying scattered about, hardly however discernible. I scratched with the end of my walking stick[;] the earth appeared fresher between the stones & finally took up a large flat stone where we discovered a white bundle, apparently a bundle of clothes." They had found "a human body doubled up in a heap entirely covered up with the grave cloathes." They proceeded to take the body out and immediately identified it as the "Body of the young Woman we was searching for."[44] Laban Smith, the father, was "almost distracted but greatly rejoiced at the discovery. The college officers, Dr. Knight, and Dr. [Nathan Smith] denied knowledge of it being brought to the College or it being there at all." Dr. Knight "sent home for a sheet & Cap had the face washed & and the sheet and Cap put on." Once the committee had reappeared with the "mutilated body, which had been found beneath the pavement in the cellar," the crowd became furious, and only the presence of the "military prevented the destruction of the edifice."[45]

With "great difficulty," Laban Smith allowed the body to be placed in a wagon to "remove it to West Haven."[46] A procession "marched to the house of Mr. Laban Smith." The following day "the remains were buried in the garden of the parent, attended by nearly the whole population of Orange, and several from the city." The *Connecticut*

Register reported that the "Rev. Mr. Stebbins, who assisted at the funeral solemnities made an appropriate address peculiarly adapted to the mournful occasion."[47]

The "grave was made within a few feet of the dwelling and there the body found rest. Members of the family watched the grave from a window of the house for a long time."[48] That week Laban Smith took out an advertisement concerning "his late peculiar affliction" and thanking all who aided him in "recovering the body of his deceased Daughter, when it had been surreptitiously removed from the grave, in which it was deposited on the late New-Years Day."[49] Mr. Laban Smith was never the same. His health declined, and "his life was believed to have been shortened by the mental anguish he had suffered."[50]

However, while the body was being borne through the town from the medical school, "crowds of People collected to view it. Bells were tolling during the procession bringing people up to a fever pitch."[51] Meanwhile, rumors spread, and "hardly a person here has lost friends for Months back but what has been to enquire of me if I did not see them at the College toNight."[52]

The crowd was not finished rioting. One local newspaper reported that "we have never known so great an excitement in the city on any occasion as witnessed during the past week. For two nights, it was necessary for the civil authority and executive officers, to be employed aided by a detachment of militia in preventing acts of violence on the part of an indignant community."[53]

Osborn wrote to his father that night that the medical students armed and "shut themselves up in the College with what they can muster" from students in the other parts of the college. The medical students expected to be attacked,

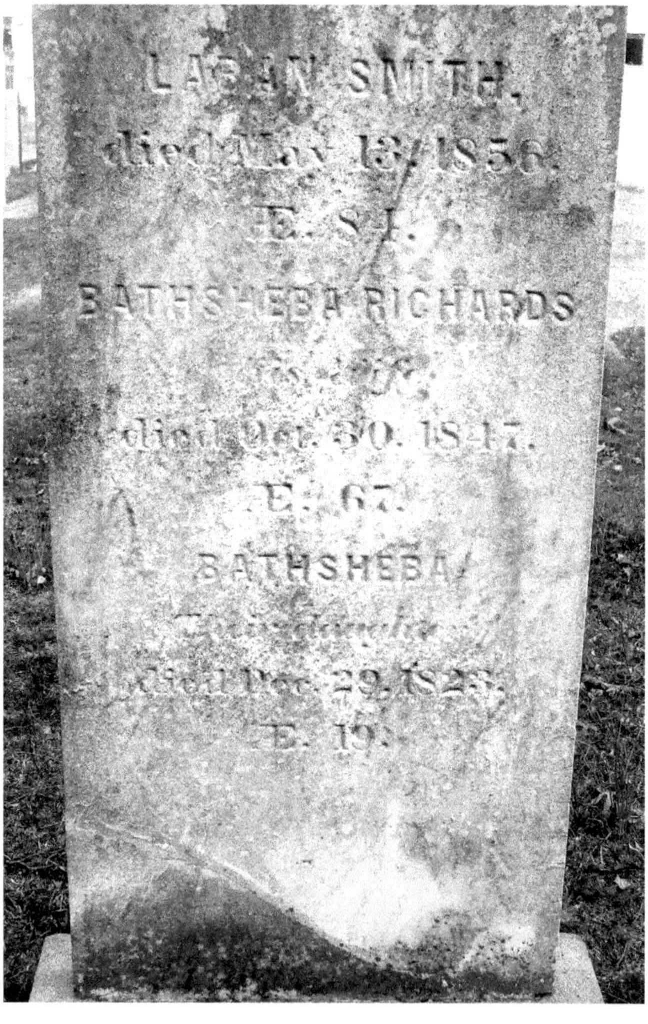

Present-day view of the gravestone of Bathsheba Smith and family in West Haven, Connecticut. Headstone reads "Laban Smith, died May 13. 1856. AE 84. Bathsheba Richards his wife, died Oct. 30. 1847. AE 67. Bathsheba their daughter died Dec. 29. 1823. AE. 19" (photograph by the author).

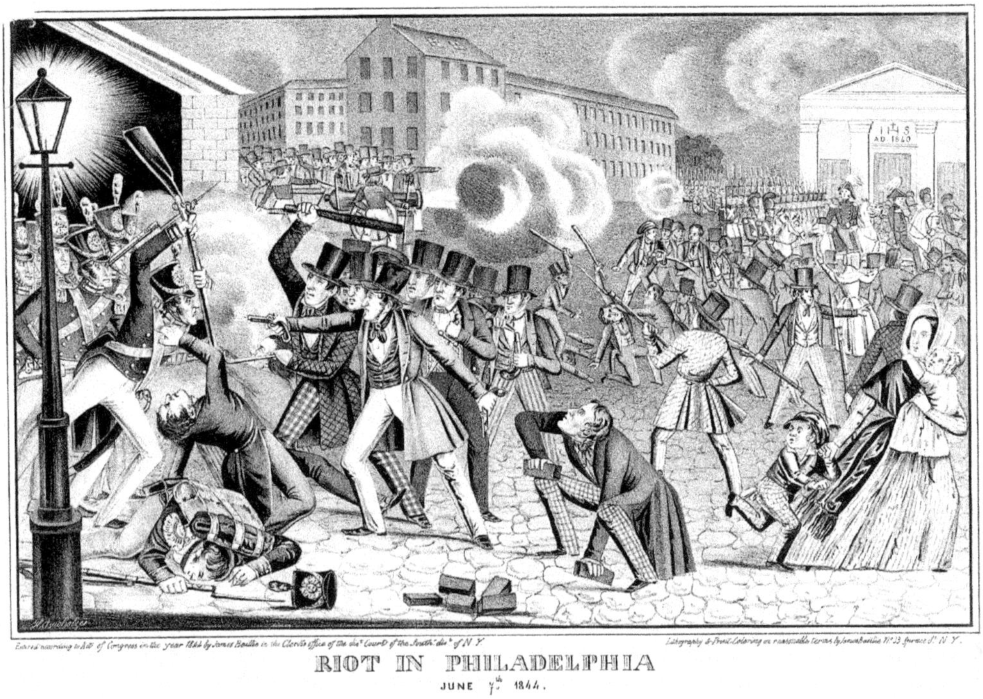

"We have never known so great an excitement in the city on any occasion as witnessed during the past week" (*New Haven Register*, January 17, 1824, 3). Although there were no deaths, there was much property damage. The print pictures an anti-Catholic riot in Philadelphia on July 7, 1844, where the state militia also had to be summoned, and gives us some idea of the fury that could be aroused in nineteenth-century urban rioters. H. Bucholzer, artist, "Riot in Philadelphia, June 7th, 1844" (Library of Congress).

because "the West Haven people, a great number, have come over & New Haven has mustered a large company. A Drum has beat & and the Streets are covered with the besieging army preparing for the assault." Here, interestingly, Constable Osborn informs his father that he intends to stay at home until the "ferment have vent or subside."[54] Fortunately for the students, militia detachments were sent to guard the medical building and were "under arms during the night completely foiling the designs of an infuriated mob."[55]

In a second letter to his father on January 19, Osborn described more of the mob's actions:

> we have had a boisterous Week since I wrote you last Monday in consequence of the removal of the Body of the young Woman from West Haven. attempts have been made (and some of them violent) upon the Medical College almost or quite every Night through the week. several Persons were committed to Jail as rioters but have since principally or all been discharged. a Watch was organized by the City Authorities Saturday & Sunday Nights & had their station near the College all Nights. The glass, a great part of it, has been broken out in the building and some of the Window frames drove in. it appears to be getting more quiet now.[56]

The authorities both civil and military seem to have been prepared to let the incensed mob riot, and the militia held their fire, avoiding greater escalation (likely to prevent the carnage as in the doctor's riot in New York in 1788 when the militia fired on the mob). At least until now, there was only property damage primarily aimed at the hated medical building. There was a sense that some of the mob's fury was justified in the eyes of the authorities because those arrested were let go, according to Osborn.

Osborn continued, two medical students have fled, "one of them accused of stealing the Body from the burial ground." This is known because he had "called upon a Man that has attended the M. College as an assistant [according to Dr. Smith the man was a sweeper; however, he was not the person charged with the crime] since the Lectures commenced to help him conceal it where it was found."[57]

The fury of the crowd is noted by the punishment the mob was willing to inflict on the accused man, Ephraim Colburn. When first charged, Colburn refused to disclose any information and was jailed. He was later let out on bond. While "the Court of enquiry was ... examining Witnesses" he attempted to leave the building and saw a group of men with a "Kettle of Hatters size [likely melted glue or gum shellac] & bag of feathers." Finding he was "exposed," he "retreated into the back part of the [Court] House."[58]

The evidence I have provided shows that the Yale Medical School riot was not a spontaneous uprising. Suspicions concerning the medical school had existed for years. When Major Tiff's body was stolen, the town of Southbury was outraged and prepared carefully thought-out resolutions to deal with this problem. The town made sure the resolutions were published in the New Haven newspapers. The ordinances provided much of the basis for the anatomy bill in 1819 that was passed in the Connecticut House but failed in the Connecticut Senate.

The Connecticut House, speaking for the people, showed the depth of outrage by the punishment it required for grave robbers and those who received stolen bodies. These would have included fines, imprisonment, time in the stocks, and disenfranchisement. The failure to pass this legislation in the Senate led to a simmering frustration among the populace and the belief that the elites would do nothing to protect the burying grounds and cemeteries in and around New Haven. Infuriated by other reports of body snatching, the people became more frustrated, and the public's rage finally exploded when Bathsheba Smith's body was taken from her grave. This exasperation was widespread and not limited to New Haven alone, because from the evidence provided, people from the surrounding towns participated in the riot to help destroy the focus of their anger, the Yale medical building.

Besides the simmering frustration of a lack of legislation to punish body snatchers, the removal of Bathsheba Smith's body provided other unique contributory factors, including an added frisson of sex and class (bourgeois respectability) that increased the fury of the public response. Michael Sappol has argued that "in the nineteenth century ... how one died and how one's body was treated after death, was a performance that fixed one's moral aesthetic, and social status." Even for poor people, the idea of a decent burial was paramount and included "placement of the body in a coffin, with some ornamentation; a respectful ceremony; and internment in a bounded plot of land with a marker." Workers and their families saved to provide funds for the burial of themselves and "loved ones." These ideas were important for all classes, although the elites had the funds to make this objective a reality. "People of all classes, ethnic groups, educational backgrounds hated the prospect of seeing their bodies, or the bodies of family members dissected, mutilated, or in any way disturbed."[59]

Generally, from a class perspective, when the indigent, immigrants, and Blacks were involved there was little outcry. When a respectable person's body was taken, there was pushback. However, when it was a young respectable woman, the outcry was considerable. All classes could sympathize, and thus the "respectability" argument as well as the idea that the youthful female body being dissected was a "violation of the body[,] ... [a] necrophiliac rape of the completely vulnerable."[60] This thinking was not absurd, because "the anatomical body did carry an erotic charge, among anatomists and the public..." especially when the body in question was that of a woman.[61]

The "desecration of bodies on the dissecting table and in the graveyard was [viewed as] an 'unnatural act' equivalent to sodomy. The affront to sexual/funerary honor was even more forcefully suggested when the body ... was that of a [respectable] woman."[62] The simmering resentment over body snatching itself, with the added elements of class and sex, no doubt inflamed the passion of the mob even more during the Yale Medical School riot.[63]

Bathsheba Smith's "respectability" was promoted by the mayor of New Haven, George Hoadley, who advertised on January 16, 1824, in "a local newspaper[,] ... which caused great discussion in New Haven and in many other towns of this state," the following:

> Whereas, on or about the 7th day instant, January, the body of a respectable female recently deceased, was unlawfully removed from its place of interment in West Haven and brought to this city for dissection: Now, therefore, by and with the advice and direction of the Court of Common Council, I hereby offer a reward of three hundred dollars to any person who will discover the offender or offenders and give such information thereof that they may be brought to justice and conviction.[64]

We note the epithet "a respectable female" used here and in other places coupled with "brought to the city for dissection." The family and friends knew that Bathsheba was a young, beautiful, unmarried nineteen-year-old woman whose body was taken from the grave to be laid on a table "to be cut to pieces by the surgical knife [phallic]."[65] The hometown papers the *Connecticut Herald* and *The Pilot* each took a different approach in describing the young lady. The latter refers to Bathsheba as a "respectable female, about 19 years of age." The former refers to her as "the corpse of a young lady of 19 years." As for dissection, the *Herald* readers are informed of the good news that "the body was found, somewhat mutilated, though [most importantly] the process of dissection had not been commenced." *The Pilot*, less thorough but likely mitigating the situation, stated that "fortunately the work of dissection had not commenced,"[66] in short, reporting that Bathsheba's body had been saved from having gone through dissection and its attendant shame, which the family and neighbors knew only too well.

The Doctors

The *Connecticut Herald* in an editorial on January 13 (before any investigation) wrote that "while we acquit the Medical Faculty of any knowledge of this base transaction, we freely accord to the perpetrators of the deed, the general execration which it has excited." The editors went on to unequivocally state that "if subjects are necessary for dissection ... the cerements of the grave ... are not to be violated with impunity, and the hand that could ruthlessly touch the hallowed spot is even more venomous than slander."[67]

However, *The Pilot* on January 15 was less sanguine and closed its editorial with "as the affair is in a train of legal investigation, we do not feel authorized after the example, of a brother editor, to acquit any class of men from all concern in the disgraceful outrage. Such a hasty judgment, to say the least, would appear indecorous to our civil community."[68] As Peck innocently concluded, the public believed that the medical faculty "of the college had no knowledge of the fact that the body was ever taken into the building, although at first, so great was the tumult that their lives were in danger of being lost. During the search of the buildings some of the medicines and other property were damaged."[69]

Notwithstanding the pass that the two newspapers gave the doctors, one irate letter on January 21, 1824, from a citizen complained that "within a few hours under cover of night, the corpse is feloniously taken from the place of sepulture and carried for dissection to the dark room of the surgeon or anatomist" and was "cut to pieces by the surgical knife … under the gaze of surrounding multitudes."[70] Those surrounding multitudes would be the professor and his male students.[71]

There is no evidence that Dr. Smith and Dr. Knight were directly implicated in this body-snatching episode though Dr. Smith did have a history of using illegally obtained bodies at Dartmouth and was quick to request bodies from his friends in Boston. Shortly after the defeat of the anatomy bill in 1819, Dr. Nathan Smith was in Maine helping to open the Bowdoin medical school. As was mentioned earlier, he blithely wrote to Dr. Shattuck in Boston asking him if he could "find some young man in Boston who would agree to furnish us with two or three subjects."[72] It seems that Dr. Smith had no problem involving perhaps a local medical student to do some grave robbing in Boston or its vicinity to obtain subjects. This does suggest that he was willing to use illegal means to obtain his subjects. It also casts doubt on his total innocence whenever there was the chance that he might have been involved in a "body-snatching incident."

In addition, as noted previously, Dr. Smith had strong relations with many of his students; "of all those who have been instructed by him, the number is small who were not his personal friends." He was praised for "his free conversation and his fund of anecdotes…."[73] It is likely Dr. Smith and Dr. Knight told their students anecdotes from their own experiences. Dr. Smith may have reminisced about his students' exploits at Hanover or regaled them about when Dartmouth's medical school moved into its own building in 1811. The "…basement was soon piled with human and non-human bones. The medical students entertained themselves with this collection by using it to terrorize the campus and the town at night."[74]

There are many examples in the literature of the "heroic" stories told of "adventure in the quest of bodies" by men who would later be leaders "of their profession" in order "to teach properly" and satisfy their own "thirst for exact scientific knowledge."[75]

On a more sober note, Dr. Smith also lectured his students that one of the greatest stumbling blocks to proper training in medicine at this time was the lack of "dissecting material."[76] Were some of Dr. Smith's and Dr. Knight's students inspired, like the young John C. Warren at Harvard or the later distinguished physician Dr. John Anderson of New York, to engage in body snatching?

"There are those still living who remember with alacrity with which 'young Anderson' went forth after the manner of 'Cruncher,' [the body snatcher in *A Tale of Two Cities*] in company with six medical students to procure a body for the use of Prof. Godman."[77]

Dr. Smith and Dr. Knight may not have been personally involved in the stealing of Bathsheba's body, but it is possible that someone was on the lookout for a "fine" specimen that would be appreciated by both professors, and the hope was that if they were successful the students would do honor to their professors as they came to the end of the term. If Bathsheba's purloined body had not been discovered, there is no doubt that she would have ended up on the dissecting table without a word being uttered.

However, it did not work out that way. Dr. Smith wrote to Mills Olcott in Hanover at the end of January 1824. "Just at the commencement of the vacation another affair took place which has given us as much trouble. Some foolish & rash fellow went to West Haven about 4 miles from this [place] & took a female subject from the grave[;] it was discovered & found in the deep cellar of the medical building where it had been placed by the person who got it & our sweeper & without the knowledge of the Faculty. This raised a mob who broke more than 100 panes of glass in the building before they could be dispersed."[78] (The previous affair Dr. Smith alluded to was the Major Tiff episode.)

Dr. Smith added, "They continued to threaten the professors ... and ... have convicted the water [waiter] for assisting & all is now quiet."[79] Presumably, the waiter he is referring to is Ephraim Colburn, who was charged in the theft (see below).

During the troublesome period that followed, Dr. Smith could point to the fact he was working with the Association of Physicians of the town of New Haven to inoculate the people against kine pock (to forestall smallpox) in the event of a breakout in the town. The association offered free vaccinations to the poor, and other funds raised by those who could pay would go to the "public library belonging to the association."

This appeal appeared during the week of the rioting and in subsequent weeks during February. Perhaps the physicians hoped this would temper the passions of the people, knowing they might be in for a smallpox epidemic. The notice assured the people that the physicians were there to help; for the poor, their services would be free, and doctors were not benefiting but instead were turning over profits to the association library.[80]

In addition, Dr. Smith was preparing for his teaching position at Bowdoin College. An advertisement appeared in the *Portsmouth Journal* on January 24, 1824, announcing that medical lectures were to begin on February 23, 1824, featuring Nathan Smith, MD, and others and extolling the "valuable Anatomical Cabinet ... equal to, if not superior to any in New England ... [and] ... contains preparations for demonstrations—with many valuable morbid specimens [for dissection]."[81]

On February 28, 1824, Dr. Smith wrote a second letter to Mills Olcott stating that "they have had a good [?] of turmoil in the academical College as well as in the medical department this winter but the storm seems to be past [*sic*] by & all is now quiet."[82]

Fear and paranoia were not completely quelled among the public. Osborn pointedly noted that people asked if he had seen the bodies of any relatives or friends in the medical building. Throughout the towns of Connecticut, the public "were greatly exercised, and in some rural cemeteries graves were re-opened to ascertain whether they had been desecrated." Perhaps to help quiet the fear, the "college authorities offered to give a bond that nothing of the sort should occur again."[83]

The Trial of Ephraim Colburn

The student or students involved in the stealing of Bathsheba Smith's body ran away from New Haven. This left the assistant (likely a waiter at the college, according to

Dr. Smith),[84] Ephraim Colburn. Colburn was arraigned and "bound over for trial with $1000 Bond surety to answer to the charge of taking up the Body, as it is suspected he assisted the Student who has absconded."[85] Colburn "was the only person indicted."[86]

The trial was held during the January sessions of the superior court in New Haven, with Judge William Bristol presiding. The state called a series of witnesses against Colburn: Horace Beach, a deputy marshal; Ely Ives, a Yale professor of materia medica, botany; Erastus Osborn, constable; and Laban Smith as well as several others.[87] Colburn was defended by Seth P. Staples, "one of the most distinguished lawyers at the Connecticut Bar."[88] (It is unlikely that Ephraim could afford this lawyer; perhaps Yale was paying for his defense.)

There were three witnesses in Colburn's defense: Luther Bradley, David Butler, and William Myers.[89] The *New Haven Register* reported that Colburn was a "labourer and sometimes acted as a Commissary General for the Medical College."[90] If the *Register* report is accurate, it is strange that Dr. Smith referred to Colburn only as a waiter. David Butler, a grocery and provisions supplier, served as a witness for Colburn along with Luther Bradley. William Myers appeared to serve for both the prosecution and the defense.[91]

Colburn entered a plea of not guilty. Unfortunately, the distinguished lawyer Seth P. Staples and the witnesses provided could not get him off on the charges. The jury returned a verdict on the "second count" but not on the first or third counts. The verdict as reported in the newspapers was as follows:

> Ephraim Colburn was tried and found guilty by the jury, for acting and assisting in opening the grave and removing the body of a female from the burying ground in Orange [West Haven], for the purpose of dissection; and was sentenced for nine months imprisonment in the county jail and a fine of 300 dollars.[92]

According to Hamlin, Colburn was likely convicted on circumstantial evidence, as there were no "actual witnesses to anything but the condition of the grave and the finding of the body." The defendant was charged for "every phase of the crime." There were three separate charges. Colburn was found guilty on the second charge, presumably as reported for opening the grave and removing the body and taking the body for dissection.[93] As for the punishment, it fell under an 1810 Connecticut body-snatching statute.[94]

Hamlin wrote that the facts of the case against Colburn were weak and concluded that Colburn was "convicted ... by the influence of outraged civic virtue, that could scarcely help being strongly represented in the jury." (Likely, the father, Laban Smith, was prominently seated in the courtroom, reminding the jurors that it could have been their daughters or wives disinterred and placed on a slab naked to be gawked at by leering male medical students and then subjected to the horror of the knife and dissection.) No doubt the outcome was a foregone conclusion.[95]

In the end the public, frustrated by the lack of cooperation on the part of the authorities concerning body snatching, had turned to violence and rioting to demand that something be done. I would argue that the rioters were successful because they forced the Connecticut legislature in the 1824 legislative session to take up, for a second time within the span of four years, the question of how to protect the burying grounds and cemeteries of Connecticut from body snatchers and how to meet the growing need of cadavers for the medical profession. The attempt at a resolution to these two issues is discussed in Chapter 6.

6

The Connecticut Anatomy Laws of 1824 and 1833

Following the Yale Medical School riot in New Haven in January 1824, the Connecticut legislature met in New Haven in May 1824. The legislature found itself under the pressure of public opinion to solve what was almost an intractable problem: how to protect Connecticut's burying grounds from body snatchers and punish them and their medical clients while finding a way to legally expand access to cadavers for Connecticut's physicians and anatomists.

A statute on the books in Connecticut passed in 1810 made it "punishable by a fine of not less than one hundred dollars and imprisonment in the county jail for at least 3 months for any one secretly to disinter the body of any deceased person for the purpose of dissection, or in any way to aid in doing, or knowingly 'assist in any surgical or anatomical experiments therewith or dissection thereof."[1]

Perhaps it was thought that this statute punishment was not strict enough to prevent grave robbing or sufficiently harsh on those who benefited from the body snatchers, the anatomy professors, and other physicians.

In the May 1819 session of the Connecticut legislature there was an attempt to pass a bill on "disinterment." One representative tried to protect the beneficiaries of the body snatchers, the "anatomists," since they could also be implicated in the 1810 statute. He argued that it was necessary to "exculpate those who may be engaged in dissection without knowing that the subject was improperly obtained." He feared allowing punishment for using a body if the anatomist did not know its origin, "introduced a novel principle in our laws that professors and students were extremely liable to be imposed upon as to the manner in which the subjects were obtained, and that the [new] bill as it now stood would equally involve the innocent with the guilty on punishment and disgrace."[2]

In the Connecticut House there was little sympathy for the grave robbers, professors, or students engaged in dissection. On June 2, 1819, as noted previously, the bill passed in the Connecticut House. The newspapers dutifully reported the punishments directed by the act and a few days later followed the terse announcement that the deceased persons bill, having passed the House, was rejected in the Senate. The opportunity to protect the dead from removal from their graves was defeated.

The attempt to solve the problem and protect the dead required an alternative solution. If professors and their students acquired subjects legally, there would be no market for illegally obtained bodies. If anyone used illegally obtained corpses, then the punishments in the statute should be harsh enough to discourage grave robbing.

The Yale episode was fresh in everyone's mind when the spring session of the

Connecticut legislature opened in New Haven in 1824. Governor Oliver Wolcott addressed several topics, including the problem of body snatching and the resulting public furor, in his opening message:

> The public sensibility has lately been highly excited in this vicinity by a discovery that remains of a respectable female had been fraudulently removed from a public place of interment to a vault in the Medical College in this city. It is with great satisfaction, I inform you that the Faculty of that Institution were not, and I believe, in any manner concerned in perpetrating or conniving at the atrocious procedure. Although it may be admitted that modern science, by prolonging the duration of life, and diminishing human suffering, has conferred benefits on mankind, many of which have been owing to anatomical examinations, yet these advantages offer no excuse or even palliation for sacrilegious violation of a private cemetery. The defense of those retreats to which we are all tending is connected with the most tender affections and amiable sympathies of the human heart. Civilized men, barbarians, and even savages of all Nations, and in every age, have consecrated to the repose of the dead, shall be inviolable in the dwellings of the living as the temples in which they worship. I therefore request you to consider on the one hand, whether any new provisions are necessary to prohibit the property of public institutions from dangerous excesses of passion and on the other to mark with punishment and disgrace, all violations of right, whether proceeding from depraved selfishness, levity, or malice, which disturb the public tranquility.[3]

Interestingly, Governor Wolcott opened with the lamentable stealing of Bathsheba Smith's body, assuring the public that the Yale faculty had nothing to do with this "atrocious procedure" (even though the other two students involved were never tracked down and made to testify.) Regarding his opinion that "anatomical examinations" were believed to have benefited mankind, there were those at the time who questioned this belief and even whether the "advance in surgery, pathological, and physiological anatomy did not necessarily benefit patients."[4]

Wolcott defended the rituals of burying the dead and their placement in burying grounds and provided a brief description of how the dead are treated by the civilized and the barbarous, asserting that their resting places should be as "inviolable" as the home or places of worship. In his conclusion he does not address the problem of "subjects" required by professors of anatomy but does look at the issue as one of defending the property rights of public institutions to find a way to inhibit these passions from being inflamed, again oddly attributing "selfishness, levity or malice" to the body snatchers who in turn then cause the peace to be disturbed. Of the three, perhaps the only appropriate motive is selfishness due to the money paid to the "resurrection men" by the professors.

During the session another high-profile attempted body-snatching episode occurred in Hartford, Connecticut. On May 8, 1824, a thirty-year-old woman, Miss Jane Benton of Hartford, Connecticut, drowned. Her earlier death notice was terse and appeared on May 11, 1824: "Died—In this City, Miss Jane Benton, age 30."[5] On that same day the *American Mercury* provided the full story of her death. She had drowned in the Little or Mill River in Hartford and was found about half a mile west of the city. "She had been subject to occasional fits of insanity" and on Saturday morning left home for a "short walk." She did not return home when expected, and the "family became alarmed, and an immediate search commenced." The next morning her body was found in the river. The inquest concluded that "she came to her death by drowning herself in a fit of insanity."[6]

The same newspaper reported following the Yale episode that it was now forced to "record another aggravated violation of the sanctity of the sepulchre which has been recently committed in our city." About two weeks ago the paper announced the death of Miss Jane Benton and "the peculiar circumstances attending her untimely exit." She was buried in the "South burying grounds" in Hartford. The following Sunday "two young ladies, acquaintances of the deceased, were walking near the grave, [and] a piece of cloth, and a tape string were found which led to the suspicion that the grave had been disturbed, and on a nearer approach their suspicions were confirmed." They informed others of their suspicions and people came to the gravesite and began "removing the earth, and horrible to relate, within a foot ... they discovered the putrid remains of the deceased with a rope around her neck."

The grave robbers had "unscrewed the lid of the coffin, and by the aid of the rope, had drawn the body from thence; but finding it not fit subject for the knife of the dissector owing to its decayed state" (given the manner of Miss Benton's death and the time spent in the water the "resurrectionists" may not have known the condition of her body beforehand). Today, forensic pathologists know that once a body in water is removed, "putrefaction is generally accelerated," and the body quickly becomes useless for dissection. "They rudely tumbled it upon the coffin, and hastily closed the grave."

The report concluded that "no event in our recollection, has created such general excitement among our citizens, and called forth such a universal burst of indignation.... Gov. Wolcott has introduced the subject to the Legislature, and we cannot believe that they will suffer the sacred depositories of the dead to be thus sacrilegiously invaded" when they have the legislative "power to prevent it."[7]

The Connecticut House appointed three representatives to form a committee concerning the disinterment of the dead. The three men were Cornelius Tuthill of New Haven, chairman; Eliakim Kimberly of Orange; and William Drakeley of Woodbury. Tuthill and Kimberly had the most interest in this committee, as both had citizens in their communities adversely affected by the Yale Medical School's body-snatching episode and the passions it inflamed. The bill they came up with as reported by the newspapers "intended, strictly to guard against the disinterment of the dead, and against all surgical and anatomical experiments upon *subjects* which have been improperly obtained." The medical institutions were to be "visited and inspected at the pleasure of the Mayor and two Senior Aldermen." The anatomical professors were put "under heavy bonds that the law shall not be violated and annexes a heavy penalty by fine and imprisonment in Newgate [Connecticut State Prison], to those who shall be found guilty of the offences described in the several provisions of the Bill."[8]

The act punished the offender "by a fine not exceeding 2000 dollars, and by imprisonment in Newgate." It prohibited "professors in the Medical Institution from performing any anatomical experiment on the body of any deceased person until they have given a bond in the sum of 2000 dollars, conditioned that no body of any deceased person, illegally obtained, shall be brought into this building belonging to the institution, for the purpose of dissection."

The statute, titled "An Act to Prevent the Disinterment of the Bodies of Deceased Persons," was finally passed by the legislature. It had not been without controversy during its three readings in the legislature. Tuthill, undoubtedly briefed by the professors and medical community, realized that a case had to be made to obtain sufficient bodies for the growing classes at Yale if the anti–body-snatching legislation was to be effective. The bill originally "reported by Mr. Tuthill, that the bodies of prisoners dying in Newgate prison, and of State Paupers, should, with the consent of the selectmen in one case, and of the overseers of Newgate prison in the other, be delivered to the officers of the Medical College for the purposes of dissection."

Representative Cyrus Swan of Sharon, Connecticut, objected at the second reading of the bill and "moved to erase that part of it which related to dissection. He said the idea of subjecting the body of a deceased person to dissection, merely because he had the misfortune to be poor, and dependent on public charity for support, was so repugnant to every principle of humanity, that he was sure it would not be tolerated for a moment by the House. Poverty was a misfortune to which all were liable, and the poor ought not only for that cause to be treated as a criminal." Tuthill argued that the penalties they were proposing were so harsh for the medical professors that the legislature should at least "take some measures to provide them with subjects in a lawful manner." Tuthill then added that "State Paupers ... were generally vagabonds, not born in this or an adjoining state." He asked that voting on the amendment be postponed so that "members might have time to reflect."

Cyrus Swan and John S. Peters of Hebron, Connecticut, opposed the postponement. They believed that the House would strike the previously mentioned clause from the bill and wanted an immediate vote. They maintained that "many of the State Paupers were respectable men, who had been reduced to poverty by sickness or misfortune, to which all men were exposed. They were sure the House could never sanction a provision which classed the poor man with the convicted felon. The amendment to strike the clause was carried almost unanimously." The bill was postponed for a third reading.

Finally, on the bill's third reading a motion was made by Minor Hotchkiss of Middletown, Connecticut, to eliminate the section requiring bonds for the medical professionals "on the ground that it was unusual and implied a suspicion" that the medical professors could not be "restrained by ordinary sanctions of the law." As the *Connecticut Herald* reported, a member of the committee stated that "the officers of the Medical institution were satisfied with the proposed measure, the amendment was withdrawn, and the bill passed."[9]

The *Connecticut Herald* later, under criticism from a *New Haven Register* editorial, corrected its account to the "officers of the Medical Institution were not satisfied with the proposed measure." However, the amendment was withdrawn, and the bill passed.[10]

Mr. Tuthill's recommendation that paupers be candidates for dissection did not go unnoticed by the national press. The Albany, New York, newspaper the *National Democrat* published a scathing editorial criticizing him on this issue. Because Mr. Tuthill was a Republican, his friends accused the newspaper of attempting to damage his reputation locally, knowing that the article would be republished in a host of other newspapers including many in Connecticut.[11]

Cornelius Tuthill studied law at Litchfield Law School. He became interested in theology and studied with President Timothy Dwight at Yale in 1815 and concluded his studies in 1816. In 1818 Tuthill became ill with "consumption" and could not preach. He also edited a Yale semi-literary magazine called the *Microscope*. He was elected to the Connecticut legislature in 1823 at the age of twenty-eight.[12] Tuthill was reelected to the Connecticut legislature in the spring of 1824, and "although feeble he was able to take part in most of the proceedings" (including as chairman of the disinterment bill).[13]

Connecticut U.S. senator Elijah Boardman died in early September 1823.[14] In October 1823, Governor Wolcott temporarily appointed Henry W. Edwards to the United States Senate.[15] When the Connecticut legislature met in May 1824, Tuthill introduced a motion to quickly vote on a replacement, and others in the legislature concurred, ostensibly to be sure that their Senator could vote in what was considered this "great national question." (There was the concern the new president might be chosen by Congress.)[16]

Representative McClellan bluntly wanted to know how the person appointed would vote on this question before voting for him.[17] Senator Elijah Boardmen had been a Republican.[18] Tuthill (a Republican) was concerned that Edwards was a democratic Republican and might "favor Andrew Jackson for the presidency" and also feared that Edwards might influence the Connecticut representatives to vote for Jackson. Tuthill fought Edward's promotion for two weeks. However, the Connecticut legislature voted in Edwards, and he was appointed to the United States Senate. Later "Edwards did use his influence, as Tuthill had feared he would, to further Jackson's presidency."[19]

Perhaps for both his opposition to a sympathetic Jacksonian senator and his proposal to dissect paupers, Tuthill was attacked in the *New Democrat* newspaper editorial (likely serving as a proxy for some local papers) for his lack of humanity, morality, and Christianity.[20] The editor accused Tuthill of making an "unprovoked attack ... of every poor man in the world, by proposing, on the floor of the Legislature of Connecticut a law, that bodies of poor men, dying in an alms house, should be given over to dissection! It was this horrible proposition, fit only to have been made in a den of cannibals that provoked me to attack the author ... when I penned that article in vindication of the insulted rights of humanity."

The editor stated that Mr. Tuthill "be[ing] a Christian ... [and] wish[ing] to make such odious and cruel distinctions between the rich and poor may be scarce among us." There is "nothing of the spirit of Christ in his proposition to dissect paupers," as he was emphatically not the poor man's friend; "it was among the poor" he "dispensed his bounty." With all of life's miseries Tuthill would add "the anticipated horrors of barbarous and bloody mutilation of their bodies after death." The editor accused Tuthill of not being a man of "sensibility ... who would not shrink with horror from the anticipation of such treatment of his relics as being given over for surgical dissection."

The editor continued with the argument that the dead deserve "decent and undisturbed repose," and even in the case of criminals he finds sympathy "when the ends of justice and public safety answered, the mutilation of the body, after execution seems irreconcilable to reason and humanity." However, the latter can be "palliated" if the object is its "utility" for a "highly important science." When it comes to the poor, he appears incredulous that "any set of men in Connecticut ... [are so] ... benighted and besotted, as to believe that pauperism sanctions the dissection of paupers" so that cures might be found for the "disorders" of the rich and prolong their lives.

The portion of the law concerning paupers did not pass, and the editor, in conclusion, hoped that the "proposition was put down with the contempt it deserved, that Mr. Tuthill has had time to reflect seriously upon it, and to feel the pang of remorse for having in the enlightened nineteenth century made such an unprovoked and cold blooded attack on the rights of paupers, and the principles of liberty and humanity, and the divine maxims of that gospel we are told he is a believer and professor."[21]

Tuthill's idea that paupers owed the state something in return for its support during their lifetime might have been discussed among elites in their salons as a solution to the body-snatching problem; however, his proposal may have been the first time this solution was offered on the floor of a legislative body. It was not supported by a wide margin.[22] In addition, Tuthill proposed it at a time when a new Democratic Party was rising under Andrew Jackson, whose party principles were in direct opposition to the elitist proposals that Tuthill advocated here.[23]

Undoubtedly, Tuthill's reputation was badly tarnished, and there is some indication that he or his friends were willing to sue the *National Democrat*, because the editor later issued a retraction on July 30, 1824. "Two respectable and distinguished gentlemen" (likely lawyers) visited the editor, Mr. Solomon Southwick of the *National Democrat*, and convinced him that his attack on Mr. Tuthill, "in relation to the dissection of paupers, was the result of an erroneous impression received from an imperfect statement in a Connecticut paper [the *Connecticut Herald*]." The editor stated that it gave him great pleasure to retract all that had been said on the subject and assured his readers that "Mr. Tuthill is a gentleman of humane and benevolent feelings, incapable of hostility to the rights of the poor."

The *Connecticut Herald* published the *National Democrat*'s retraction but retorted that the editor, "Mr. Southwick," may have suffered an "erroneous impression" from the *Herald*'s reporting but "that no such statement can be pointed out, and that everything we have said on this subject can be fully substantiated."[24]

Whether Tuthill got his entire reputation back is not known, but as in all these matters even today the damage was done, and few read the retractions. Cornelius Tuthill died at the age of twenty-nine in April 1825 from consumption. If Hamlin can name Ephraim Colburn a martyr to the cause, then perhaps Cornelius Tuthill deserves to be recognized as one who had his reputation sullied in the attempt to provide more "subjects" for the professors in Connecticut.[25]

The Act to Prevent the Disinterment of the Bodies of Deceased Persons, June 4, 1824

The "Act to Prevent the Disinterment of the Bodies of Deceased Persons" passed in the Connecticut legislature on June 4, 1824. It was divided into six sections. Section 1 concerned itself with the disinterring and removal of deceased persons from their grave or place of "sepulture."

> Sec. 1. Be it enacted by the Senate and House of Representatives in General Assembly convened, [sic] That if any person or persons shall open the grave of any deceased person, or the tomb where the body or bodies of any deceased person or persons have been deposited, or shall remove the body or bodies or remains of any deceased person or persons from their grave, graves, or place of sepulture, for the purposes of dissection or any surgical or anatomical experiments, or for any other purposes without the consent of the near relatives of the deceased; or shall in any way aid, assist, or procure the same to be done; or shall receive, conceal or secrete, any such body or bodies, or shall aid or assist in any such surgical or anatomical experiments or demonstrations ... or dissections ... knowing said body or bodies to have been so taken or removed from place or places of their sepulture; ... every such person so offending shall forfeit and pay a fine not exceeding two thousand dollars, nor less than two hundred dollars, and shall be further punished by imprisonment in Newgate prison for a term not exceeding ten years, nor less than one year, at the discretion of the Court having cognizance thereof.[26]

Clearly, this was purposely a harsh punishment meant to put a stop to what people believed was a horrific practice. The punishment of consigning the malefactor to Newgate prison for not less than one year was especially important, particularly if one knew of the conditions in that Connecticut prison. One traveler, Edward Augustus Kendall, in the early part of the nineteenth century wrote, "This establishment ... is designed to be, from all its arrangements, an object of terror."[27] He described what prisoners could expect when being incarcerated there:

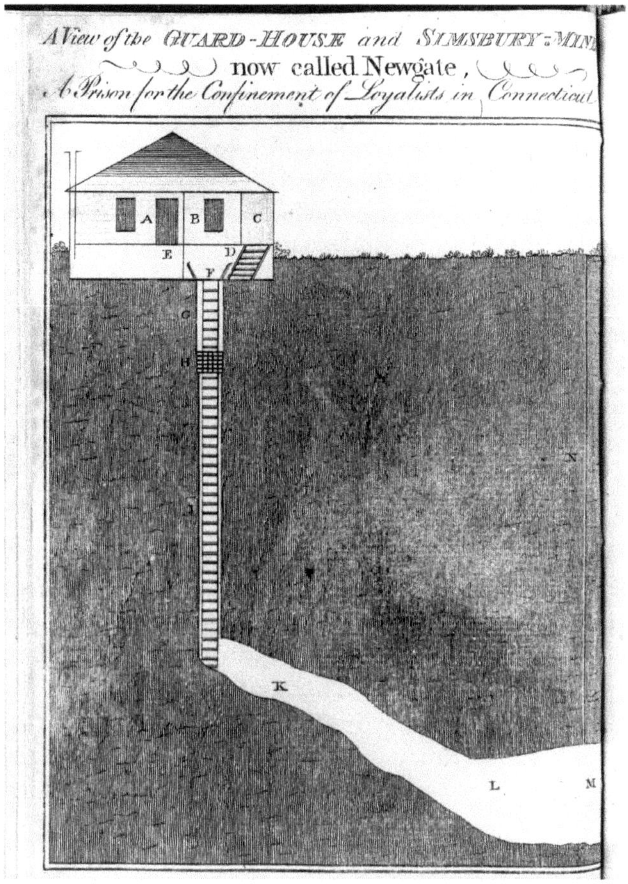

This 1781 print shows a view of the guardhouse at Newgate, originally a prison for the confinement of Loyalists in Connecticut that subsequently became the state prison. Note the shaft from the guardhouse leading to an underground chamber. There was a "strong trap door" that opened to the shaft leading to a descent to the underground area "commonly called Hell." ***The Political Magazine and Parliamentary, Naval, Military, and Literary Journal*****, London: J. Bew, Pater-Noster-Row, 1781 October, 596–597 (Library of Congress).**

> A bell summoning the prisoners to work had already rung; and in a few moments they began to make their appearance. They came in irregular numbers, sometimes two or three together, and sometimes a single one alone; ... the soldiers were ordered to present, in readiness to fire. The prisoners were heavily ironed and secured both by hand-cuffs and fetters; ... [they were] unable to walk, could only make their way by a sort of jump or a hop. On entering the smithery, some went to the sides of the forges, where collars, dependent by iron chains from the roof, were fastened round their necks, and others were chained in pairs to wheelbarrows. The number of prisoners was about forty; and when they were all disposed of in the manner described, sentries were placed within the building which contained them.[28]

Kendall continued, stating that the prison was an "object of terror; and everything is accordingly contrived to make the life endured in it as burdensome and miserable as possible[;] ... the place chosen for the prison is no other than the mouth of a forsaken copper mine.... The cells are areas previously excavated in the mine. The prisoners descend by a shaft, which is secured by a trap door, within the prison house, or goaler's house, which stands upon the mine."[29]

Kendall visited the cells of the prison:

> The trap door being lifted up, I went down an iron ladder, perpendicularly fixed to the depth of about fifty feet. From the foot of the ladder a rough, narrow, and low passage descends still deeper, till it terminates at a well of clear water, over which is an air shaft, seventy feet in height, and guarded at its mouth, which is within the gaol yard, by a hatch of iron. The cells are ... at different depths beneath the surface, none perhaps exceeding sixty feet. They are small, rugged, and accommodated with wooden berths, and some straw. The straw was wet ... [and he was assured that the cells] ... were in general dry, and that they were not found unfavorable to the health of the prisoners.

Kendall recounted how the prisoners move about from their cells. "The prisoners are dismissed at four o'clock in the afternoon, every day without exception, and at all seasons of the year. They descend in their fetters and hand-cuffs, and at four o'clock in the morning they ascend the iron ladder, climbing it as well as they can by the aid of their fettered limbs." There were no women at Newgate; they were consigned to county jails.[30]

Finally, he described the feeding of the prisoners who were served "pickled pork for dinner." Pieces of the pork were given separately to the prisoners "at each forge." The food was "thrown upon the floor and left to be washed and boiled in the water used for cooling the iron wrought at the forges. Meat had been distributed in like manner for breakfast. The food ... consists in an alternation of pork, beef, and peas."[31]

The aim of making body snatchers and those receiving bodies for dissection, surgery, or demonstration incarcerated in Newgate was to deter these practices. There was no hint at reform, and the punishment was extraordinarily harsh and cruel. Kendall concluded that "such is the seat and the scene of punishment provided by Connecticut for criminals not guilty of murder, treason, or either of a few other capital offences.... I cannot get rid of the impression, that without any extraordinary cruelty in its actual operation, there is something very like cruelty in the device and design."[32]

Section 2 of the act ensured that anyone engaged in dissection had to be bonded. "No professor, teacher or lecturer, in any academy, school, or medical institution, shall perform any anatomical or surgical experiments, on the body of any deceased persons" until those persons have given a bond "with sufficient surety to the Treasurer of the State, on the sum of two thousand dollars" as long as the body was legally obtained. If not and the body was illegally procured and the person was convicted before the "Superior Court," the person would have to [forfeit and pay to the Treasurer of the State a fine not exceeding two thousand dollars, not less than five hundred dollars, at the discretion of the Court." Obviously, these fines were set extraordinarily high to prevent the illegal use of bodies in certified medical establishments and by requiring "surety" inhibiting independent "demonstrators" setting up shop and offering dissection classes without any oversight.

Section 3 gave the mayor and two senior aldermen of any city and the selectmen of any town in which "such college, academy, school, or medical institution may be located ... authority, at all times to enter, and inspect every part of such building."

Section 4 was probably the most controversial of all the sections, stating "that the bodies of criminals who shall be confined to Newgate prison for crimes hereafter committed, and shall die in said prison, who have no known relatives, shall with the approbation of the overseers of said prison, be at the disposal of the Professors of Anatomy and Surgery in the Medical Institution in this State, to be used for the purpose of

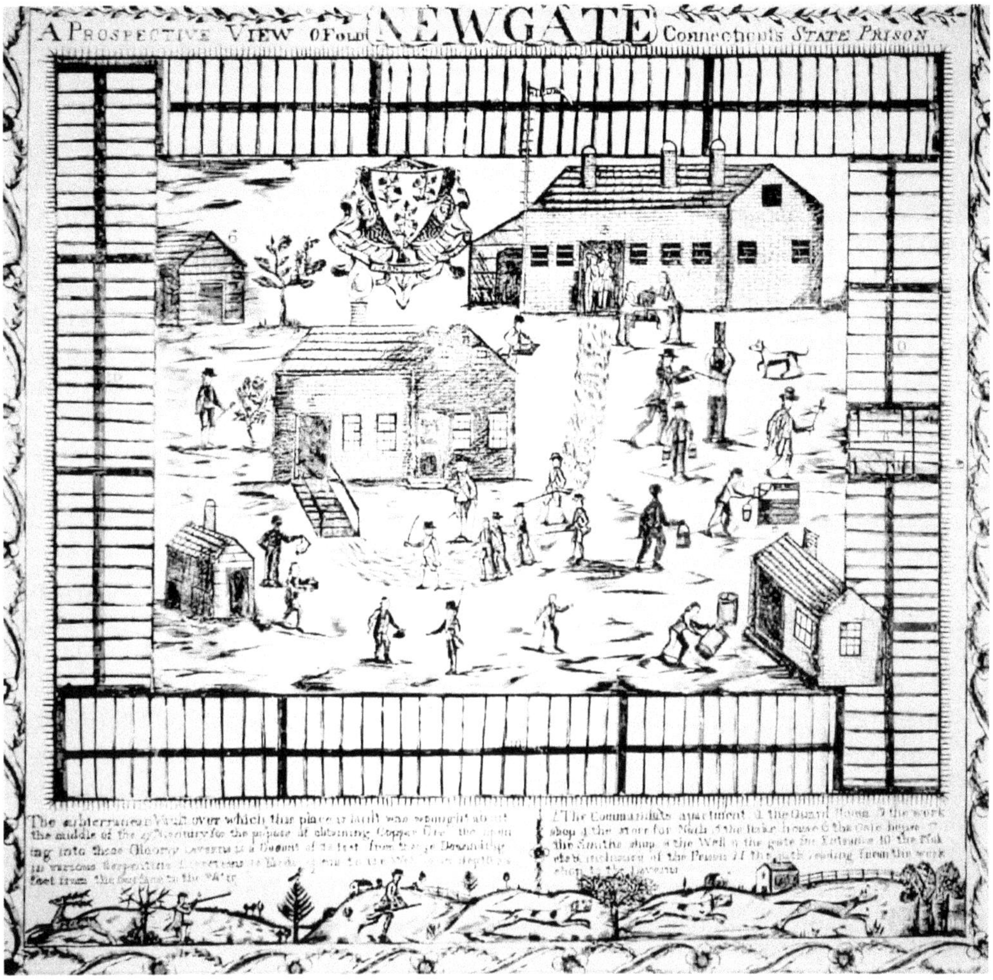

"A Prospective View of Newgate Connecticut State Prison," by Richard Brunton, a counterfeiter who served two years in Newgate from 1799 to 1801 for this crime. The engraving was probably made around 1802. Albert C. Bates, *An Early Connecticut Engraver, and His Work, Hartford*(Case, Lockwood and Brainard Company, 1906), 26.

advancing medical science, and shall at all times be subject to their orders; and also the bodies of persons capitally punished under sentence of the law, at the discretion of the Court before whom the conviction of such persons takes place."[33]

Only the Newgate state prison was mentioned in this act, and presumably those without relatives would likely be immigrants or strangers with no local family. Also, according to the historian of Newgate, most of the prisoners were incarcerated for a variety of crimes, and not all were hardened criminals. This act did not apply to those held in local jails. And as we have seen previously, courts in the past did have the ability to sentence criminals but only those convicted of capital crimes to dissection after execution.[34]

Section 5 simply stated that in the event of a breach of "section 1 of the first section of this act," the governor, on a request from the selectmen where the breach took place, was authorized to offer a reward not "exceeding two hundred dollars," to be paid by the state once "the offender or offenders" had been "apprehended and convicted."

Section 6 repealed the seventy-second section of an "Act concerning Crimes and Punishments," except for "offenses now committed, nor any prosecutions pending."[35]

The Connecticut Anatomical Law of 1824 Controversy

The Connecticut Anatomical Law of 1824 is considered notable by Hamlin and others because it was the first legislation in the United States regarding "disinterment" and provided the means of obtaining human material other than from murderers and duelists for dissection.[36] This may be accurate but, in a sense, this law according to one contemporary and others was seen as a disgrace to the medical profession and hobbled progress in this area. In 1824, following the enactment of the new law, an article appeared in the *Westminster Review* by William Mackenzie of Glasgow, Scotland, that referred not to the Yale riot but to the curious circumstances of Jane Benton's disinterment. Without referencing the Connecticut Anatomical Law of 1824, he implied criticism of the law, as he concluded directly after referring to the Benton episode the following: "We maintain, it is both absurd and criminal to make the practice [of exhumation] a felony, without providing in some other method for the cultivation of anatomy."[37]

Dr. Elisha North of New London, Connecticut, wrote a series of newspaper articles under the pseudonym Vesalius. He admitted being influenced by Mackenzie's 1824 article and recommended it to his readers. In his book *Outlines of the Science of Life*, North included a chapter based on his newspaper articles titled "The Rights of Anatomists." He boldly criticized the Connecticut Anatomy Act of 1824. His reason for why his book was "delayed a considerable time [until 1829], so that those humane but injudicious passions might subside, which occasioned the law complained of; otherwise, one could not expect to be candidly heard or coolly attended to."[38]

North did not mince words about his essays' intention "to show the great mischief insidiously done to the whole community by public law, more particularly the one recently made in Connecticut, in relation to the exhumation of the human body, which law converts the slight offence of trespass, into the heinous one of felony."[39]

North argued, for example, from Section 1. What if a human body falls into the possession of a surgeon, "whose professional duty might require that he should perform surgical experiments upon them" and then finds out the person who furnished the body "had broken the law respecting exhumation; does such knowledge subject the surgeon to the punishment of the State Prison, for ten years or less, and to pay a heavy fine?" According to North, "such a law would be unjust and unreasonably severe. And yet it is believed that such must be the operation of a law in Connecticut, unfortunately passed in 1824."[40]

How effective was this law in providing subjects for the medical college? According to North, anatomical dissections were made "indisputable" by the provision in the law, "but ... said provision is completely inadequate to the purpose for which it was designed, for not so much as one dead body could be yearly had by that provision from the whole State. This will undoubtedly create ... a kind of monopoly in favour of a few surgeons, who are now in actual practice. They, of course, in general, will keep silent on this subject."[41]

What of missed opportunities for the education of young promising physicians? North informed us that "it remains to be ascertained, whether a court and jury can be found, who may be willing to execute so cruel a law, as the one under consideration." He was aware that several persons "innocent of the crime of real felony ... have been caught in the meshes of the cruel laws of this country, in relation to anatomy." One of these, "after lying in a county jail many cold winter nights, was, by the powerful aid of highly respectable friends, with much difficulty ... at last saved from suffering the penalties of the state prison [Newgate] for ten years, as the case might have been. This person wisely concluded, if such were some of the evils of the mysterious, or secret art of surgery, to quit the business; and the next we heard of him, he was calculating to become a seafaring man."[42]

As for North's opinion of the legislature in Connecticut, "there is so much intelligence of a particular sort, and nice discrimination needed in the management of medical affairs, and human health ... that mankind, even in a highly intelligent state of society, make innumerable blunders, when they undertake to conduct such business without the advice and aid of the most intelligent medical men." Laws concerning anatomy and surgery should not be made without "first seeking professional advice."[43]

North understood how such a law was passed because the "surgical and anatomical professors in Yale College, were unreasonably compelled, by the law ... to submit their daily conduct in the anatomical theatre to the public authority." Otherwise, they would lose "a profitable business" and, in addition, "give a heavy bond to the government" to prevent them from violating "a statute made for them and others." North concluded that "justice would seem to require, that other people should give bonds, as well as those gentlemen, not to violate a penal law.... For how can one perform the duties of teaching anatomy without the means [subjects]? And such means cannot always be imported, on account of the very great difficulty in the case."[44]

North blamed the weakness of the professors, especially Dr. Nathan Smith and Yale College. "Perhaps the incumbent professors, upon a principle of good citizenship, were excusable for a submission to an unjust penal statute, made by impassioned and ignorant persons." Those who made the law were "undoubtedly ignorant on the subject of anatomy, and likewise highly impassioned, if we have been correctly informed."

North argued that perhaps we should have some sympathy for the "incumbent professors in the Medical College for patiently sustaining the indignity put upon their feelings by the Hon. Legislature of Connecticut." However, Dr. Nathan Smith was "submissive to the laws. It may well ... be made a question, whether the Doctor would not have done more good, if he had possessed less humility in regard to the oppressive law under consideration."[45]

Dr. North was especially incensed that the public authorities had legal license to inspect the dissection laboratories. Did not the humblest of citizens, he asked, have the "right secured to them by the highest of all laws, the Constitution of the State, to occupy their own houses or buildings in such a way as they may choose, without being annoyed by daily or hourly visits from the public authority, to see whether they may not be doing mischief? Whether giving the public authority access to a secret dissecting room, without a reasonable and legal process, is a violation of the Constitution of the State, is left to the inquiry of intelligent lawyers."[46]

North also considered the Connecticut Medical Society a major problem. He explained the shortcomings of medical men during this early period, and the one "principal evil, which has originated from our medical society," was that they are "too officious, for all concerned." (By his description, they were concerned about too many trivial matters.)

Of greater concern and with direct bearing on the 1824 act was the mistake in "making a medical institution succumb to a mere literary, moral, or religious one [here he means Yale].... If, thirty years ago, the medical society had been formed in the best possible manner, and if its members had possessed intelligence, decision, and energy enough, that society might now have had a medical school or college of its own.... Such a noble institution ... [serving as a] promulgating point for medical science.... If such had been the case, the associations of intelligent men in general would have been such, as to have prevented the cruel law complained of."[47]

In conclusion, North wrote, he had "foreseen, about twenty-five years ago, some of the evils the medical profession are [*sic*] now experiencing in this State." He argued that if "the powerful Yale College interest ... would address the people, or otherwise act efficiently, even at this late period, in favour of removing the deadly blow struck at the very foundation of correct medical science, by the Hon. Legislature of the State, it might operate against the unfavourable opinion of many ... in relation to the union of the Medical Society with that institution."

North believed that the union of Yale and the medical society acted against the interests of the medical community ("that society might now have had a medical school or college of its own"). If it had a medical school of its own, it might have been more effective in influencing the legislature in making anatomy law friendlier to the medical profession. He did not hold out much hope that Yale and the medical society would disassociate themselves; "the powerful, and sometimes durable influence of what we consider wrong associations, induces us, however, almost to despair of living long enough to see such a desirable act as is now alluded to."[48]

The Connecticut "Act regarding Anatomical and Medical Sciences of 1833"

On April 15, 1832, the New Haven Medical Society argued for modifying the 1824 Connecticut "Act to Prevent the Disinterment of the Bodies of Deceased Persons," stating that the "the science of Anatomy is greatly impeded by the difficulty of procuring subjects for dissection ... and the high price of subjects has, in some instances led to unprincipled and overt acts by which public feeling has been justly exasperated." The writer then expounded the merits of the anatomy act passed in Massachusetts 1831 and the Warburton Act by Parliament in England in 1832.[49]

Influenced by North's writings concerning the plight of anatomists and the passage of the Massachusetts and English anatomy acts, in May 1832 the Medical Society of Connecticut recommended a change in the 1824 legislation. "It may be presumed that the legislature of Connecticut will be willing to give the subject a calm and deliberate consideration and we feel assured that an enlightened and rational view of the subject will lead to the same results as in the legislature of Massachusetts and the Parliament of Great Britain."

The article made many of the same claims that North did in his book: the role of dissection in medical education, the lack and expense of subjects, and the conundrum of the medical man with laws condemning him to the severest penalties to become acquainted with anatomy yet affording him no legal means of acquiring "competent knowledge." The dilemma was that the law said you must "dissect dead bodies" to qualify as a physician, but if you make a mistake, you will be sued for malpractice and deprived of "property and reputation." However, if you "disinter a body for dissection your property shall be sacrificed, your body shall be committed to a State's Prison, and your family after doomed to poverty and disgrace."

The solution offered by the physicians in their article was modeled after the Massachusetts law, as "it continues penalties for disinterment," and provisions were made the "persons required to be buried at the public expense, may in certain cases, be taken for dissection." The law accounted for the "feelings of friends" and the disposition of strangers. To the heart of the matter was where these subjects would come from. They would come from

> that vicious and abandoned class of the community, who have during life become a public nuisance and have no friends or acquaintances to lament their death.... [T]hey are a burden to the community, a pest to society—after their death their bodies may thus be rendered subservient to humanity.

The article concluded that the Massachusetts act "has proven advantageous to the cause of science and salutary to the public. The Warburton Act in Great Britain was also praised as advantageous and in a quote from an unnamed periodical 'the business of the resurrectionists is destroyed.'"[50]

The medical society made its proposal to the Connecticut legislature in the spring of 1833. The bill for a public act regarding anatomy and medical science was advanced in committee. Six of the eight members voted for it, and it passed and then went before the Connecticut House and Senate. The "Act regarding Anatomical and Medical Sciences" became law on June 5, 1833.

The act stated that "whenever any person shall die in any town in this State, who may be at the time of such death, supported by the State, or by any town in this State, or whose interment must be at the expense of this state ... it shall ... be lawful for any professor ... surgeon or physician, duly licensed ... to apply in writing to the select-men of the town in which such person may die for the body of such deceased person."

Friends and relatives had thirty-six hours to claim the body (hardly time to get to the deceased, given the mode of transportation and communication in 1833), and then the selectmen could deliver the body to any "licensed physician or surgeon" officially entitled to receive the body. In addition, a $500 surety was required. The deceased body must be used for the "purpose of advancing anatomical and medical science," and after use the "remains ... shall be interred." Finally, the act gave priority to any professor in a county where there existed a medical college in the state, giving the professor "preference over other applications in the same county."[51]

Some representatives later recalled that "the feelings of the community were strongly against it. Many people feared that they might have friends subjected to the law, without their knowledge, until they had been given up for dissection." Still "the act was passed with a large majority."[52]

If the Connecticut physicians thought they would finally be able to reap the benefits of their Massachusetts and English anatomy colleagues with the passage of this act, they were to be sorely disappointed. The drumbeat to repeal the act began immediately. On July 20, 1833, the *Columbian Register* stated the act's passage was without "good and sufficient reason."[53] The *Courier* on July 24, 1833, stated the act

> rendered quite uncertain whether those who are desirous of a decent Christian burial are to have one, especially if they die poor, or whether their bodies, after death, are to be dissected, cut, and mangled, and exposed by some surgeon, physician or professor to the view of hundreds of young medical students.

The editorial asked what right the legislature had "to say that the bodies of their fellow citizens, who have been guilty of no crime, but ... poverty and destitution ... shall be thus dealt with after death?" Further, it argued that the law was "objectionable in the extreme and will never suffer to exist by a free and enlightened community.... [T]he pains and horrors of death were sufficient, without increasing them by human legislation." If physicians and anatomists are determined "to have subjects for dissection ... for the benefit of science ... let them voluntarily surrender their own bodies for dissection, instead of compelling their fellow citizens, by legislation, to be exposed, cut, and mangled, because they happen to die poor or destitute of kindred and friends."[54]

The citizens of New London were so incensed that they held a town meeting on October 7, 1833, and voted unanimously "that all persons dying in the Almshouse, and all poor strangers dying in this town, should be decently intered [*sic*] at the expense of the town." The object of the vote to remove "the discretionary power" given to the selectmen by the state that permitted them to give up a "body for the advancement of anatomical and medical science" if the person had been "supported by the town or state and whose interment must be at the expense of either...."[55]

The complaints continued into the spring of 1834, with those authorized to turn over cadavers refusing to participate in this endeavor. On April 30, 1834, the *New London Gazette* complained that "this law is so revolting to the feelings of the public, that Selectmen refuse to obey it," and called for its repeal: "why continue a law obnoxious to the public sentiment?"[56] In May just prior to the legislative assembly meeting, the *Connecticut Courant* in an editorial called for the repeal of a number of laws passed in the last session, including the anatomy act because it "created an odious distinction between the poor and the rich, and we believe the public voice calls for its repeal."[57]

That spring the Connecticut Assembly found itself reconsidering the 1833 act. In the meeting of the House on May 19, 1834, representative Amariah Kibbe of Somers, Connecticut, "observed [that] the bill had created much feeling in his section because the town poor of every town were liable after death to dissection. He thought it went farther than any law ever passed before on this subject. The Massachusetts law, from which this bill in most of its features is copied, expressly excepts town paupers from its operation, and he thought it right that our law should also be stripped of this objectionable feature."

Representative Isaac Townshend of New Haven suggested that the medical convention now being held, having appointed a medical committee, should be consulted to obtain "information necessary for a deliberate opinion." Mr. Kibbe replied that "everybody in the House was qualified to make up his opinion immediately, without waiting for the interference of any foreign power. The law he said, smelt of blood." He reminded the House members that "anyone of them before another year might suffer poverty, sickness, and death, and thus be subject to the law. At that very moment some of their friends might be under the dissection knife of an anatomist." He urged the immediate repeal of the law "because he looked upon it as a foul blot on the moral escutcheon of the State of Connecticut."[58]

The House of Representatives met again, and the bill "To Repeal the Anatomical and Medical Science Act" was read a second time. Mr. Kibbe "thought the law of a barbarous nature, and reflected no great honor on the State." Representative Elisha Haley of Groton, Connecticut, "thought last year, as he thinks now[,] that it was an injudicious law." Representative Charles McCurdy of Lyme noted that there had been much excitement over the law in some areas of the State, "but not so much in his quarter, as in others." The act had been passed with a large majority, "but if the people disapproved it, it ought to be repealed or modified." Later he and another representative suggested that more information was needed to proceed. Representative Samuel Robinson of Madison, Connecticut, suggested "let[ting] the bill lie" and consulting with the medical convention's medical committee, "where the most objectionable features could be done away with and render it acceptable to the House."[59]

On June 5, 1834, the members of the Connecticut Assembly repealed the contentious 1833 "Act regarding Anatomical and Medical Sciences."[60]

Besides public opinion being against this act, political and economic conditions had changed dramatically in Connecticut from the late spring of 1833, when the 1833 Anatomical Act had been voted into law.

Summary

The Connecticut "Anatomical and Medical Science Act of 1833" was first seen in Connecticut by the medical community as an important breakthrough in providing subjects for surgeons, physicians, and anatomists.[61] As we have seen, it fell short of this mark and was a public opinion disaster for the Connecticut Assembly. Although modeled on the Massachusetts Anatomy Act of 1831, it lacked the wording and safeguards that the Massachusetts act contained to tamp down opposition.[62] The Massachusetts act, to avoid the stigma of targeting the poor, "used the term unclaimed rather than indigent bodies" and "limited its application to those living in…" Boston "and provided an exception for poor people who had been long time residents of the area [called town paupers]."[63] Immigration increased over the decades to Boston and Charlestown, and it was the "unclaimed" immigrant dead that provided most bodies for the anatomists.[64]

The problem with the "Connecticut Anatomical and Medical Sciences Act of 1833" was twofold. The act named the indigent poor as candidates for dissection after death. This was quickly seen as morally depraved, as noted above. A second factor was that the poor law system in Connecticut was almost entirely based on a town system without any state aid to the communities. The state government's policy was to shift the responsibility for the poor to the towns, with the generally uncontested view that the "local selectmen knew more about individual case histories than state officials could hope to learn without considerable effort."[65]

Unlike Massachusetts, the statute was not limited to an impersonal large city with an expanding immigrant population but also applied to the local communities with people who had been the responsibility of the community over the years.[66] In 1821, the poor law in Connecticut was revised and ordered that "paupers be cared for by towns in almshouses."[67] Many also felt it was their obligation to help the poor, as anyone could fall into poverty given the right circumstances. The Connecticut law was too broad and uncaring for it to be effective, given the unique circumstances of poor relief in Connecticut. Unlike Massachusetts, Connecticut did not have a large impersonal immigrant population to draw from for its anatomical subjects.

In addition, economic conditions in Connecticut had changed since the 1833 act. Several areas of the state were in the throes of a "business depression." Manufacturing plants in the New Haven area and mills around Hartford had closed, and men were "going begging for employment." After the elections in April 1834, the new governor, Samuel A. Foote, in his message to the legislature said it "might be advisable to abolish imprisonment for debt due to the unfavorable business conditions of the time." This change in business conditions would have also sensitized the population to the anatomy law and may account for the repeated fears of anyone falling into poverty and becoming a victim of this "odious" law.

As the Connecticut historian Jarvis Means Morse wrote in his book *A Neglected Period in Connecticut History, 1818–1850,* the Whig Party (formerly the National Republicans) coming to power in the Connecticut assembly in 1834 "set about the pleasant task of undoing the work accomplished by the late Democratic assembly" by repealing two acts, one of them being the act "which permitted surgeons to use bodies of deceased paupers for anatomical studies."[68]

As I have shown, this was not a mere whim of the Whigs undoing a Democratic reform but instead was necessitated by public opinion opposed to what was considered a barbaric and odious law against the poor.

7

Under the Dark Vermont Moon

One could argue that in the early nineteenth century Vermont suffered from an embarrassment of medical school riches, although the three medical schools recently founded needed illegally obtained cadavers to make them a growing concern. Consequently, their establishment and operations over time were resented by the public and the legislature and eventually led to competing poems over the infamous body-snatching saga of the Hubbardton Raid in 1830, both published nearly fifty years later. One was considered laudatory by some, and the second was an answer to the first poem considered offensive and injurious to the good people of the town of Hubbardton.

The first medical school established in Vermont was Castleton Medical Academy in 1817 in Castleton, Vermont. The nearest school for medical instruction was Dartmouth's medical school, a mile from its eastern border. The next closest school was in Fairfield, New York, 150 miles away. The Yale Medical School was about the same distance, while medical schools in Boston and New York were approximately 200 miles away. These distances represented "three to five days" of travel at the time if the roads were in good condition; travel took much longer during the winter months.[1]

The decision to establish the Castleton medical school originated with two doctors, Dr. Selah Gridley and Dr. Theodore Woodward, "popular preceptors" who had "more applications of young men that wished to study under them than they could accept."[2] In July 1820 an article appeared in the *Rutland Daily Herald* reporting that "it has long been a subject of regret that young gentlemen were obliged to go to some of the neighboring states in pursuit of those advantages in the study of Medical Science which are essential to qualify them for the profession. We can now congratulate our readers on the growing respectability and usefulness of the institution established by the legislature at Castleton in this county."[3] The founding document refers to the school as the Castleton Medical Academy.[4]

To establish the college, a charter was required. The Vermont legislature convened in mid–October 1818 to address a "a petition seeking a charter for Castleton Medical Academy." Interestingly, there was no objection, and "the charter was granted on October 29, 1818."[5] In order to "excite emulation among the students" and confer degrees, "application was made to the trustees of Middlebury College … [and on] … August 16, 1820, the affiliation was approved."[6] In October 1822 the academy changed its name to Vermont Academy of Medicine, and the name was legally changed by the Vermont legislature in November 1822.[7]

In January 1821 a committee at the previously named Castleton Medical Academy was established "to solicit subscriptions" for a new medical building. The building was soon completed and stood at two stories, "fifty feet by thirty." It contained a turret for a bell and a skylight. The first floor had a "spacious lecture room with ascending seats, a chemical laboratory and apparatus, and a study and library room." Located on the second floor was the "anatomical theater and lecture room directly under the skylight." In addition, there was a "dissecting room, and another room … occupied for a valuable anatomical museum, various minerals, and natural curiosities." The building was opened for the fall "session" beginning on September 20, 1821. It was truly "a commodious building for a country medical college."[8] The new building was necessary because a good medical building demonstrated "prosperity" and helped to attract students and their fees critical for the financial viability of the college. "Therefore every medical college endeavored to be able to state within three years that it had a building of its own."[9]

It was not long before other competitors began to establish medical schools in Vermont. They included the University of Vermont Medical Department in Burlington, Vermont, in 1820 and the Vermont Medical College in 1827 in Woodstock, Vermont.

Besides the competition for students and their fees, a second important difficulty for the early medical institutions was the supply of anatomical material. Even prior to the establishment of the three medical schools in Vermont, in 1804 Vermont enacted "An Act, Against Disturbing the Remains of the Dead." The act contained the following penalties: "Any person or persons shall dig up, or remove, or disturb the remains of any dead person … shall pay a fine … not exceeding one thousand dollars; or be publicly whipped, not exceeding 39 strips; or imprisoned, not exceeding one year or any or all punishments, at the discretion of said court."[10]

The legislation went further to protect the dead: "if given a license to dig up the body" it must be "in the day time, in the presence of five good witnesses of the Vicinity."[11]

This early Vermont grave-robbing law was enacted because the Vermont border is approximately a mile from Dartmouth College. Vermonters "felt it necessary to take precautions against resurrection, by agents representing the school, so the assembly enacted a statute with penalties similar to those in New Hampshire."[12]

By 1827 with the establishment of a third medical school in Vermont, the people of Vermont "were inclined to suspect very strongly that their dead might rest none to[o] securely in their graves" while the medical schools "were in session."[13]

For example, the "Medical Department of the University of Vermont began teaching in 1822 and graduated its first class of four men in 1823." The "rise of two rivals, each within one hundred miles also brought competition for students in western Vermont, western Massachusetts, and eastern New York."[14] In 1827 a third rival appeared at Woodstock, Vermont, "only forty miles distant … under the name the Clinical School of Medicine and the Vermont Medical College as a competitor to the other two medical colleges in Vermont." The "application to the legislature for a charter was vigorously opposed by the friends of the two existing medical colleges in the state and the charter was refused, forcing suspension of the institution after one session, to be revived later."[15]

It was during the attempt to incorporate the Vermont Medical College of Woodstock that body-snatching concerns were raised in the Vermont legislature. "Mr. Bradford of Sunderland replied on a bill to incorporate the Woodstock Medical College hoped it would not pass 'for although the gentleman last up painted and varnished it up so far it appeared like a white sepulchre, yet he suspected that it was in fact full of dead men's bones.' Mr. Ransom of Townshend proposed an amendment fixing the location of the said school at Brattleborough [*sic*]. The man from Chelsea … wished the institution to be placed as far from him as possible and regretted that the amendment did not designate Vernon which was still further off."[16]

Initially most "medical students dissected a human body while studying with their preceptors, this being secured from some country burial ground in the dark of the moon and dissected in the hayloft of the preceptor." As a result, early medical colleges did not "have to provide practical anatomy for all their students." Dissection was not mentioned in their catalogs, as it "would indicate participation in the felony of grave robbing because it was evident that cadavers for dissection could be secured only through illegal channels."[17]

Dissection is first mentioned at Castleton in the 1828 catalog, where an "opportunity to pursue dissection is provided." Some evidence suggests that "dissection was done at Castleton before 1828, and probably beginning with the first session." However, in early January 1824 a Rutland, Vermont, newspaper reported "the arrest of three students of the Vermont Academy of Medicine for alleged robbing of a grave at Poultney, eight miles distant from Castleton. Their case was discharged for lack of evidence."[18]

This latter event, because it occurred in Vermont, likely "resulted in the following resolution by the trustees of the Vermont Academy of Medicine in January 1824: 'Resolved by the corporation that no subject for the use of this institution shall be taken from any graveyard or burying ground in this County: but such as may be necessary shall be procured from the great seaports of the neighboring states.'"[19] The "nearest seaport was two hundred miles distant when wagons or sleds were the only means of transportation and each of the seaports had its own medical college seeking all available dissecting material. This resolution was for public consumption to allay suspicions of the inhabitants of neighboring towns."[20] More likely, it was easier and there was less liability in Vermont if they obtained their cadavers close by in New Hampshire. For example, a Connecticut newspaper reported in December 1824 that two students at the Vermont Academy of Medicine in Castleton were accused of stealing a body from a grave in the village of Acworth, New Hampshire, on November 29, 1824.[21]

In 1829 while the medical school in Woodstock was attempting to incorporate, there was much bad feeling in the town of Woodstock due to the "unwarrantable disinterments which had been practiced in the neighborhood, and as the Faculty professed a just abhorrence of the unlawful and immoral methods pursued by some for obtaining subjects for practical anatomy they pledged themselves to the community not to use, nor suffer to be used, so far as might come to their knowledge, any human body that might be disinterred *hereabouts*," adding somewhat piously that "it may be invidious to set limits, but we are willing to say the State of Vermont."[22] The pledge concluded that "we are well assured of securing competency of the means from remote parts and in a manner that ever will be justified by the well informed and judicious part of the community."[23]

A plan like Dartmouth's and Yale's was adopted by the faculty to relieve the public mind. On this issue, a "committee was appointed consisting of three persons entirely disconnected from the school, who were at all times to have access to the premises, and to whom keys were delivered whenever demanded, and whose duty it would be to disclose any improper proceedings on the part of the faculty in this direction."[24]

No doubt these promises to mitigate grave robbing by students "did not preclude resurrections in New Hampshire, the border which was only thirteen miles distant." Also, suspicions were continually aroused, and the "medical college building was often searched by a constable, who was sometimes accompanied by a committee of citizens, in search of a body removed from a grave in some neighboring village. The resolution by the trustees of restriction of grave robbing to areas outside Rutland County was marked more by violation than by observance."[25]

According to Frederick Waite, it was likely "that nearly all cadavers used in each medical college in New England before the Civil War were disinterred in the immediate neighborhood." He "collected a considerable number of records of disinterred bodies having been recovered from medical colleges, in every case from the institution nearest the site of the disinterment."[26]

Unfortunately, the latter proved true as the following two events attest. Following the pledge from the Woodstock Medical College, the following year "the body of Polly Chamberlain was stolen from her grave in Barnard, ten miles away. When the loss was discovered, irate citizens marched on to the medical school, searched the premises, but were unable to find what they were looking for. Because of circumstantial evidence, four students were arrested, then taken to Barnard for questioning by the justice of peace. Two were released, the other two were held for trial in the County Court at Woodstock on June 10, 1830. The trial continued from early morning until 11:00 p.m., in a jam-packed courtroom. The verdict rendered was not guilty."[27]

Yet, what was to follow in November 1830 was one of the most disturbing and gruesome body-snatching episodes in New England history and occurred in Vermont in the nearby town of Hubbardton, an event that continues to haunt the people of the town even today.

The Hubbardton Raid

Phineas Penfield Churchill was born in Hubbardton, Vermont, on September 14, 1804. At age twenty-three he married Marilla Gregory on September 27, 1827. The two had a son, Henry, who died in infancy. Marilla, or Mrs. Penfield Churchill, died from consumption and was buried on Saturday, November 27, 1830. It was soon discovered that some marks left on the grave were "removed which induced the belief that the body had been stolen—on examination, the supposition proved to be correct; the grave contained nothing but an empty coffin. Suspicions were excited that the body was brought to this town… [Castleton] … and on Monday last a warrant was issued."[28]

The idea of leaving secret marks on the graves of the newly buried was said to have come about as the result of a botched grave robbery in the town of Benson, about twelve miles from Hubbardton. Two students, pupils of Dr. Cooley of Benson, Vermont, were in training to become physicians. One evening the students stole the "corpse of a lady from Westhaven," a neighboring town. They "proceeded to a secluded place in some woods where potash was made and in the night proceeded to boil the flesh from the bones; the lye causing the eyes to open in a ghastly light; and the baying of the dogs, roused by the scent, frightened them from their purpose, so that they fled from the spot in terror, leaving proof of their guilt, which was discovered and reinterred a few days after." After this incident, the graves of the "newly buried were now guarded or secretly marked, which last measure" led to the following, "well remembered by many in Hubbardton fifty years after the event."[29]

On Monday, November 29, 1830, from the poem the "Song of Hubbardton Raid," we sense the feelings of the townspeople and their reaction when the coffin was discovered empty:

> The sexton raised the coffin lid, …
> The coffin was empty! The body stolen!
> The awful fact of resurrection
> Fired the wrath of the beholders,
> Fired them all to vengeance,
> Fired these rustics of the forest,
> In the wildwoods of Hubbardton.[30]

Immediately "a large party was secretly organized, …with the proper authority and the sheriff … Dan Dyke." The citizens "proceeded to Castleton in two parties by two different roads" and were "to meet and surround the college" once the medical students assembled "at the ringing bell on Monday morning."[31]

The crowd appeared at the medical building with the sheriff at its head demanding Mrs. Churchill's body. The dean insisted that he did not have the key to the building (it was in his pocket); he told the sheriff that he would have to send for the key at his home. While the dean delayed the mob, the students decapitated the body to avoid identification and concealed the remainder under a board in the floor. A committee was admitted, making a search of the building.[32]

While the search was under way the dissecting room was ransacked. The students inside began to leave the building. "Some in the cloaks of those days were narrowly watched." Hidden under a student's overcoat was Mrs. Churchill's head. The student carrying this bundle "sauntered … through the crowd" and went "to a neighboring barn, where he deposited her head in the haymow."[33]

The following newspaper report was less dramatic than later reports; undoubtedly some of these were later recollections of participants, as discussed below. As reported initially in the *Vermont Statesman*, following a general search of the medical buildings at Castleton, "the remains of a person with the exception of the head, were discovered, which the husband recognized as those of his deceased wife, and which were taken to Hubbardton to be re-interred. Two students attached to the medical institution were immediately arrested on suspicion. Their examination we understand took place yesterday. We have not heard the result."[34]

According to a later report found in the *Vermont Historical Gazetteer*, the search of the medical building continued throughout the day until the party decided they had been "outwitted and began to think of giving up the search, when one of them happening to cast his eyes up to the ceiling (most accounts refer to a floor board), observed some nails in a large board partially drawn out." The searchers reached up to the board, removed it, and found "the headless trunk of a female partly dissected." Mr. Churchill recognized "it by certain marks, as the body of his wife" but hesitated to take it, "intimidated by the threats and questionings of the students, when he was promptly told by Dyke, if he was satisfied in his own mind, as to the identity of the body, to take it, as in law any other claimant must prove whose it was…. Unable to find the head, the party proceeded home-wards with the body, when they were overtaken by a citizen" carrying the head, "having found it in his haymow. It appeared one of the students had carried it out under his cloak suspended by a string around his neck."[35]

Another source giving further information on the Hubbardton Raid is the poem "Song of Hubbardton Raid," mentioned previously, first read at an oyster supper at the residence of Dr. James Sanford in Castleton on November 29, 1879. Those attending included members of the Castleton Medical and Surgical Clinic.[36]

The poem gives additional details on the grave-robbing incident, the search, and the identification of the body of Mrs. Churchill. Below are edited portions of the poem concerning the search for Mrs. Churchill's body in the medical building describing what the husband and searchers were confronted with when they entered the building.

> The doors were opened, the search began,
> The horrors of the dissecting room appeared, ...
> Such ghastly sights! such human merchandise!
> Long rows of tables of mangled remains!
> Dirt and filth, saws, knives and forceps,
> Bones, muscles, and parts of flesh, lay in piles, ...[37]
> No learned anatomist in any college
> Could tell a youth from an adult;
> Could tell a Negro from a Yankee;
> Could tell a Squaw from a Scotchman;
> Out of such a motley mess of human debris.
> So the sheriff told the husband,
> This husband filled with sadness and sorrow, ...
> To identify his beloved wife,[38]
> He groped about among the tables,
> Squinted here and there among the subjects,
> And picked out one from certain marks
> That he could call his wife, under oath;
> And was ready to pack it up and start ...
> When the professor, learned and wise,
> Told him that subject was a burly Negro,
> And wore a number fourteen boot, ...
> The students offered these raiders
> Bones and flesh enough to make a wife
> If they would quietly take them and depart....[39]
> This jocose remark provoked [the searchers] wrath,
> And after hours of fruitless search,
> They swore they would burn the town
> If the stolen body was not produced,
> If not brought forth from its lurking place....
> The search was renewed by these raiders,
> A closer search by these citizen-soldiers, ...
> A suspicious nail-head revealed the secret,
> Told the story of human resurrection,
> Disclosed the hiding place of the body,
> The body of the wife stolen from the graveyard,[40]
> They pulled up a board from the floor, ...
> And saw the body of the missing wife,
> The headless body of the exhumed woman,
> Thrust into a cramped-up corner.
> These rustic raiders stood horrified
> Before this awful spectacle!
> This awful deed committed by the students ...
> By the students of Castleton Medical College.
> The husband identified the remains,
> Could say they were his wife's, under oath,
> The body that was stolen from the graveyard.
> From the sacred graveyard in Hubbardton, ...
> By way of compromise with these raiders,
> The students offered to throw in the head

If they would leave this land in peace, ...[41]
They picked up this human merchandise,
This batch of stolen property,
Stolen from the graveyard in Hubbardton
Packed it in a box on some straw, ...
These three mighty armies fell into line,
They formed one grand procession,
They took up their long line of march
To the wild woods of Hubbardton.[42]

One historian concluded that the "searchers demanded the missing head, and the dean said it would be delivered if the sheriff made no arrests. They agreed and she was apparently reburied in the East Hubbardton Cemetery, but there is no record of her burial."[43] However, arrests were made. In an initial report the students had only been identified as "two young men from Windsor [Vermont] formerly students in the Vermont Academy of Medicine, ... arrested on suspicion of being the authors of the outrage in the disinterment of the body of Mrs. Churchill of Hubbardton."[44]

The following article appeared in the *Brattleboro' Messenger* on January 29, 1831. "Two young men, Almon Lull of Hartland, [Vermont] and Mr. [Thaddeus] Phelps have been bound over for trial in Rutland County as the perpetrators of the late grave robbery in Hubbardton."[45] On February 1, 1831, the *National Gazette* of Philadelphia reported the following: "Almon Lull of Hartland, Vermont, one of the young men apprehended at Castleton, charged with disinterring the body of Mrs. Churchill, has been held in $1,000, to appear for trial at Rutland."[46]

It is not clear whether the two men were fined. However, according to school records, both men were students at Castleton, having enrolled in 1830. Both left Castleton designated as nongraduates and later enrolled forty miles away at the Clinical School of Medicine and the Vermont Medical College in Woodstock, Vermont, receiving their MDs in 1832.[47]

According to family lore, Almon continued his body-snatching activities in Vermont. In 1846 he and two medical students came to Windsor, Vermont, to disinter a recently buried body to use in anatomical instruction. They spent most of the night digging up the corpse and decided it would be too risky to move it in a wagon during the day. They decided to hide the corpse "under the steps" of the nearby church. The next evening, they returned to acquire the body, but

> unfortunately for them, the crime had been discovered and the bushes were alive with sheriffs, constables, and irate citizens. All three were arrested. The following day the two students were released but Almon, as the ringleader, was dragged before a local justice of the peace. He was bound over for trial at the next session of the County Court at Woodstock and given the choice of spending the intervening months in the county jail or posting a cash bond of $500. His brother somehow managed to come up with the money and Almon was released.

As a result of his nefarious activities, it was said that his "name was mentioned only in whispers by his Vermont relatives, if his name was even mentioned at all."[48]

Family lore is usually inaccurate, and there are newspaper accounts and advertisements that place Almon Lull in Madison, Wisconsin, in 1838, where he was offering his services as a "Physician and Surgeon."[49] He married in Madison, Wisconsin, on June 7, 1842.[50] By 1850 he had partnered with another physician, D.M. Holt, in a new establishment offering "Drugs and Medicines."[51] However, in an article dated June 7, 1881, Dr. Lull and his wife returned to Madison, Wisconsin, to visit old friends. The article noted that he was the "first physician of the city" but indicated after a short time that "he removed to some other place but returned to Madison in 1850 for a few years and left in 1853."[52] Dr. Lull signed on as a surgeon during the Mexican-American War (April 25, 1846–February 3, 1848), and this probably explains why he left Madison during this time.[53] It seems unlikely that he was involved in the body-snatching episode related above based on the "recollections of Col. Thomas Lull (1883–1960). Dr. Almon Lull was his great uncle."[54]

After leaving Madison, Dr. Lull traveled to California and settled in Berkeley, California. During the gold rush he did not pan for gold, but due to much sickness, lack of doctors, and the exorbitant fees he was able to charge treating the sick, he became rich. He seems to have invested wisely in many enterprises and became a wealthy man. "He sent recruiters to Windsor, Vermont, and neighboring areas to enlist young men for his various enterprises and many apparently left Vermont on that account."

Dr. Lull continued his connections with Vermonters and supported the "Vermont Relief Committee" while in California, helping to raise funds for the "Patriot Fund" aiding families of Vermont volunteers in the Second War of Independence (the American Civil War).[55]

Almon returned to Windsor, Vermont, toward the end of his life. His "sudden departure nearly 50 years before [was] apparently long forgotten by the authorities," and presumably, his relatives hoped later to receive a sizable legacy.[56]

Almon's partner in crime, Thaddeus Phelps, was born in Windsor, Vermont.[57] He graduated from the Clinical School of Medicine and the Vermont Medical College in Woodstock, Vermont, in 1832. According to one brief biography in the *Proceedings of the Tioga County, Pennsylvania Historical Society* immediately after graduation, he was invited to visit his friend Dr. Lewis Darling, Sr., to locate in Knoxville, Pennsylvania.

There were several physicians educated in Vermont who went to Pennsylvania, including Dr. Darling. The information in this short Tioga County biography notes that Phelps was "born and educated in Massachusetts." This was not accurate, as we saw above. It seems more likely he left Vermont immediately after graduating under the shadow of the body-snatching accusation and found refuge far away with a friend who gave him an opportunity to practice medicine, his true background unknown to his patients. However, he could "not conform to the backwoods setting" and within two years returned to "civilization" hoping his reputation would not follow him to Massachusetts.[58]

His reputation secure, Thaddeus Phelps went on to a long and distinguished medical career. He first settled in Milford, Massachusetts, and later in Cumberland, Rhode Island, and finally in 1838 in Attleborough, Massachusetts. There he built up a "lucrative practice." He attained a "considerable eminence in his profession."[59] He was a founding member of the Bristol North District Medical Society in 1849. Over the years until his retirement from the society he held numerous offices including president in 1856 and 1857.[60] In 1865, toward the end of the Civil War, he was appointed surgeon at the Portsmouth Grove Hospital in Rhode Island. Soon after, he met with a "severe accident." He was able to return to his practice with great difficulty and died on May 31, 1879, his accident likely the "predisposing cause" of his death.[61]

Ironically, Dr. Phelps passed away only thirty-nine days before the annual meeting on July 9, 1879, of the Rutland County Medical and Surgical Society in Pittsford, Vermont. At the meeting Dr. James Sanford of Castleton gave a talk titled "Reminiscences of Castleton Medical College." He "referred to the raid of the citizens of Hubbardton on the Castleton Medical College to recover the body of Mrs. Penfield Churchill." His speech was printed in the *Rutland Herald & Globe.* "Many of the old students who had attended this once famous institution read the address, and some of them at once challenged the doctor's date of the raid and wrote to him accordingly."

At the next regular meeting of the society, held in Castleton, on October 9, 1879, Dr. Sanford proposed that Dr. John M. Currier investigate the matter. Shortly after the meeting Dr. Currier informed Dr. Sanford he had found several newspaper articles from 1830 containing the exact date of the raid. On November 28, 1879, forty-nine years after the event, Dr. Sanford gave an oyster dinner not celebrating the Hubbardton Raid but instead hoping his guests might be "inspired by the event." The inspiration was the threats and physical harm doctors and students had to endure to train for their profession before the advent of liberal (progressive?) anatomical laws now being passed in some states.

After dinner Dr. John Currier read his poem "Song of Hubbardton Raid," written after the manner of Longfellow's 1855 poem *The Song of Hiawatha.*[62] Of the guests at the dinner, Dr. Sanford was a graduate of the Castleton Medical Academy in 1840. Dr. Josiah Norton graduated from the same school in 1841, and Benjamin F. Adams was a former member of the School's Corporation beginning in the middle 1850s. These were men who were close enough to have known people familiar with the described events.[63]

The poem was received so heartily that on December 15, 1879, at a meeting of the Castleton Medical and Surgical Clinic, the members requested that Dr. Currier publish his poem. The publication of Currier's poem sparked a visceral reaction in the people of Hubbardton, causing another poem in reply to Currier's poem to be written by a local Vermont

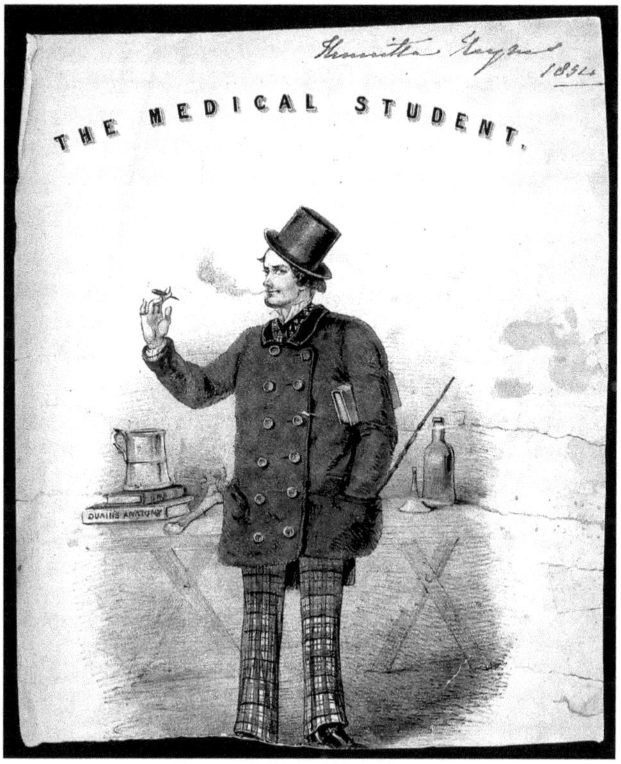

Doctoring had fallen "to such a low estate that it was said medicine was the career for those who were too lazy to farm, too stupid for the law, and too immoral for the pulpit" (U.S. House of Representatives, *Subcommittee on Health, Panel Discussions on National Health Insurance* [Washington, D.C.: U.S. Government Printing Office, 1975], 27). Shown is an English medical student, smoking, with a tankard and *Quain's Elements of Anatomy* on the table—what the typical medical student was thought to look like. American medical students enjoyed the same reputation as their English counterparts. The date on the original is 1854 (courtesy Wellcome Library, London).

poet, G.D. Spencer, titled "A Poem of the Hubbardton Raid Read in the Congregational Church Hubbardton May 12, 1880…."

At the reading of Spencer's poem, Reverend J.C. Edgar was invited to first read Currier's poem "upon the *Hubbardton Raid*" that described "all Hubbardton going to Castleton for the body of Mrs. P. Churchill, which was exhumed from the burying ground in Hubbardton in 1830 and taken to the Vermont Academy of Medicine in Castleton." Afterward, G.D. Spencer read his poem. After the readings, two resolutions followed; the first thanked Mr. Spencer for his poem and requested the poem be published. The second resolution demonstrated the true feelings of the community regarding Currier's poem: "Resolved, that for the insinuating, sneering, and lying slang contained in a poem called the 'Hubbardton Raid,' that the author shows himself destitute of the finer feelings of a gentleman and merits the scorn and contempt of this community."

For the Hubbardton community, an old wound was torn open. The community may have come to terms with the event, but it had continued to haunt the community over the years. Currier's poem was seen as an attack on the town and not to be celebrated or remembered in the manner of his insulting and "sneering" poem.[64]

Spencer's poem began with an insult to the caliber of members of the medical profession. It should be borne in mind that medical schools at the time of the raid had a "poor reputation" as nothing more than diploma mills. Doctoring had fallen "to such a low estate that it was said medicine was the career for those who were too lazy to farm, too stupid for the law, and too immoral for the pulpit."[65]

The poet began his poem, disparaging the medical profession by introducing the parents of a young man with little ambition and few prospects. They complain their son John is "too lazy to work," lacking brains to even be a "cobbler" or, in the poet's words, a "follower of St. Crispin." His clever wife tells her husband "our John, Knows [*sic*] enough to grasp the head of a snake." The husband asks, "Where, tell me where, dwells the snake He can grapple." The wife replies "In Castleton, Before" [*sic*] it was a "land of slates and quarries" (a refrain used throughout the poem the "Hubbardton Raid."[66]

The poem continued:

> Lived a snake of dirty brown.
> Its shape was hideous and repulsive
> Around this snake there gathered
> Those who had failed
> By honest toil to earn their daily bread.[67]

The medical school is described as a snake pit (the snake a medical symbol) where those who cannot earn an honest living go to "to bleed, to purge, to puke; Perchance 'a seminary girl meet."[68] The medical students are contrasted with the "honest men" and "noble women" of Hubbardton who "…kept the law of God."[69]

John, referred to as "This would be Esculapius [Asclepius]" arrives in Hubbardton, and though a stranger, is welcomed into a home, fed, and treated with "kindness."[70]

The poet continued to lambast the medical profession. John "was filled to the brim," and on "To Castleton …' the land of the lancet that bleeds,' The lancet made of steel for the vein and a misrepresentation for the pocket…." Here he implies that doctors are quacks and only in it for the money by not offering a real cure.[71]

As John traversed Hubbardton he came across a procession, "a wife … whose sands of life had run out." Following the procession making its way to the house, he sees the husband and children weeping.[72]

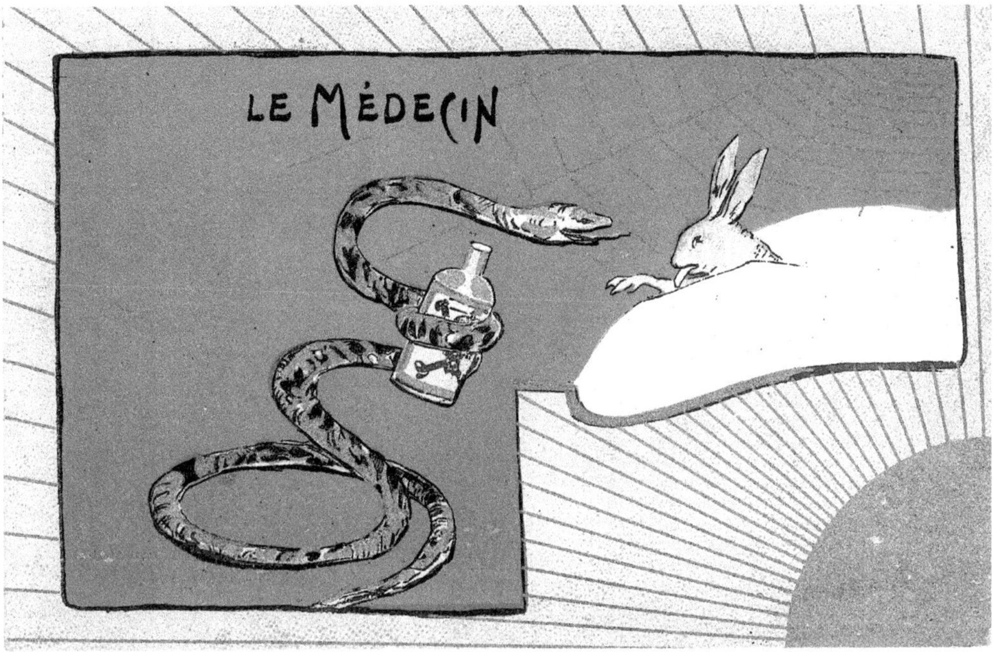

"Lived a snake of dirty brown its shape was hideous and repulsive." This image is from a French postcard, "Le Médecin" (the doctor), ca. 1910. However, the sentiment expressed was common in caricatures of doctors in many countries throughout the nineteenth century. Here the doctor is imagined as a snake poisoning his frightened patient with his medicine (National Library of Medicine).

At the house "this disciple of Esculapius" hid himself from view and saw the coffin, heard the mourners weeping, and the minister preach on "The resurrection day.... God shall raise the just and unjust." He saw her remains buried, and when "The dead was left with God" and everyone went home "The snake upon his belly Peaked, watched; all was clear.... To Castleton."[73]

> Hither the disciple of Esculapius wended his way.
> He met a chum, too lazy to work ... ,
> "In Hubbardton, the land of honest men....
> A woman died.
> I know where they laid her;
> I saw the husband and children weep;
> We can steal her; make fifty dollars."
> "Oh, how can you, John!"
> We must have her—science demands it—
> We need the money badly.[74]

Here the poet illustrates the callous nature of the medical students. John has witnessed the entire funeral, the outpouring of grief from the family, and the minister's words that promise the resurrection of the body. He still plots to steal the corpse for the money. When questioned by his friend he justifies it further by saying "science demands it," but this appears secondary, and his primary reason is no better than that of an amoral professional body snatcher who does it for the money alone. (Is the poet suggesting that the medical students were compensated for the bodies they delivered?)[75]

The two students started for Hubbardton "To steal … from the grave.… The wife, mother daughter sister; … Mourned by all who knew her … who … Lay in her narrow house Waiting the judgment day." In the next few lines, the poet contrasts God's plan for the resurrection of the body at some future time and the "resurrectionists" who hurry the process along, foiling God's plan.[76]

> When in an instant, in the twinkling of an eye,
> The dead should be raised.
> The decrees of God were slow,
> Too slow for these pukers;
> So, with shovel and spade,
> Dark Lantern, black hearts.…
> They wended their way to
> Hubbardton.[77]

Upon reaching the burying ground the poem becomes more dramatic, and the removal of the corpse is described.

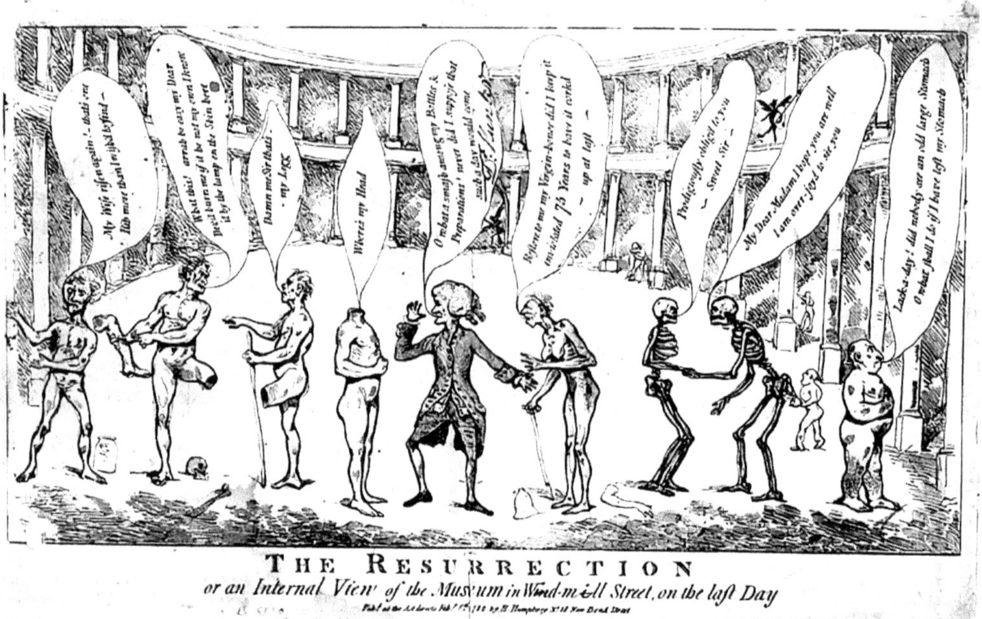
THE RESURRECTION
or an Internal View of the Museum in Wind-mill Street, on the last Day

As described by the Wellcome Library, this anonymous caricature, published in 1783, shows "on the day of resurrection" when all will be raised again, in their "whole bodily form, to be judged. This has been the cause of the breakage of the jars of preserved body parts" with the English anatomist, William Hunter, "at the centre of the print while on either side figures demand the return of their missing parts." The text bubbles (from left) read: "My wife risen again! that's one rib more than I wish'd to find"; "What this! arrah be easy my dear devil burn me if it be not my own I know it by the lump on the shin here"; "Damn me Sir that's my legg; Where's my head"; "O what a smash among my bottles and preprarations! never did I suppose that such a day could come (Dr. Hunter)"; "Restore to me my Virgin-honor did I keep it inviolated 75 years to have it corked up at last"; "Prodigiously oblig'd to you sweet Sir"; "My dear Madam I hope you are well I am over-joyd to see you"; "Lack-a-day! did nobody see an odd large stomach O what shall I do if I have lost my stomach" (courtesy Wellcome Library, London).

Hark! The stillness of the midnight
  Is broken by the shovel of the Marauders.
  They dig, dig, dig,
For a loved one.
... Deeper, deeper they go.
The coffin is reached.

There is no prayer nor asking for "God's protection" but,

An uplifted hand holds the axe;
The axe falls;
The coffin is broken;
The wife, mother,
... Was enshrouded for the grave,
Was again brought into the world.[78]

The poet speaks of the feelings of the father and children for the dead wife who they do not know has been removed from her grave, but her body is now on the dissecting table being mutilated.

Where now are the mortal remains
Of her who when in life
Was an affectionate wife,
Loving mother....
On the dirty table surrounded by thieves,
Thieves of the human body,
Sat the men too lazy to work; ...
Cutting and slashing
The wife, mother sister[79]

The poet explains how the missing body was discovered. The sexton had heard that the medical students in Castleton had stolen bodies. He made "Marks" over the grave. When these were "obliterated" he knew the grave had been robbed and aroused the men of Hubbardton. Everyone dropped what they were doing, knowing they had been "insulted by the body snatchers." Why should their family and friends have to contend with this women's "ignominious descent to the grave ... be all the more painfully sensitive to the thought of violence to her remains." The townspeople gathered and marched to Castleton and "Demanded the return of the dead."[80]

The poet initially referenced "In the barn of the deacon ... was the head of the woman." In other reports they searched for the body first in the school building, saying "Give us back our dead." The medical students cried, "Why don't you find her?" The "honest men" of Hubbardton demanded her body or they would bring down the medical building. The medical students "knees were weak ... and cried ... Wait a moment." The professor who had helped defraud the mob using his cloak as a cover revealed the body (the poet differs here from other reports that the body was found under the floorboards) and returned it to the mob, and her "mortal remains" were returned to the burying ground.[81]

The remaining third of the poem is a criticism of those responsible for writing and publishing "Song of Hubbardton Raid." The poet excoriates the doctors who brought up an event that had been long buried, though hardly forgotten, by the forgiving folks of Hubbardton. The wound was reopened with the publication of "Song of Hubbardton Raid."

Fifty years have gone since the brutish act....[82]
  Was it an intended insult? ...
  Who would want the mortal remains of
  Wife, mother daughter, sister
  Upon the block, with veins, arteries,
Nerves, muscles, exposed to view?[83]

The poet speaks of the bastardization of Henry Wadsworth Longfellow's 1855 epic poem "The Song of Hiawatha."

Again after fifty years is the wound opened afresh;
Its sting strikes all alike, old and young.
Hiawatha! Hiawatha! Better never had been born
Than to have been brought to so base a use!

The poet goes on to ask the people of Hubbardton to show they can "forget, forgive."[84] At the dinner in which "Song of Hubbardton Raid" was first read aloud it was a tradition to serve oysters, the poet wrote.

There should be no resurrection
Of the bad to season the bivalves
Furnished by the doctor.[85]

He makes a pointed reference to the insult the husband had to endure from the students while hunting for his wife's body.

The good is traduced;
When the husband
Is offered old bones, putrid flesh,
From which to "gather his affectionate wife?"[86]

The poet is even more incensed by the callous treatment of the husband when he thought he had identified his wife, reducing her body to a good to be bought and sold. There is a sense of irony here, since at the time of the raid a "negro" in life and death was considered merchandise to be bought and sold. Was the poet implying that all human bodies in death are converted into an equivalent "human merchandise" as well?[87]

'Twas not enough to rob the grave....
But when the sorrowful husband
Had gathered his flesh and bones
"The twain shall be one,"
He knew it to be his loved wife.
Tell him it was a negro!
Call a wife "human merchandise!"[88]

The poet tells the audience it has been fifty years, and they met that evening not to "feast" and not to stir up trouble but instead to feel their "fathers were insulted." They feel obligated to "repel the insult."[89]

The final lines of the poem summarize the feelings of the community, especially the religious meaning of the burial of the dead and the heroic men of the community who came to defend the honor of Mrs. Churchill.

Let our dead remain
  Until the trumpet's sound;
Leave to God the disposal of the dead;
  Seek not to belittle honor;

Strive not to exalt dishonesty.
We meet to repel the insult....
So think the disciples of Esculapius [*sic*]....
The noble deeds of Hubbardton....
Will be forgotten
When Mt. Zion vanishes,
When yonder monument crumbles....
When America raised the red, white, and blue,
Are forgotten.[90]

As a finishing touch and for the benefit of the audience, the poem concluded by accusing a third medical student, William C. Fox, of being involved in the Hubbardton Raid.

> May 25, 1880, W.C. Fox, M.D., of Wallingford [VT] died.[91]
> Thus has departed the last of the medical students who were in the "Hubbardton Raid." It would be well could the raid never be referred to.[92]

The feelings expressed in Spencer's poem were widely shared, as the editor of the *Vermont Historical Gazetteer* in 1877 concluded in an article on the Hubbardton Raid.

> The dissection of the dead to promote the arts of surgery and the knowledge of human anatomy, and the robbing of the grave, their sacred resting place, is in the first instance, is repulsive to all feelings of human sensibility and decency; the last, a harmless offense when undiscovered; is properly by law a felony; The depredations of the students of the Medical College at Castleton on the burying grounds convenient were frequent in the vicinity, although probably exaggerated, and were stimulated by the faculty of that institution for many years.[93]

We can contrast these later feelings engendered and expressed in the reply to the Hubbardton Raid and the editor of the *Vermont Historical Gazetteer* with the body-snatching response earlier in Vermont in 1834 from an account of the missing body of Mrs. Holbrook of Burlington, Vermont.

"Two brother students" at Woodstock "were accused of body snatching, in March of 1834" in Burlington, Vermont. John Daggett, aged eighteen, and his elder brother were arrested and brought before a magistrate, who bound them over to the grand jury. Two indictments were returned against each for digging up the dead. "When the disputed body was returned, one indictment against each was quashed by order of the attorney for the state." Both were convicted and sentenced on the second count, to serve three years in the Vermont State Prison, "pay a fine of $500 and the costs of prosecution." "The older brother completed the full term, whereas the younger was pardoned and discharged after a little more than two years."[94]

In a letter addressed to the faculty of the Woodstock Medical College signed by 125 citizens of Burlington, the following requests were made following the trials of the two brothers. What can be derived from this letter is from the court proceedings. They knew the body of Mrs. Holbrook was at Woodstock College and had been stolen by the students. Mrs. Holbrook and "her family are highly respectable," and "the disinterment of her remains has occasioned to her relatives ... distress" and "is universally regarded as a vile outrage." The letter continued, stating that it is likely "the dissecting knife has not been used upon her remains." Here the letter does not blame the faculty, as the response to the Hubbardton Raid and the *Vermont Historical Gazetteer* stated, but cannot believe that such respectable men would have anything to do with this outrage, as the following shows:

> We are unwilling to believe that Gentlemen so respectable as the Faculty of the Woodstock Medical School would countenance in the smallest degree an outrage of the kind—and although we fully believe that the true character of the outrage was unknown to you at the time, and would be indignantly reprobated by you at any time, yet we can have little doubt that your endeavors to procure the restoration of the body would be successful, and probably would be the sole means of effecting it.[95]

Surprisingly, looking at the Woodstock College today, it would appear that it had a penchant for accepting and graduating individuals previously accused of body snatching, for example, Almon Lull, Thaddeus Phelps, and the convicted John Daggett who graduated from Woodstock in 1837.[96]

As the *Vermont Historical Gazetteer* noted, stealing bodies in Vermont was "properly by law a felony." In 1804, Vermont had enacted a law that made body snatching a "felony and indictment and trial were in the hands of the higher county courts." Between 1820 and 1840, there were only seven indictments for disinterring dead bodies. Only two individuals, the Daggett brothers, were accused, convicted, and punished.[97]

In 1852 a committee of the Vermont Medical Society was appointed to propose legislation for "legalizing the study of anatomy." According to the physician Bingham H. Stone, "in what way it intended that this be done the record fails to state." He mused "presumably by giving physicians and colleges a legal means of obtaining unclaimed bodies for anatomical purposes."[98] As late as 1880 in Vermont with the revision of the Vermont laws, there was no statute expanding access to bodies for the study of anatomy. There are three sections: the first section is against grave robbing, the second section allows for a warrant to search for dead bodies, and the third section reads as follows: "The preceding section shall not prevent a surgeon or physician from having in his possession a dead human subject for anatomical investigation and instruction of students if such subject was obtained without violation of the law of the state."[99]

Presumably this means either a criminal body or one legally obtained from out of state. In summary, in Vermont it is a "fair estimate that the more than 1,600 students who did dissection in Vermont from 1820 to 1840 used at least 400 cadavers." Allowing for the fact that the "legal acquisition of cadavers furnished only a negligible number at this time, one or two a year. Practically all of the cadavers had to be secured illegally, and most of them were secured within the boundaries of Vermont.... There must be in the cemeteries, churchyards, and private burial plots in Vermont far more empty graves than was [ever] suspected."[100]

This makes sense. As noted previously, the nearest seaport was over two hundred miles away, and the medical colleges in these seaports had enough difficulty obtaining subjects for their own students.[101]

One physician at the time did allow that after the construction of the canal from Albany to Whitehall finished in September 1829, "many human bodies were received from Albany and Troy, New York, the bodies being in barrels and in brine marked 'pork' and shipped by canal to Whitehall and from there to Castleton by wagon. They were consigned to a grocer at Castleton who was a trustee of the medical college."[102] However, given the expense and demand for cadavers, it is unlikely this route ever came close to meeting the demands of the three competing Vermont schools.

With the inability of the authorities to prevent and prosecute body snatching, there is ample reason to understand the intense suspicion and bitterness held by Vermont natives toward the medical schools and colleges. They undoubtedly were not so naive as to underestimate the impact of the three medical schools on the sanctity of their buried dead.

By 1884 the Vermont Legislature finally reformed its anatomical laws and removed the confusing and difficult problem for physicians: how to obtain cadavers legally to practice their profession.

The 1884 anatomical law was divided into two sections and was similar to the earlier anatomical law passed in Connecticut. In the first section, poor law officials in the towns and cities were ordered if requested by a physician resident in Vermont to turn the body of an indigent over to the requesting physician for anatomical research if the individual was to be buried at public expense. However, there were exceptions; specifically, "no such body shall be so delivered, if the deceased person, during his last sickness, has made request for the burial of his body or if a person claiming to be kindred to the deceased, and satisfying such overseer of the poor or superintendent, thereof shall, within forty-eight hours after such person's decease, require such body to be buried...." The law also authorized the burial of a "stranger or traveler who had died suddenly, and before making himself known..." as well as any "deceased person" who had "served in the army or navy of the United States."

The second section ordered that the body could not be removed from the state or used in any way other than for "anatomical research." Also, the body must be decently buried either by the overseers of the poor or if relatives "of the deceased person require the same for burial." If this section was violated, the penalty was a "fine of not more than five hundred dollars or be imprisoned not more than five years or both."[103]

As we have seen in other cases, the latter was only a partial solution and did not always supply enough corpses to meet the demand, as either the noncooperation of officials or the actions of families and friends often kept the poor or strangers from the shame of the dissecting table.

8

Grave Robbing Comes to Washington, D.C.

When Dr. Thomas Sewall left Essex, Massachusetts, for Washington, D.C., following his conviction for receiving illegally obtained corpses, he did so at the invitation of Daniel Webster. In 1800 the population of the city of Washington was 14,093. There were two other well-established towns bordering Washington: Georgetown on the Maryland side and Alexandria on the Virginia side.

On his arrival Sewall found a newly organized city with a limited medical establishment. In 1816 in the city of Washington there were nine physicians and two apothecaries (both physicians), in Alexandria there nine or ten physicians, and before 1800 there were five physicians in Georgetown.

Given the population the numbers seemed sufficient, but some physicians did not practice medicine full-time. One physician was an Episcopal minister in Georgetown, and another operated a brewery near the Naval Yard. In addition, there were charlatans and quacks. The education of physicians "fell far short of the standard." Incomes for attending the sick were minimal; the general fee in Washington was one dollar. Physicians made up for this by selling drugs. Obstetrics was generally left to old women, and in addition "surgical cases were rare."[1]

Based on this description of the medical environment, there would be plenty of opportunity for Dr. Thomas Sewall to make a name for himself in the city of Washington, especially in the teaching of anatomy and surgery. He found this opportunity when he was appointed a professor of anatomy and physiology at the newly established Columbian College in 1824 (today's George Washington University).

The Columbian College of the District of Columbia was chartered by an act of Congress on February 21, 1821. At a board of trustees meeting on November 21, 1821, the decision was made to add a medical department. In the summer of 1824, the medical department was inaugurated, and professors were appointed. In March 1825, a course of lectures was begun on the different branches of medicine. Dr. Thomas Sewall had been appointed professor of anatomy and physiology. In addition, there were five other professors in the medical department. In the first circular printed by the medical department, one paragraph read as follows: "Such arrangements have been made as will furnish the Professor of Anatomy with materials for demonstration and the class with ample opportunity for the cultivation of Practical Anatomy."[2]

The description of the material to be used is vague and could mean anything including pictures and charts, wax figures, animals, and human bodies. It would have been interesting to know what these specific arrangements were, although as we will see we can hazard an informed opinion. It was not uncommon for college catalogs and other printed communications to be circumspect and "not mention dissection." Any reference was to the "opportunity for such as desired to dissect." To protect the medical schools, many medical students depended on independent instructors (preceptors) to "teach practical anatomy."[3]

Dr. Sewall delivered the opening lecture of the medical department at Columbian College on March 30, 1825. It was a remarkable and well-received lecture. He outlined the early history of medicine (such as it was in America), with the revival of the interest in medicine in Europe that led to the founding of two schools in Philadelphia, and discussed the history of sixteen medical schools now established and the rise of medical societies in the states. He went on to discuss the great progress in medicine during the past sixty years, the rising importance of the nation's capital, and the hope that the medical school would someday produce physicians like "a Sydenham, a Harvey, a Hunter, or a Bichat or to give to the world a Bard, a Rush, a Warren, a Barton, or a Wistar."[4]

Sewall discussed anatomy and dissection, providing a brief description of two early dissections. The "first in 1750 on the body of Hermanus Carroll, a criminal who had been executed for murder, was dissected in the city of New-York, by Dr. John Bard and Dr. Peter Middleton, two of the most eminent physicians of that day." Additionally, in 1756 "a course of lectures on Anatomy and Surgery, accompanied by dissections of the human body, … [was] delivered at Newport, in the State of Rhode Island, by a Doctor William Hunter, a distinguished Scotch [*sic*] physician, who had been educated at the University of Edinburgh." Sewall concluded that these "dissections and lectures were only temporary, and no plan was matured and carried into operation, for instituting a regularly organized medical school, till the one of Philadelphia, in 1765."[5]

Sewall continued, stating that today courses on anatomy are "illustrated by demonstrations on the recent subject, by the exhibition of models and drawings of the different parts of the body, by dried preparations, and specimens of morbid structure. The course on Surgery is accompanied by operations on the dead body.… Private dissecting classes are established, which give the student an opportunity for a more minute examination of the parts displayed in the lecture room and familiarize him with surgical operations by the habitual use of his own knife."[6]

Again, no one seemed to question where the specimens for the dissecting rooms originated or for the students to "familiarize" themselves for surgical operations.

Given Sewall's background as a convicted receiver of the stolen dead, it is ironic that in 1827 he stood in for the president of the college at the medical school's commencement on March 22, 1827. Usually, the president spoke to the students on "their moral deportment," and the dean of the medical faculty spoke on their "professional conduct." Sewall was required to speak on both issues. He said that the "parchment roll" they were receiving was an acknowledgment of their professional skill. As to the moral charge, Sewall emphasized their moral duty to the medical profession, to be gentlemanly, to attend to the suffering of the poor, to cultivate a gentle manner and kindness of heart, keep the Sabbath," guard "against infidel sentiments," limit the drinking of "ardent spirits," and "do not gamble and do not duel."[7]

Columbian College Medical Department Challenged

Following the establishment of the Columbian College, it soon found itself in a serious financial situation. However, the medical department "was not materially involved in the financial woes of the institution" except on the matter of prestige. The medical department was financially independent from the college, with all the risk being taken by the faculty. Shortly after the medical department's founding, its existence was challenged.[8]

Whenever a second medical school or more was proposed in the same area, the lay public feared that its establishment would create competition among the faculties and students for bodies for their instruction.[9] However, sometimes the faculty attempted to establish a second medical school because faculty "dissension" over the "defense or condemnation of students involved in resurrection" simply could not be resolved any other way.[10] Besides medical schools, bodies were also needed for "instruction for preceptors and for the use of practicing physicians." The latter two were "little suspected by the general public, who connected grave robbing almost entirely with dissection in the medical colleges."[11]

Earlier when Harvard wanted to build a new medical building in Boston, the public demanded that something be done "to prevent the robbery of graves."[12] And in 1827 when the medical school in Woodstock, Vermont, attempted to obtain a charter from the legislature, it was denied over "four successive sessions." One of the primary reasons is that people feared it would lead to grave robbing in the neighboring towns near the medical school. The Woodstock medical school only received its charter after affiliating in 1829 with a local college of arts with the power to "to confer medical degrees."[13]

Oddly enough, if we look at how the Columbian College Medical Department was established, it came into existence like the first medical school in Castleton, Vermont, under auspices of a College of Arts (Columbian), without a direct charter. Initially, there was some question of whether the medical department was lawfully established and whether it operated on a "dignified basis."

A group of petitioners in Washington wanted to establish a medical college in competition with the Columbian College Medical Department. They applied to the U.S. Congress for a charter in terms of a memorial to establish a second medical college in Washington, D.C., with the "advantages" that could be "derived from well-regulated medical colleges." The request was made by many of the leading worthies in Washington as well as seven physicians.[14]

Sewall represented the Columbian College Medical Department and replied to the memorial, noting that the charter for Columbian College authorized it to establish the medical department. He described the professorships, the value of the medical department, and how it was financially independent of the college as well as the legislature's establishment of the medical society in 1819 with specific powers, including the granting of licenses to practice and "to repress ignorant and empirical pretenders."[15]

Sewall discussed the problems encountered in Philadelphia and New York City when there was an attempt to establish a second medical school. This created a spirit of competition between the two schools in each city as student enrollments increased. As for Washington, Sewall wrote, a second medical school "here in this city, might not tend to create a spirit of professional discord and result in fatal embarrassments to both."[16]

Sewall's statement was rhetorical, and he did not have to go back to the early founding of the schools to highlight the difficulties that might be encountered even in Washington by the establishment of a second school. What might he have implied by "fatal embarrassments"? He argued "that the population of Washington does not compare with that of the two cities of the era alluded to."[17]

The early physicians of Washington only had to look to the city of Baltimore and the experience of Dr. John B. Davidge, who in 1807 established a small anatomical building in the city. The fact that he had acquired a corpse (illegally, because Maryland did not pass an anatomy act until 1882) aroused suspicion as well as the fact he was using it for teaching. As one newspaper reported, Dr. Davidge received the illegally obtained body of Zoroaster Miller on November 16, 1807. He opened the body in the presence of his students and gave lectures and dissections until the end of the week using Zoroaster's body.

On Saturday morning Mrs. Miller arrived and requested her husband's body. She was refused. On Sunday, some boys went to the top of the building and looked "through the sky-lights" and saw a "skeleton and the mangled remains of Miller." The boys spread the alarm, and soon a crowd gathered. Some bricks fell from the building, and "panes of glass were broken." The neighbors confronted Dr. Davidge and said they thought the house was a "nuisance." Soon after Miller's son appeared and knocked down the door to the building, he entered, along with the crowd and, when he saw his father's remains, "fainted on the floor." The "putrefying body" was carried from the house and placed in a coffin to be taken away for burial.[18]

It seems clear from the events as reported that the body stolen from its grave and the mangled corpse resulting from dissection of the dead father caused untold anguish to the son. The final insult to the family was Dr. Davidge's refusal to cooperate with the family and return the body, "ordering the widow away in a peremptory manner."[19]

Undoubtedly, the Baltimore experience was behind the thinking in a letter to the editor of the *Metropolitan* (Georgetown) newspaper on March 26, 1826, signed by "Civis," discussing the second medical school controversy. Civis "declared that it is well known to most of the citizens of the District of Columbia that the oldest practicing physicians in Washington had contemplated the establishment of a medical school long before 1821 but had 'deferred to a more auspicious period' because the sparseness of the population would make … difficult the securing of material for an anatomical branch."[20]

Civis might as well have added what a Boston newspaper had stated in its report on the Baltimore riot: "prudence might tell the Anatomist, that in the present state of Society, dissections should be performed in a retired place, or in a private manner,"[21] presumably not in the open arena of a medical school with illegally obtained cadavers.

The "lack of population" is code for the inability to obtain enough anatomical specimens for teaching and research. It was probably not that an additional medical college would have been competitive in most areas of teaching except anatomy and clinical medicine but instead that the additional students and faculty as well as preceptors competing for a limited number of bodies would have caused the "fatal embarrassments" Sewall alluded to, negatively affecting the reputation of both if a second medical school was established in Washington.

Sewall had good reason to fear that this issue would become an embarrassment for his school because it had already become a problem for other schools, especially the schools he alluded to in his memorial. He knew that any medical school that wanted to be credible and succeed had to offer courses in anatomy and dissection. Recently the demand for "material" for anatomy had caused intense competition among the most prestigious medical schools. The early 1820s had seen a growth in the number of medical schools. These medical students were now demanding "instruction in anatomical dissection" along the lines of the Parisian model.[22] As a result, the schools simply could not keep up with the demand for bodies for dissection.[23]

In Philadelphia, the competition for bodies was so contentious that a secret agreement among the anatomists was reached on November 22, 1828. The intent was to ensure a "fair distribution of bodies."[24] The agreement contained euphemistic language, but reference to anatomical specimens is obvious: "All members of the Profession in the city of Philadelphia, of fair standing shall have equal facilities for the acquisition of anatomical knowledge or for teaching it to others, as far as these facilities depend on the public places, etc."[25] In addition, "with a view to sustain the medical interests of Philadelphia and prevent the public scandal and excitement incident to the cultivation of anatomy, the written agreement drawn up by Dr. Horner … [should] be adopted as a code by which anatomists shall be governed…."[26] Even with this agreement, the fighting over corpses continued.[27]

The second conflict Dr. Sewall mentioned in the memorial concerned the College of Physicians and Surgeons and the Rutgers Medical College (1826–1831), both located in New York City. The former was chartered in 1807 and became part of Columbia University in 1860. In the 1820s a large portion of the faculty seceded; the conflict included personal animosity and the concern that the school was too slow in adapting to the Parisian model. In 1826 the New York legislature refused to give the defecting professors a charter. Unable to secure a charter, they used a "dormant New Jersey state charter … for the never viable Rutgers Medical College to set up shop in New York City." They hired John Godman, "an avid supporter of pathological anatomy," from Philadelphia. This led to an increased interest in "practical anatomy" among the medical students.

The demand for bodies had always been high, and obtaining them had been difficult for one school. The solution to obtaining more cadavers in New York was to bribe "public officials and burial-ground employees to gain unhindered access to the Potter's field." For those with friends and family, they would be buried in field No. 1 and were not to be dissected. Those in field No. 2 were "plundered … for the medical colleges."[28]

This still did not satisfy the need for cadavers, especially when the College of Physicians and Surgeons and the Rutgers Medical College competed to cut off the supply of corpses. One student, Edward Dixon, wrote about his adventures in grave robbing in the early 1830s. As a poor student at Rutgers, he wrote that the "supply of material for the dissecting room" was cut off when the other school paid off the officials to supply corpses for their use alone, and he and a few of his classmates would "turn to become resurrectionists themselves." In his memoir, he related stories of his grave-robbing adventures.[29]

Dr. Sewall was aware of the shortage of bodies for anatomical courses even among the most prestigious medical schools in the country and the potential impact on acquiring corpses for the Columbian College Medical Department if a second medical college was established in Washington.

The response to Sewall and the dean of the college was the "Counter Memorial of Sundry Citizens of the District of Columbia praying That a Charter may be granted by Congress to Enable them to Institute a Medical College in the City of Washington, February 20, 1826." The counter memorial, an eight-page document, argued that Columbian College was a college, not a university, and was only authorized to offer "honorary academic degrees in the liberal arts and sciences." Much of the document is concerned with distinguishing the difference between a college and a university and why the formation of the medical department was illegal. Also, the "Professors" attempted to establish a monopoly, and the comparison to schools in Pennsylvania, New York, and Massachusetts was invalid. The counter memorial concluded that the medical department at

Columbian College is illegal, and if the "Professors" had not objected and allowed their project to go forward they "never would have been induced to raise questions or difficulties upon the subject if they had been permitted to proceed without molestation and opposition in the fair legal acquisition of this object."[30]

In its conclusion, the counter memorial contained bitter and threatening language with such words as "illegal," "monopoly," and "molestation." It is not hard to imagine what was going on behind the scenes. However, for the "professors" the very existence of the medical department was at stake, as was their income. Their ability to attract first-rate instructors and students and raise the status of the medical department depended on an adequate supply of corpses at a reasonable price for the anatomy department.

Dr. Sewall and his colleagues must have explained the underlying causes of the conflict and professional squabbling at the medical schools in New York, Pennsylvania, and Massachusetts in forceful language, because two days later Congress received the following memorial signed by thirteen doctors and eighty-eight prominent citizens: "We, the undersigned physicians, and citizens of said District, desiring that the injurious effects of rivalry and division in the early periods of medical instruction, experienced repeatedly in other parts of our country, may not create the same embarrassments here: and moreover, impressed with the belief that the institution at present existing is fully adequate to the present exigencies of the profession and the community, do humbly pray that another Medical College may not be incorporated."[31]

As the examples above demonstrate, the addition of a second medical school even when the original schools were highly prestigious led to a shortage of corpses, the rise of body snatching, and the exposure of this underground economy in the popular press, embarrassing the medical schools and the doctors.

Although the Columbian College Medical Department catalog advertised its anatomy courses, there was no mention of how bodies were obtained for these early courses. The first mention, although much later, is interesting. J.M. Toner wrote, "There have been some individual efforts in the teaching of particular branches of the science of medicine by physicians in Washington that are worthy of being noticed. The first of this character was by Dr. J.C. Hall, who, in 1828, opened a private dissecting room.... His efforts were so well patronized that he continued the course for some years to good classes, and until he was elected professor of surgery in Columbian College" in 1839.[32]

Although dissection was being done at Columbian College, it is interesting that Hall set up his private dissecting clinic in 1828. As we saw earlier, people were aware that dissections were done at the colleges but seemed unaware of these private dissecting facilities. It is likely that after the Burke and Hare trial on December 31, 1828, that gained worldwide attention when it was learned that these men were murdering people in Edinburgh, Scotland, to supply bodies to physicians, the teaching colleges had to be more cautious in obtaining bodies for dissection. Private facilities were not in the public eye, which likely explains the popularity of Hall's "private dissecting room."

As we have seen, the "underhanded practice of obtaining bodies for dissection and demonstrator purposes was rife during the first quarter of the nineteenth century." Burke and Hare had introduced a method that avoided the middleman by delivering the dead person directly to the customer rather than obtaining the body from a grave site. This gave rise to the term "burking," "which now means to smother another human being."[33] The method they used did not leave any violent marks on the bodies. The murders by Burke and Hare likely began in January or February 1828 and culminated in

December 1828 with their arrest and subsequent trial on December 31.[34] The impact of this trial in England and in the United States was immediate. The effect in Scotland and England led to a "reign of social terror." Newspaper reports, graphic enough, were supplemented by tales of horror published in broadsides and sung about in "ribald ballads," eagerly sought by the populace." These "inflamed the mind of the public…every household gathered its members within doors before dark and working men walked home from their night's toil in groups."[35]

The newspaper reports were international news and were reprinted in American newspapers. This information reached legislators here in America "as well as all members of the American public." Perhaps some of the broadsides and ballads likely made their way to the United States as well. For the medical profession, it "seemed like a good time to push for reform." The impact of this event even seemed to awaken legislators to the need for reform on the acquisition of bodies for medical education.[36]

As a direct consequence, Massachusetts enacted a law in 1831 legislating that unclaimed bodies of paupers from state institutions in Boston could be provided to medical colleges. New York (1854) eventually followed with its own anatomy law. The New England states of Connecticut and New Hampshire passed anatomical laws like the Massachusetts law, but as we saw earlier the Connecticut law was repealed the following year in 1834 and the New Hampshire law passed in 1834 was repealed in 1842. Most other states did not pass such measures until after the American Civil War. Only the Massachusetts and New York anatomical laws "enacted before 1860 had continued in force."[37] As late as 1881, Congress had passed no such law for Washington, D.C. "In order to punish body snatching, [the District was] obliged to fall back on the common law penalty."[38]

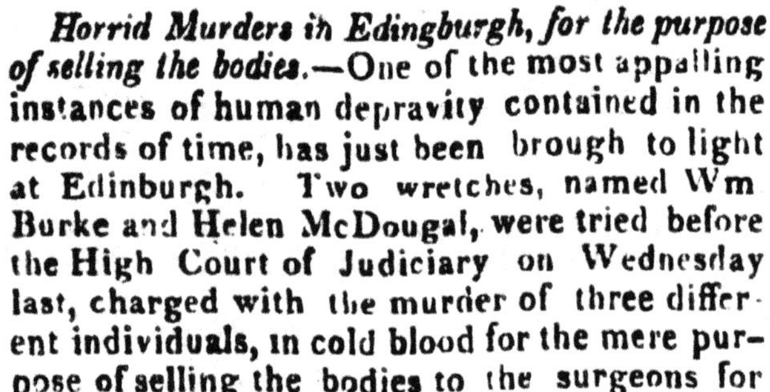

Horrid Murders in Edingburgh, for the purpose of selling the bodies.—One of the most appalling instances of human depravity contained in the records of time, has just been brought to light at Edinburgh. Two wretches, named Wm Burke and Helen McDougal, were tried before the High Court of Judiciary on Wednesday last, charged with the murder of three different individuals, in cold blood for the mere purpose of selling the bodies to the surgeons for dissection! So unnatural and incredible did the case seem, that we believe it has scarcely gained credit in England, and it has been declared in some of the newspapers, to be a mere ruse to favor the introduction of a bill for supplying the surgeons with subjects in some legal way. The trial, however, exhibits all the facts of this horrible trade in blood, so as to silence and appal the most incredulous.

Wm. Burke and Helen McDougal, who are both Irish, & who lived together in Edinburgh, as man and wife, were indicted together for the murders of Mary Paterson or Mitchell, James Wilson, known by the name of 'Daft Jamie,' and Mary Campbell or Docherty, by strangling them. The last of the three cases was taken first; and the following are the facts

Newspaper reports on the trial of William Burke and William Hare were international news. The above account was long and detailed. After several paragraphs, Dr. Knox's assistant David Paterson provided a quote that said Burke and Hare had "frequently brought subjects that had not been interred for dissection" (*Phenix Gazette*, Alexandria, VA, March 3, 1829, 2; Library of Congress).

Ironically, in 1830 when the Massachusetts legislature was looking to initiate a new anatomy law to repeal the 1815

"Act to Protect the Sepulchers of the Dead," the committee proposing new legislation wrote to Thomas Sewall along with other prominent physicians and asked the questions enumerated below in his letter of support:

> Sir.
>
> In reply to your interrogatories—"Are the study and knowledge of Anatomy essential to the understanding and safe practice of medicine, and is not the dissection of dead bodies essential to this study and knowledge?" I answer first that the study and knowledge of Anatomy are not only essential, but indispensable to the safe practice of medicine; and anyone who attempts the Healing Art without this knowledge, can have no correct idea of the seat and nature of disease and the operation of remedies, and must daily see his patients, falling victims to his ignorance. Second, I answer that there is no other source from which knowledge of Anatomy can be acquired, but that of dissecting dead bodies. I can add from experience and observation, that just in proportion to the acquisition of Anatomical knowledge and consequently in proportion to the facilities of acquiring that knowledge by dissection, will be the skill and respectability of the medical profession. The truth of this position is established by the experience of every age, and every country.
>
> Very respectfully yours,
> THOMAS SEWALL.[39]

Interestingly, Sewall's letter is dispassionate and terse. Other letters of support were longer and gave examples of the necessity of why this new law should be passed and the negative impact of the 1815 act on the education of physicians in Massachusetts. Likely, since Sewall had been convicted under the 1815 act and heavily fined, he did not want to call more attention to himself than was necessary or he would have shown more enthusiasm to have the 1815 act repealed. For example, George C. Shattuck wrote a letter in support of the new legislation referencing Sewall's experience:

> Massachusetts speaks as hard a language to her practitioners of the Healing Art; bind up these wounds and heal these diseases, for both your reputation and your fortune are at stake on the issue, but do not dissect a human body to learn your art. Of her statute, the hard hearted oppressor takes advantage, he drives the houseless vagrant hungry from his door, and when he has perished in the street from cold and hunger, and after he shall have been interred at the expense of the town when the aspiring son of medical inquiry, as he supposed, had secretly disinterred for the light of anatomical science the unfortunate wanderer, gripes all at once, when there is to be nothing out of pocket, feels a touch of humanity for the corruptible body, and calculates on both a harvest of applause, and money for this patriotic zeal. The unfortunate tyro [novice] in physic is immured in prison, is sentenced to pay a fine to which he is unequal, and consequently expiates the offended law by protracted imprisonment to the loss of health and life.[40]

Or, as others wrote in reference to Burke and Hare, "a minute knowledge of anatomy is unattainable but by the dissection of dead bodies, some provision I think should be made by the Laws for the attainment of this object. And this would have the good effect of preventing the violation of the graves of the dead, which is so revolting to the friends and relations of the dead; as well as serve to do away the temptation to murder, which has disgraced some of the capitals of Europe."[41]

Another wrote that "the laws are now, certainly, prohibitory of dissection, since they punish the taking of a dead body, under any circumstances, with little less severity than felony.... [T]he present laws, likewise, consigns the actual procurement of bodies to desperate and unprincipled men, who alone are willing to take the risks attending the occupation, and who are thus preparing themselves to become the terror of peaceable and virtuous citizens. It must of necessity be that ... every school of anatomy in the country, must depend on such men for their supply of subjects. In other countries these men have committed murders which chill the blood to mention; why may they not do the same in this?"[42]

The following was later written about Sewall: "Anatomical Research, almost driven in labor, watch and peril to rob graves was ever brought to the criminal dock. To meet pecuniary costs of such sorrow, esprit du corps was appealed to; but self-reproach, wounded spirit, who could bear [it]?"[43]

Sewall's colleagues in the medical profession saw him as a martyr to their cause in pursuit of legislation in both Massachusetts and other states to free up their access to human bodies to continue their teaching and research. The Massachusetts Anatomy Act of 1831 was sold to the public by appeasing the concerns of the religious by Christian rites of burial. The goal was to remove the previous stigma that only executed criminals were dissected. Now that unclaimed indigents (in Boston) were eligible for dissection, the seemingly insatiable needs of physicians for bodies would put an end to grave robbing by putting the "resurrectionists" out of business, thereby protecting burying grounds and cemeteries from their ravages.

The Impact of the Cholera Outbreak in the City of Washington in 1832

In 1832 the Asiatic cholera appeared on the American continent. During the summer and fall it spread over the greater part of the United States and was first noticed in New York City on June 26, 1832. The first case in Washington appeared on August 10.[44] The city government of Washington quickly organized against the cholera. The Board of Alderman and the Board of Common Council appointed individuals within the six districts to serve as police commissioners and be associated with the Board of Health for four months. The mayor was authorized "to appoint such additional members as scavengers as he felt proper."[45]

During the cholera of 1832, three temporary hospitals were established in the city. They were called the Western, the Central, and the Eastern. The medical staff of the different hospitals was appointed by the Board of Health on August 7, 1832. Dr. Sewall was a consulting doctor at the Central.[46]

In 1832, physicians did not understand the cause of cholera. Therapeutic treatments administered to the victims were ineffective in many cases, and some exacerbated the progress of the disease, especially bloodletting. The disease is caused by the cholera *vibrio*, which disrupts the exchange of sodium and chloride ions in the small intestine, leading to watery stools and eventually dehydration and death.[47] Although cholera is still a deadly disease, oral hydration restoring the proper balance of electrolytes in the victim is the recommended remedy to prevent death.

Because treatments were ineffective and the cause was unknown, the response to cholera primarily consisted of public health measures of quarantine (not imposed in Washington) and recommendations concerning diet and morality. Some doctors considered cholera to be contagious, while others believed it was due to miasma or "bad air."

The Board of Health in Washington did not support quarantining individuals, but it did order restrictive public health ordinances concerning entertainment, trade, and diet. It also suggested to the public that anyone with loose morals was an excellent candidate for the disease. Those in Washington opposed to the Board of Health's restrictions supported a completely free market and advocated that cholera arose from a poisonous effluvium.

On August 14, 1832, the Board of Health advised religious groups not to hold nighttime meetings. A second recommendation that had been earlier discussed by the board was to forbid the sale of ardent spirits; this did not include beer and wine.[48]

Thomas Sewall, a member of the District of Columbia Board of Health since 1824 and a member of the D.C. Chapter of the American Temperance Society, was in a perfect position to influence the resolutions of the Board of Health concerning the belief that intemperance was a major cause of death from cholera.

Many reports in the newspapers of cholera deaths "mentioned that the victim was an alcoholic." Other accounts merely stated that those who died were "intemperate."[49] Cholera provided physicians "with the evidence" that alcohol was, as Sewall had put it in 1830, "a vice ... attended with so many circumstances of suffering, mortification, and disgrace, that it seems difficult to understand how it should ever have become a prevalent evil among mankind."[50] Later he wrote that cholera, "wherever it appeared, singled out the intemperate for its victims, in a marked and most extraordinary manner."[51]

The board unanimously passed a resolution urging the city council to enact a law that "will effectively close all the dram shops, or drinking houses, throughout the city, and to restrain as much as possible, intemperate drinking."[52] "Closing the bars did not solve the problem and on August 14, the Board voted the sale of hard liquor be discontinued for the space of ninety days from this date."[53] On August 16, the "Board banned all theatrical shows ... and exhibitions."[54] Its reasoning was to prevent large gatherings. The board opposed quarantine restrictions "as tending to create a false confidence ... to the neglect of more important preservatives from the cholera."[55]

Ironically, on August 16 the Board of Health also banned various foodstuffs, and it was this ban that caused the most trouble for the board. Beginning on August 22 and for ninety days hence, the only food crops that could be sold in the city were "tomatoes, potatoes, beets and onions." All others were forbidden as well as "fish, crabs, oysters, clams, lobsters and crawfish."

One item led to a long caustic letter that was published in the newspaper the *National Intelligencer* accusing the Board of Health and the city authorities of not "having the corporate authority ... or legal authority to prohibit the sale of watermelons in the City." The author argued that it would be right to exclude watermelons if the facts showed that "watermelons produce cholera." Since physicians have no knowledge of "the disease and it's cause," they cannot know what can or cannot be eaten during the cholera epidemic, and "this they are perfectly ignorant of, and every opinion expressed by them is speculation and conjecture."[56]

Many others had the same opinion. (This was not only an agrarian society, and the ban overlapped with the fall harvest. Clearly, many farmers and fishermen would have been ruined with nowhere to sell their crops or their catches.) On the evening of August 21, 1832, a public meeting of the citizens was called at Washington City Hall. The citizens wanted an accounting for the measures "to be imposed upon the production of the earth and honest industry" ordered on August 16, 1832, by the "despotic proceedings of the Board of Health." The agenda was to include the "caterers of our markets; and a free discussion of the merits of the subject so deeply involving the reserved and inalienable rights of freemen, is particularly invited." The Board of Health was accused of turning away from the "real nuisances" of refuse and stagnant water and instead trying to "paralyze industry and superinduce famine, which is as bad as the plague." The "moderate use of production of the season is eminently conducive to good health," and "total abstinence from them is highly injurious to digestion and invites disease." Besides, the foodstuffs found favorable by the "sage Board of Health, are not produced in sufficient quantity to substitute for the twenty or thirty" other proscribed items, "nor are they more wholesome than most of those which their sapient heads have forbid."

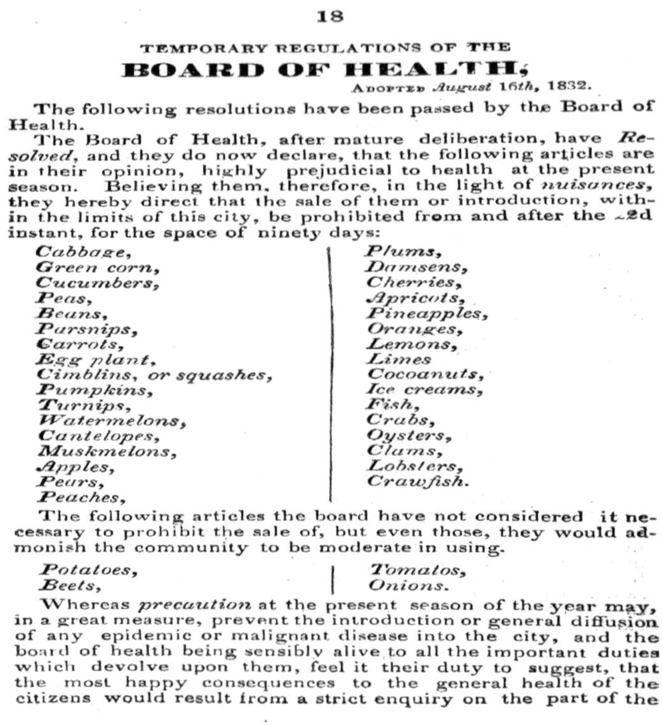
18

TEMPORARY REGULATIONS OF THE

BOARD OF HEALTH,

ADOPTED *August 16th*, 1832.

The following resolutions have been passed by the Board of Health.

The Board of Health, after mature deliberation, have *Resolved*, and they do now declare, that the following articles are in their opinion, highly prejudicial to health at the present season. Believing them, therefore, in the light of *nuisances*, they hereby direct that the sale of them or introduction, within the limits of this city, be prohibited from and after the 22d instant, for the space of ninety days:

Cabbage,	*Plums,*
Green corn,	*Damsens,*
Cucumbers,	*Cherries,*
Peas,	*Apricots,*
Beans,	*Pineapples,*
Parsnips,	*Oranges,*
Carrots,	*Lemons,*
Egg plant,	*Limes*
Cimblins, or squashes,	*Cocoanuts,*
Pumpkins,	*Ice creams,*
Turnips,	*Fish,*
Watermelons,	*Crabs,*
Cantelopes,	*Oysters,*
Muskmelons,	*Clams,*
Apples,	*Lobsters,*
Pears,	*Crawfish.*
Peaches,	

The following articles the board have not considered it necessary to prohibit the sale of, but even those, they would admonish the community to be moderate in using.

Potatoes,	*Tomatos,*
Beets,	*Onions.*

Whereas *precaution* at the present season of the year may, in a great measure, prevent the introduction or general diffusion of any epidemic or malignant disease into the city, and the board of health being sensibly alive to all the important duties which devolve upon them, feel it their duty to suggest, that the most happy consequences to the general health of the citizens would result from a strict enquiry on the part of the

During the cholera epidemic in 1832, the board of health of the City of Washington established a series of controversial ordinances. The regulations established on August 16, 1832, regarding foodstuffs, fish, and shellfish elicited an especially caustic reaction. Washington, D.C., Board of Health, *Laws of the Corporation, and Regulations of the Board of Health of the City of Washington: In Relation to the Removal of Nuisances and the Preservation of the Health of the City* (Washington, D.C., 1832), 18. National Library of Medicine.

At the meeting, Dr. Robert Mayo read the ordinances adopted by the Board of Health. The meeting produced three resolutions:

1. That we the citizens of Washington in a general town meeting assembled, hereby enter our solemn protest against the authority of the above (Board of Health sanitary measures) assumed, and positively forbid any attempt to execute the edict above quoted.
2. That we will contribute our individual and united aid to abate nuisances in masses of putrid matter and stagnant water.
3. That we request the mayor and corporate authority of the city to interpose on behalf of the citizens in vindicating the freedom of markets.[57]

A second public meeting was held at city hall regarding the edicts of the Board of Health. On the same day of this meeting the Board of Health reported four cases of cholera.

On August 22, the Board of Health published an address to the citizens of Washington and stated the board had been "appointed by the constituted authority of the city without solicitation; they were aware that ignorance and selfish cupidity and vicious propensities find themselves thwarted and opposed and from these sources, opposition was to be anticipated to any measure that might be proscribed. Measures were being taken calculated to cast odium upon the actions of the board, which if successful, would render the exertions of the board fruitless and unavailing, and, left without the support of public opinion, the consequences would be chargeable to others, not to them."[58]

When cholera broke out in Washington it "swept principally through the ranks of Irish and the Negroes and raged unchecked until the frost in the fall."[59] Reports indicate that it had dissipated by October 1, 1832.[60]

According to Toner, "no complete report of the epidemic cholera as it existed here at that time was ever published. The minutes of the Board of Health show that such a report was ordered to be prepared, but it was not published; and, if prepared, is now lost from the archives of the Board."

The following is a synopsis of a preliminary report made by the doctors Henry Huntt (head of the Board of Health), Thomas Sewall, and Nathaniel Pope Causin and published in the *National Intelligencer*. Deaths from cholera were males, 269; females, 190; whites, 251; Blacks (free), 160; and Blacks (enslaved), 46. Total deaths were 459.[61]

During the cholera epidemic in 1832, cholera riots did not occur in the United States but did in Britain and on the European continent.[62] The riots in Britain especially were related to the new anatomy act. The mob cried out against doctors, dissection, and body snatching. On April 7, 1832, William Cobbett reported that in Manchester, England, when cholera victims were put in isolation in the cholera hospitals, it was thought that "cholera was merely an excuse to get the sick into special hospitals where they could be dissected."[63] Specific to body snatching and cholera, the historian R.J. Morris related an event in Paisley, Scotland, in which "two small shovels and a hook on the end of a piece of cord were found by two boys playing under a bridge on the way to a cholera burying ground on Paisley Moss. The tools of the body-snatching trade." The "coffins at the burial ground were opened.... Six out of seven coffins were found empty." The crowd became uncontrollable and began to riot, smashing the "windows and shops of all the doctors in the town.... The gates of the cholera hospital ... were forced and the cholera van carried away and broken up."[64]

In the United States, all was quiet in the Washington cholera hospitals during the epidemic. However, there were newspaper reports from Philadelphia that "the doors of cholera hospitals have been beset by crowds of persons, who have in many cases prevented the admission of patients."[65]

However, even in this case there was nothing equivalent to the body-snatching concerns in England. According to one report, the cholera epidemic in Philadelphia in 1832 produced an "alarm equal" to yellow fever in 1793 and 1798. The first case to enter the asylum of the Philadelphia Almshouse and Hospital was on July 21, 1832. The president of the Board of Guardians and the mayor of Philadelphia arranged "for the admission of a number of cholera patients to the asylum." Cases increased dramatically, and a "general panic" occurred. The nurses requested higher wages, and "the demands were met." However, between "the terror and want of moral sense" the nurses were "seized with a kind of mad infatuation. They drank the stimulants provided for the sick, and in one ward where the pestilence raged in its most fearful forms, and where between the dead and dying the sight was most appalling, these furies were seen lying drunk upon or fighting over the dead victims of the disease."

Order was restored after a local bishop gave permission for the religious order of the "sisters of charity" to enter the asylum and tend to the sick. The sisters remained there until May 20, 1832.[66]

The fact that there were no reports of body-snatching accusations at American hospitals can be attributed to several factors. America was rural at this time; there were few hospitals, and those that existed were seen as warehouses for the dying poor. Nearly all people who could afford a physician were treated and operated on at home. They were taken care of by their families. It was only the poor and those without resources who found their way to hospitals. The poor feared hospitals, thinking "they might be used for surgical experiments or, even turned over to medical students for dissection."[67] This did not appear to be an issue during the cholera epidemic. Unlike in Britain where body snatching was tied to the teaching hospital, in America dissection and body snatching were primarily attributed to medical schools, not hospitals. The first and only body-snatching riot initially targeting a hospital occurred in 1788 in New York City as part of the "Doctor's Riot."[68] Since the founding of medical schools in America, the stigma of body snatching was transferred to them, with a series of riots imputed to them for this reason. However, during the cholera epidemic there were no known cases connecting cholera victims with body snatching at hospitals or medical schools.

The cholera epidemic and cholera deaths were not as dramatic in Washington, D.C., as in other cities in the United States. Ironically, the one thing the cholera epidemic did highlight was the need for a public hospital in Washington. The members of the Board of Health spent the next six years appealing to Congress to establish an appropriation for the city to establish a hospital. As we will see below, the Columbian College Medical Department and its faculty would be instrumental in making the hospital a reality.

The Medical Department of Columbian College Suspends Lectures, 1834–1839

The next major event following the end of the cholera epidemic to affect the medical department of Columbian College and Dr. Thomas Sewall was for some unknown reason the suspension of lectures from 1834 until the faculty was reorganized and lectures began again in November 1839.[69]

Although there are no records concerning this lapse in lectures, I believe there is the implication of an internal conflict in the department over what the faculty should teach based on the failure of the French physician François-Joseph-Victor Broussais's system of "physiological medicine." Early in the century it had rapidly become the most popular medical philosophy in Paris and influenced American physicians. Broussais insisted that "all disease originates as an irritation of the gastrointestinal tract that passes to other organs sympathetically." His treatment for all diseases included exsanguination. In the case of cholera this treatment is especially deadly because it contributes to the dehydration of the body, which is the cause of death from cholera.[70] Unfortunately for Broussais, he was one of history's most notorious "bleeders." His medical system fell into disfavor during the 1832 Paris cholera epidemic when his bleeding treatment ended in an excessive number of deaths of his patients.[71]

To regain some credibility, Broussais appears to have turned to phrenology (another popular a priori medical system) and in 1836 published his book *Cours de Phrénologie*. In his introduction he wrote, "I will only mention one utility of phrenology in this foreword, the others will be deduced enough from reading the work: it is about medicine. This science now has a pressing need for cerebral organology; madness is not the only disease which demands it; all cerebral affections, all neuroses, all acute inflammations of the great viscera ... all diseases without exception must draw from it."[72]

Thomas Sewall published the following critique of phrenology in 1837: *An Examination of Phrenology: In Two Lectures, Delivered to the Students of Columbian College, District of Columbia, February 1837.* Sewall wrote that phrenology should be investigated because it is popular in many circles and claims to be a science, the "knowledge of which is all important to the well-being of society." He wrote that the object of his lectures was to investigate this new science by presenting the chief tenets of phrenology: "to ascertain how far these are sustained by the anatomical structure of the parts more immediately concerned."[73]

Sewall criticized phrenology, using his knowledge of anatomy, writing that the structure of the parts of the brain "show the absurdity of the idea of organs as described by the phrenologist. The notion then of the division of the brain into phrenological organs is entirely hypothetical, is not sustained by dissection, and is inconsistent with the whole formation."[74]

Sewall also assailed phrenology's belief that intelligence could be equated with brain and skull size. He made his argument using drawings of brains illustrating his criticism. He concluded that historically, men have sought the means to suggest something that will "reveal all secrets ... which savors of mystery or a miracle. Something to supersede tedious observation, and laborious research."[75]

To his students, Sewall wrote (with a nod toward the need for opening the body) that the phrenologist cannot know the human mind by examining the skull. He quoted Napoleon, stating that "nature does not reveal her secrets by external forms. She hides and does not expose her secrets." To attempt to "seize or penetrate human character by so slight an index (as the development of the head) is the part of a dupe or an imposter."[76]

Sewall concluded by telling his students to "beware, gentleman of that delusive science[;] ... distrust its application to yourselves as well as others."[77]

Sewall investigated the basics of the system of phrenology, believed to be scientific in nature. Phrenology had gained great popularity in the 1830s and 1840s in America and become accepted among many leading intellectuals and doctors at the time. As Sewall discovered, it was an a priori and hypothetical system that did not stand up to empirical evidence easily obtained by the dissection of the human brain.

This idea of not depending on a priori and nonempirical medical systems to understand the cause and the treatment of disease is taken up by Dr. John F. May's inaugural lecture to the opening class of Columbian College on November 4, 1839. This lecture followed his and Dr. Sewall's reorganization of the medical department at Columbian College in 1839.

Dr. May was a student at Columbian College in 1831; he graduated in medicine in 1834 and completed his studies in Paris in 1837. In Paris he attended the lectures of Dr. Alfred Velpeau, who advised his students to distinguish fact from opinion (ironically, he was trained early in anatomy by dissecting corpses "he obtained by body snatching from cemeteries"), and the celebrated physiologist Dr. Francoise Magendie, who advocated the experimental method and expounded the same medical doctrine.[78] As we will see, May's relationship with Dr. Sewall and his further training explain his forceful advocacy of pathological anatomy, observation, and experimentation in medicine.

The issue over utilizing the now flawed medical system, that of Broussais (or any earlier system since disproven), versus the strict empiricism of the anatomists was revealed in two lectures given in 1839 and was featured in the medical journal the *American Medical Intelligencer.* The lecture in support of the value of a grand medical system (even if flawed) was argued by Dr. Thomas Hun before the Albany Medical College and published at the request of the class. The lecture advocating the view of the anatomists (likely approved by Sewall based on his previous writings), was delivered by Dr. John F. May of the newly reorganized medical department of Columbian College.[79]

Dr. Hun argued that although grand medical systems had their failings, they have had "their utility." "The absurdities into which men have fallen by blind adherence to systems have been eagerly seized upon by the enemies of reasoning to give plausibility to their empiricism. Currently we have no system[;] ... we witnessed the downfall of Broussiasm[;] ... it fell under the rude attacks...[and] ... criticism of the anatomists." Although it "contained great truths[,] ... I know there were many who never comprehended the system when it was in vogue ... [and] now applaud themselves for their sagacity in its downfall." Today "no system exists in medicine."[80]

Dr. May in his welcoming lecture to the students of the medical department of Columbian College in November 1839 was almost triumphant when he wrote that he would like to extend "the application of the important study [pathological anatomy] to almost every ramification of medical science." He criticized "false facts" and "theoretical delusions" in medicine "even today." There are those who live in a world of "abstractions" and would rather "invent for nature" rather than "learn from her teachings.'" For them "*a priori* is a point of departure." Past systems have been "speculative" and "teach with absurd dogmas"; these same systems have fallen like alchemy or "the absurdities of humoralism, solidism and vitalism; ... or other superstitions ... [such as] ... theosophy, magic, and astrology."

May informed the students about the "influence of pathological anatomy, and the inductive character of the age; this speculative tendency is wearing away fast." However, there will always be some teachers and students who look to the "great names" for authority; "it will never be eliminated from our profession." He admonished new students to respect those authorities whose "labors and research have 'thrown light on the truth'" but not to trust authority completely; to use your own reason: "if you cannot comprehend" something "do not accept it blindly but reserve it for further inquiry and for future investigation."[81]

It is unusual that such a strong message opening a reorganized medical department would not have been influenced by debates within the Columbian faculty and the medical associations in Washington. The opening of the department was continued under the leadership of Thomas Sewall, and there was no doubt that anatomy and instruction in dissection would continue to be prominently featured in the revived Columbian College Medical Department.

The Establishment of the Washington Infirmary

As noted above, one outcome of the cholera epidemic was the collapse of the Broussiasm medical system and the justification of "pathological anatomy" as a more scientific mode of inquiry. It was certainly more important for the development of medicine than, as pointed out earlier by Sewall, the pseudoscience of phrenology. For the Columbian College Medical Department this was a continued justification for the importance of teaching anatomy and dissection. This increased the demand for corpses over time and led to the growth of body snatching in Washington, D.C.

A second outcome of the cholera epidemic for the Columbian College Medical Department was the founding of an infirmary under the auspices of the latter and a new home for the medical department.

Following the end "of the cholera, at the suggestion of the Board of Health, several public meetings were held, with a view to encourage the establishment of a general and permanent hospital in the city." Unfortunately, the hospital was "not encouraged" or "patronized by Congress or the Corporation, [and] the project for the time fell through." However, the Board of Health from 1832 to 1837 continued "to appoint a committee to memorialize Congress to obtain an appropriation to establish" a public hospital in the city of Washington.[82]

On August 29, 1842, Congress passed a law authorizing the old jail in Judiciary Square to be altered and fitted up for an insane asylum. But in 1844 "when the alterations had been completed, it was decided by Congress it was not a proper place for an institution of that kind." The medical faculty of Columbian College applied to Congress for the use of the building for an infirmary and other purposes.[83]

On June 15, 1844, a law was passed by Congress and approved by the president of the United States:

> That the Commissioner of Public Buildings be directed to allow the Medical Faculty of Columbian College, District of Columbia, to occupy the insane hospital, with the adjoining grounds, situated in the Judiciary Square, in Washington, "for the purpose of an infirmary, for medical instruction, and for scientific purposes." Professors Thomas Sewall, Harvey Lindsly, Thomas Miller, John M. Thomas, William P. Johnston, and Charles G. Page of the Medical Department of Columbian College signed the bond.[84]

The first patients were admitted into the infirmary in mid–July 1844. The infirmary was opened "upon the most liberal terms to the public, the first general hospital in Washington City." The infirmary "was well sustained by the public, and in a short time Congress, upon the petition of the faculty and influential citizens, made a

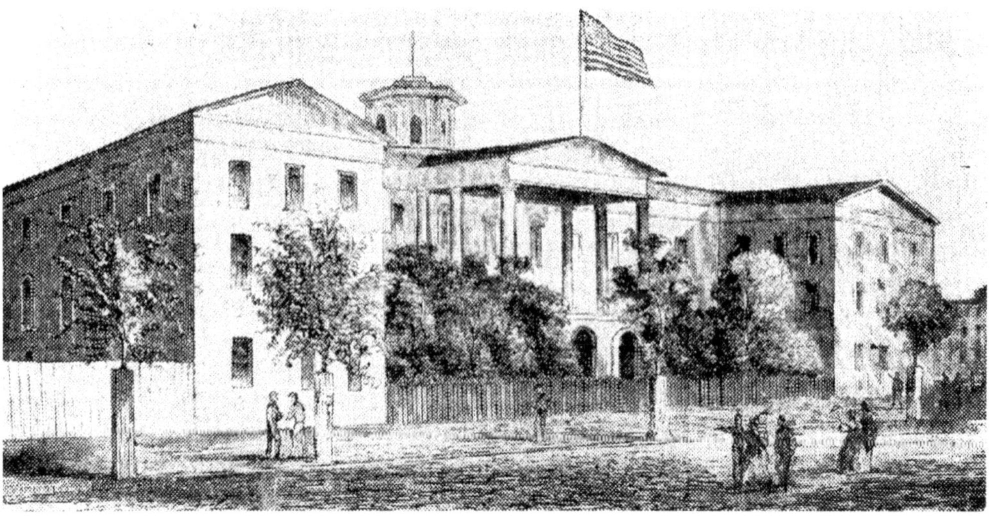

"Washington Infirmary Hospital, destroyed by fire in 1861" (National Library of Medicine).

yearly appropriation of at first, $2,000, then $3,000, and it was finally raised to $6,000, for care and medical treatment of the transient paupers of the District of Washington." The Washington Infirmary also became popular with the growing District population including strangers, mechanics, and laborers.[85]

Although this might have appeared to solve the hospital problem in Washington, there was continued opposition by the medical community because the facility was "under the exclusive control of the medical faculty of Columbian College," and later access "to the facility was not open to members of the other school," specifically the Georgetown College School of Medicine established in 1851. None but members of the Columbian faculty could "send a private patient and retain management of their care."

At the outbreak of the Civil War, the War Department took over the Infirmary as a military hospital. On November 3, 1861, the infirmary building was destroyed by fire.[86]

Legislation establishing the Washington Infirmary included the phrase "medical instruction and for scientific purposes." No doubt "scientific purposes" could be interpreted as meaning dissection. Ironically, it could be argued that by acquiring the infirmary and exclusivity the medical school had obtained its own hospital, an institution that in America had not previously been tainted with the stigma of body-snatching riots.

Body Snatching in the City of Washington Supplying the Doctors in the Columbian College Medical Department

Some of these transient paupers and strangers likely ended up on the dissecting tables of these eminent professors in charge of the infirmary if their bodies were unclaimed by friends or relatives. Additionally, there is evidence that body snatching was going on in the District in support of the activities of the doctors at the Columbian College Medical Department at the Washington Infirmary initially under the authority of Dr. Thomas Sewall. With the addition of new medical schools in Washington, the Georgetown medical school, and the Howard University Medical School (1869), the demand for the services of body snatchers increased well into the 1890s.[87]

Dr. Llewellin Eliot wrote that his father was a body snatcher, a demonstrator, and afterward a professor of anatomy. In 1844 he worked under Dr. Thomas Miller, professor of anatomy in the Columbian College Medical Department, and continued until 1849, when he became professor of anatomy in the Georgetown medical school. As we saw, Dr. Miller was one of the signers of the bond to establish the Washington Infirmary in what had been the old jail. Dr. Sewall was the chief administrator until his death in April 1845. There is little doubt that those doing the body snatching (early on they were probably doctors and medical students) were experienced at grave robbing, and this had probably been occurring from the school's inception under Sewall's leadership. Elliot proudly related the following anecdote:

> When the Columbian Medical College was located in the old jail, the Demonstrator gently and quietly and carefully lifted the body of a brother Mason from its final resting place, and promptly entered it in the student class of anatomy. In some manner suspicion was aroused; the Lodge ordered an investigation. The grave was reopened; the committee found the clothing and other belongings in the coffin, but the brother had left for parts unknown. The chairman of the committee visited the Demonstrator and requested permission to make a search of the college; this permission was freely granted. Immediately afterwards the Demonstrator

> hurried to the college, had a section of the flooring taken up, the body placed, and the flooring replaced. The committee arrived; they were assured most positively that they would not find the body; they searched into every place but failed to find the body. They left, the flooring was again removed, and the body carried to the dissecting table.[88]

This tale suggests even brother masons (who likely took an oath to protect each other) were not off limits to the doctors at the Columbian College Medical Department. The story confirms the location where the body was received, formerly the old jail and now the new infirmary where the Columbian medical faculty were located, and body snatching was done by students and staff at the newly opened infirmary under the authority of Dr. Thomas Sewall. The culprits were well versed in the art of obtaining illegal corpses and sequestering bodies so they could not be found if the facility was searched. Once the authorities left, the culprits returned immediately to the business at hand. This cold professionalism suggests to me that these doctors and their students had a long history of body snatching. Most likely even with the patients at the infirmary there were simply not enough of those who died without friends or relatives to meet the demands of the doctors for dissection.

In 1861 Dr. Miller became professor of anatomy in the Georgetown medical school and was soon transferred to the chair of surgery. Here we have evidence that the medical school at Georgetown College was also engaged early on in body snatching, as the following account shows. "Although the duties of bodysnatching were given to another [Dr. Miller] remained the friend and protector of the legitimate body snatcher until his death."[89]

Dr. Sewall's Death

Unfortunately for Dr. Sewall, following the acquisition of the infirmary for the school, "at 1 o'clock on Thursday morning, April 10th, [1845] at his residence" in Washington, "after an illness of three weeks duration, in the fifty-ninth year of his age, Thomas Sewall, M.D. succumbed … to an inflammation of the lungs and stomach." However, most authorities subscribe his death simply to his twenty-year battle with "consumption."[90] His obituary is laudatory, and there is no mention of his earlier conviction of "grave robbing." The writer mentions Sewall's move from Essex, Massachusetts, to Washington in 1820, as well as his "lucrative practice" and his appointment as a member of the medical faculty of Columbian College. Highlights included his *Tract on Temperance* and *Essays on Phrenology*, both of which enjoyed wide circulation. "He never allowed his judgment to yield to the fascination of theories or to the authority of systems … yet his constitution was feeble; several of his organs were chronically disordered and for the last twenty years of his life he was fighting off the fatal consumption."

Ironically, based on his profession and dark past, in 1828 Sewall joined the Methodist Episcopal Church and became a Methodist minister. "In the discharge of his duties as an officer of that Church he was scrupulously regular. It was his rule to attend public worship twice on every Sunday, however exacting might be his professional engagements."

Sewall's found faith must have been galling for those who read his obituary and had their family members missing from their graves in Essex, Massachusetts. The following lines must have been especially upsetting: "The faith which he professed was his guide through life and his consolation in death. From an early period of his malady, he despaired of recovery; but that despair of life here was brightened by the hope of life hereafter and by his lively but humble trust in the promises of the Gospel."

Based on the current beliefs of the time, the resurrection of the body was a core belief, and for someone who had created such sacrilegious acts in his training and early practice and supported body snatching throughout his professional career in Washington, this suggests to me an intense feeling of shame that he attempted to assuage through intense religious devotion, and he perhaps saw his "malady" as punishment that had to be overcome through the latter.

Throughout Sewall's life, his "natural benevolence ... expanded and regulated by the precepts of Christianity, showed itself in the extent of his charities and in his zealous agency in the philanthropic enterprises distinguishing the age in which he lived. To the cause of missions foreign and domestic, he contributed liberally his means and counsels." For example, in 1834 he was "elected a manager" of the American Colonization Society; "the legitimate objects of the society" were seen "as the source of incalculable advantages, moral and political, to both the white and black races."[91]

In addition to the care Sewall sought for his patients and other personal merits described in the obituary, he was also "the personal physician of three presidents of the United States."[92]

With all Sewall had done for Washington, his death did have a profound effect on the community. Besides the members of the medical profession, medical students, the faculty of Columbian College, and the Medical Society of the District of Columbia, "public grief was attested by the mourning multitude, which followed the corpse to the grave. The funeral took place at half past three o'clock on Friday afternoon, 11th April, from the Wesleyan Chapel, where the religious ceremonies were performed and an appropriate and impressive address was made by the Reverend Norval Wilson; after which, the remains were conveyed to the Methodist Episcopal burying ground. The number of persons present is supposed to have been greater than on any previous occasion, in Washington."[93]

Dr. Thomas Sewall did not leave his body to be dissected by his colleagues, nor do we know if he made any arrangements to prevent it from being stolen by body snatchers. However, Dr. Sewall was later buried with his wife, Mary Choate Sewall, in Washington's Oak Hill Cemetery.[94] This cemetery opened as a new "Rural Cemetery" in 1849 as part of the progressive cemetery movement, "intentionally designed, and formally laid out ... secular[,] ... meant to be a peaceful respite ... [with] meticulously designed landscape with meandering roads and foot paths ... [and] elegant monuments and thoughtfully arranged vistas."[95] In a supreme irony, when the philanthropist William H. Corcoran gave ten acres to establish the Oak Hill Cemetery, he became the corporation's president. He imposed an "iron-clad regulation ... that every grave should be bricked in and cemented on all sides and at the top." He did not want any "resurrection scandals so frequent in the District" to be attached to the Oak Hill Cemetery.[96]

This was a true disparity compared to the run-down and ill-served cemeteries found in Washington and exploited by the grave robbers in Washington, D.C., well into the latter part of the nineteenth century.

This also contrasts with an observation made in 1871 by a visitor to the Washington Asylum burial grounds, who observed that "amongst the graves of the Almshouse dead ... we felt the sobering melancholy of the spot." The burial grounds were "scattered about with little stones and mounds … a dead-cart and a spade sticking up as symbols and the neglected river, deserted as the Styx[;] … we felt the sobering melancholy of the spot."[97]

Dr. Sewall's Mixed Legacy in Washington, D.C.

With Dr. Sewall's arrival in Washington and the opening of the Columbian College Medical Department the need for cadavers to meet the demands of the faculty and students for the anatomy classes was initiated. There is little mention of the business of grave robbing in Washington, likely because at first there was no competition for bodies and only the faculty, students, and staff engaged in the practice. In some respects, the stealing of cadavers may have been an open secret in Washington when there was only one medical school, and there were many in the community who sympathized with the need if these doctors were to be trained properly. However, with the establishment of a second medical school at Georgetown in 1851, the competition for bodies intensified and is illustrated by the following event that occurred prior to 1859. "A man had died of some peculiar disease; both medical colleges wanted the body, and the Superintendent of Washington Asylum knew it." To protect the corpse, he "had the body brought from the dead house and placed in his back office." The "dead house was a secure place, with windows barred, door locked and chained, almost impossible of burglarious entrance; the body would have been safe there."

After dark the superintendent was visited by two students, and as the evening progressed more guests showed up. The party finally broke up at midnight. While the superintendent was entertaining his guests, the body in the dead room "was lowered from the window into the arms of waiting students and carried away."[98]

The Unforgotten

The man whose conscience feels no wound
Is not alarm'd to hear the sound
Of Satan's jarring strings.[99]

While Dr. Sewall was praised in Washington for his contribution to medicine, his "sin," betraying his family, friends, and patients in the small community of Chebacco, Massachusetts, had not been forgotten. The town historian Duane Hamilton Hurd wrote that when he came to live among the people of Essex twenty-two years after the event, there was still a "pungency and acerbity" in every occasioned allusion to it by the majority of the adult population, "who freshly remembered the circumstances."

What occurred, the "tradition of it, more or less minute in detail, has been and is continuously transmitted from one generation to another of the resident population of the town and its vicinity."[100]

In the 1930s Maidee P. Polleys, a member of the Essex Historical Society, presented an undated paper titled "Robbed the Graveyard." Polleys was born in Essex in 1873 and grew up among townspeople who had memories or were the children of those affected by the grave-robbing event. To outsiders, "Yes. 'A great scientist!' learned beyond his day!' but to the people of the little Chebacco village branded as an unfeeling monster."

She knew whereof she spoke and referred with authority to eyewitness sources and the event's continuing effect on the town. "So, the queer gruesome story has come down to us whose forefathers lived in the little town and who remembered the far-off day … when again came the citizens gathered in the old burying ground for a funeral service over empty caskets which were buried in one grave near the entrance."[101]

The event is still remembered, and in the "Old Burying Ground" in Essex (established in 1680) stands the "Hearse House," and under it is said to be buried the empty coffins memorialized in Reverend Crowell's July 23, 1818, sermon.

9

The Diary of a Body Snatcher in the District of Columbia

Medical education in America in 1860 had not improved much since 1830. Admittedly, there were some basic standards, low as they were, but the "great majority of medical students in America had no legal systematic hospital teaching and little or no legal access to cadavers." Specialization was rare, and most American physicians were general practitioners.[1]

The American Civil War influenced improvement in the areas of medicine and surgery. Medicine went through a period of rapid growth, especially anatomy. Now, for the first time, physicians who had little or no experience with cadavers in the past had access to "thousands of bodies created by the war," leading to new educational opportunities. Now, pathology in medical care "promised intellectual vitality, professional legitimacy and perhaps superior medical care."[2]

The experiences by practitioners during the Civil War led to progress in the teaching of "anatomy and operative surgery on the cadaver." The demand for cadavers in post–Civil War instruction in medical schools was brisk throughout the country.[3] As late as the 1880s and 1890s, the anatomy laws were not entirely effective. Northern schools participated in this "far-flung, interstate business. Southern body snatchers, for instance, regularly shipped the bodies of Southern blacks to Northern medical schools."[4]

The Diary Exposed

Immediately following the Civil War, the business of body snatching increased dramatically in Washington, D.C. Strangely, with the high demand for cadavers for teaching, there was no strong impetus from the public in D.C. to implement an anatomy law. Washington cemeteries, white, Black, and mixed (though carefully divided by race), became sources for the three medical schools in Washington, D.C. (the Howard University Medical School was founded in 1869) and medical schools in the South and Midwest. There is much evidence that medical schools in Washington did business with these new grave-robbing professionals, the "resurrection men."[5]

As one observer noted, "The history of the District of Columbia is in this respect a truly disgraceful one.... We have had the demoralizing spectacle of some five hundred students among several schools, almost under the shadow of the Capitol, dissecting bodies that everyone knew had been illegally obtained. Washington, especially at the close of the war and for some years after, was a great field ... for these resurrection men."[6]

Not only had "the professional body-snatcher flourished, but a new figure [had] arisen,—the dealer in human bodies, who, procuring corpses, either by theft or by corruption, [was] able to distribute them at a high rate of payment to colleges throughout the country. Sometimes the same man ... combined the two professions." These men "did a large business in several States."[7]

One of the most prominent men of this description was George Christian, arrested for body snatching in December 1873. Remarkably, he had been keeping a diary of his grave-robbing activities, and it was found on him when he was apprehended.

Christian was a clerk in the surgeon general's office and operated his grave-robbing and corpse-shipping business out of that office. "He associated himself with a bad gang—Percy Brown and his sister Maude; 'Workhouse' Kate and Margaret Harrison." This gang "did a big and profitable business ... that included a shanty, where they ... accumulated a great quantity of clothing, shrouds, and other graveyard things." Christian moved their storage facility to a local medical college, and there "Christian

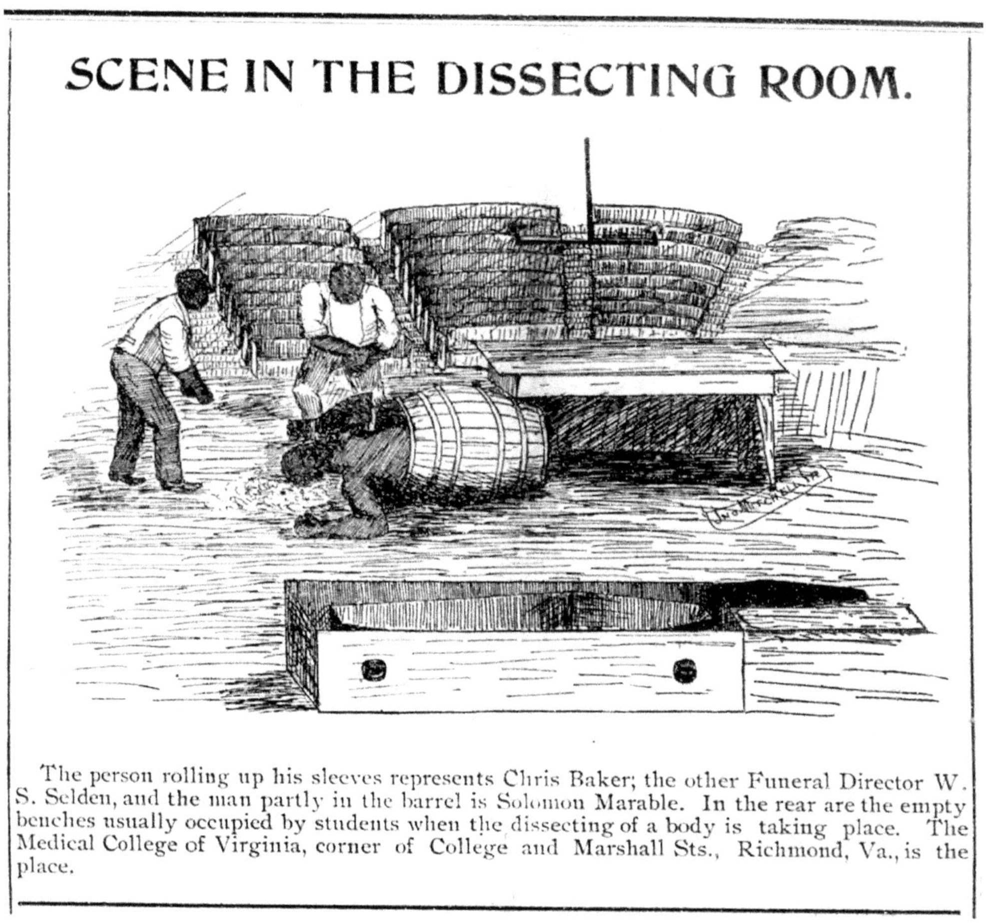

"Christian would inject and pack the bodies in whiskey barrels and ... roll these barrels up in front of the Army Medical Museum, where the express company would call for them." We see the final stage of the shipping process, the barrels containing the bodies as well as a body half out of a barrel on the dissecting floor to be made ready for dissection. "Scene in the Dissecting Room," ***Richmond Planet*****, August 1, 1896, 1, Richmond, Virginia.**

would inject and pack the bodies in whiskey barrels and ... roll these barrels up in front of the Army Medical Museum, where the express company would call for them; Christian was always on hand to pay charges and direct the shipments; in this way the company did not suspect the fraud. The price of bodies fluctuated with the demand and the weather. When the demand was great it was a common thing to charge one hundred dollars for a good subject; when the market became glutted the average price was forty dollars."

Christian was described as "a man of medium build, athletic ... [and] a good worker in the cause; his hair and beard were black. His clothing was always that taken from the grave; he, therefore, was usually well dressed. His frequent raids and his sullenness when drinking were the causes of his undoing."[8]

The Washington newspaper the *Evening Star* gave a full account of the arrest of George Christian and two of his accomplices. It is of interest for the detail it provides of the arrest and prosecution of this "resurrectionist" and for what is generally not mentioned in a description of this event, the reaction of people who felt their loved ones may have been victims of this ring. Note that the crowd is described as both white and Black. In the diary found on Christian, most of the burial grounds he and his gang robbed were Black burial grounds.

Arrest and Trial Reports

The report of the arrest and trial of George Christian and his colleagues reads as follows:

> **Arrest of Alleged Body Snatchers**
>
> The attention of the officers of the 4th precinct (Lieut. Greer) was attracted last night by a horse and buggy standing for a long time near the circle at 22nd Street, with a woman in the vehicle. The officers kept their eyes upon the vehicle until after midnight, when one of them approached it and inquired of the woman the occasion of her being there so long, when she said she was waiting for her husband who was in a house near by engaged in transacting some business.
>
> **Two Men With Shovels**
>
> This was accepted as a satisfactory explanation, but watch was kept on the horse and buggy and later in the night a man was seen to approach the team, holding in his hand a shovel, which he placed in the vehicle. Soon afterwards another man come from the same direction as the first; also with a shovel, and when the men were seated in the buggy, they all drove off in the direction of New Hampshire Avenue which thoroughfare they followed out towards Boundary Street. The officer suspecting that they were conveying stolen goods or engaged in some way with thieves arrested them while they were crossing 20th street and drove the buggy with all it contained to the station-house on K street, and conducted the two men (one white and one colored) and the woman (white) into a private room, when they were questioned but returned evasive answers.
>
> **A Graveyard Kit**
>
> In the buggy were two shovels which had the appearance of having been recently used, about a half dozen large strong bags, a bottle of liquid, a syringe, and a ball of string twine. It occurred to the officers that from the kit found these persons might be engaged in grave robbing, and Sergeant Kneass with Officers McGlue and Hawkins started to visit the graveyards. There was also a screw-driver in the buggy.

A Dead Body In A Sack

On taking a circuit of Holmead's burying ground they discovered on the 19th-street side, by the fence a large bag and on closer inspection found that it contained the dead body of Thomas Fletcher, colored, who was buried yesterday from his late residence on L street. The body was doubled up in order to get it into the sack, with the head and hands at the mouth of the same, and on each end of the bag were fixed strong hand holds, for the purpose of carrying it with more ease. Leaving one of the officers in charge, the sergeant stationed the other officer at a distance, to see if any party or parties should take the body away, while they returned to the station house and telegraphed to lieut. Noonan, of the second precinct, to send his men to take charge of the body it being in his precinct.

The White Man [sic]

who was arrested gave his name as Dr. George C. Archer. He was searched, and a six-barrel revolver, loaded, found in his pocket, together with papers and a memorandum book, from which it would appear that his right name is George A. Christiana [*sic*], formerly a clerk in the Surgeon General's office, now residing on Capitol Hill, and that he has been carrying on an EXTENSIVE BUSINESS AS A BODY SNATCHER for some time, the dates showing his transactions with several medical institutions in Cleveland, Ohio, Virginia, and the District, to which he has sent bodies for about six months, and during that time he must have sent away several hundred bodies. A recent order from an institution in Virginia directs him to pack two bodies in whiskey barrels tight and use sawdust for packing. One from Cleveland tells him to use strong boxes instead of barrels, as the barrelheads get loose, and might occasion suspicion, one memorandum shows that he went to Potter's Field for Henry Young's body [who was recently hanged], and was disappointed by digging up the body of a women instead of Young's. The book shows that he has taken bodies from the graves in almost every cemetery, Holmead's, Mount Zion [Black], Potter's Field, and Young Mens Benevolent Association Cemetery [probably Young Mens Baptist Cemetery, a Black cemetery] burial grounds being frequently noted and that the University of Virginia and other medical departments have been customers of his [including of course the three medical schools in Washington, D.C.].

Christiana's [*sic*] diary contains notes for every day in this year from January to December 8th, from which it appears he has been attending medical lectures, but no mention is made of the subject until August last then there is a reference to the body of Beau Hickman. On the date of Monday, Dec'r 1st, it is stated—"visited Potter's Field shipped two subjects in whiskey barrels to Virginia; Dec'r 4th,—visited Holmead's and Young Men's grounds and failed"; Dec'r 6th, "visited Ebenezer," [another Black cemetery] Kate and I, got a subject; Dec'r 7th, "went to Mt. Zion and got a subject"; Dec'r 5th, "visited Holmead's" and "Young Men's grounds and failed." Under the date of Tuesday September 9 is written: "Dr. and I went out this evening and succeeded in getting (illegible) Beau. It was a lovely moonlight night, and everything went off lovely." Under the date of September 10th, the excitement caused by the discovery of Beau's body having been tampered with is referred to and he states, "I have found no one who suspicions who did it." In some of the entries is mentioned, "I paid [blank] his share" and in one or two "went to [blank] and returned the keys."

The Price For Dead Bodies

A correspondence show[s] that the price demanded by him [$40 per corpse] was considered too much by some of his customers, who thought $30 ought to be enough to satisfy him. In his pocket was also found a card of membership in the Young Men's Christian Association. The woman who was with him is young and keen looking and gives her name as Margaret Harrison. The colored man, who is doubtless hired by Christiana, is a young man, slender built, with dark hair and complexion, and it is said has a wife and children living in this city. He gives his name as Charles Green. They are all in custody at police headquarters.

EXCITING SCENES AT THE POLICE STATION

This morning early the station house was besieged with many persons who were much excited, and later this morning some four or five hundred colored and white people were in front of the doors and had to be driven away by the police. All the prisoners are at headquarters awaiting an investigation by the proper authorities, but what form the investigation will take is not yet determined upon. It is understood that as there is no local law covering the case the old Maryland laws will probably be brought into requisition.[9]

Night Doctors

The hysteria generated by the arrest of these body snatchers, likely at the station, was part of a groundswell in the belief that not only were the graves of "colored folks" robbed in larger proportion than white folks but also in stories of the "night doctors" who prowled the Washington streets. For example, the *Evening Star* on January 15, 1872, published an article titled "'Night Doctors' A Curious Superstition among Some Colored People How They Think Castor Oil Is Made." Although the night doctors mentioned here were after the living to deliver them to the dissecting table, for some they served as material to supply doctors in other cities, and these folk tales undoubtedly contributed to the general hysteria.

> According to popular report among the class referred to, these "night doctors" perambulate the streets in pairs about midnight, and between that time and daybreak searching for victims for the dissecting room. Armed with adhesive plasters piaster, they are believed to lie in wait for "subjects" in dark alleys, from which they stealthily but quickly emerge when a colored person of suitable proportions passes. Advancing with muffled steps behind unsuspecting victims one of these terrible "night doctors" reaches his hand over the shoulder of the colored man or woman, and dexterously claps the adhesive plaster over his or her mouth. In order to prevent any outcry, the confederate quickly ties the arms with a cord, with which he is prepared.

Once in the hands of the night doctors,

> the poor victim is placed in a covered carriage in waiting nearby, and carried to the dissecting room, where he or she is chloroformed into insensibility, and then BLED TO DEATH by the heartless students. The dissection of the body then follows, after which the fatty parts of the body are "tried" in caldrons, for the purpose of obtaining the oil, which ... afterwards appears at the drug stores in the form of castor oil. So firmly are many of the colored people impressed with this belief that they venture on the streets after nightfall with fear and trembling and take to their heels whenever they notice anything suspicious in the movement of the passers-by. Of late they assert that the number of colored people that have disappeared is much larger than usual, and they are convinced that the doctors of Washington are not only supplying the dissecting rooms of the city with subjects but are furnishing "castor oil" manufactured from colored adipose matter to the large cities throughout the country.

The following example given in the report states the real problem, that there is no law against body snatching in Washington, so it is difficult to obtain redress. However, if the stories were true, certainly the charge would be murder.

> A solitary horseman was seen on the Island by some colored people, with a body thrown across the horse in front of him and some colored persons who saw him imagined, from the limberness of the corpse, that it was some poor fellow, with his mouth effectually sealed with a sticking plaster, on his way to the dissecting room, there to be hacked into mincemeat, or to

be boxed for export to some other city. There who saw him were afraid to tackle the man but notified the police. There being no law against body snatching in force, and no way to reach the offender, no action could be taken.

Finally, the report singles out one type of body in demand, humpbacks who were "especially desirable on account of their peculiar physical conformation, which renders their dissection of particular interest to medical students. Indeed, it is reported that as high as $150 each [a significant sum] for first-class hump-backed subjects is offered by the night doctors."[10]

The fear of night doctors and body snatchers turning to the living to acquire cadavers for medical schools was exacerbated in December 1886 when newspapers began to report on the murder of Emily Brown with headlines such as "Burking in Baltimore: Old Woman Killed for Her Body." The report explained the origin of the term "burking" and noted that it was rare, which made the crime "all the more startling."[11]

Multiple newspapers reported the story. Emily Brown (white), once a respectable woman, had fallen on hard times and had taken up residence in cheap lodgings in the Black section of Baltimore with a Black family in the home of Mary Blockson, which included her stepson John Thomas Ross, Sarah Blockson and her eleven-year-old daughter, and Anderson Perry, a janitor at the University of Maryland School of Medicine. Emily was generally "under the influence of drugs and liquor." She obtained funds by begging. She drank most of her income and fell behind in her rent. Perry saw Emily as a "salable corpse" and convinced Ross that her body could be sold for dissection.[12] One evening John Thomas Ross arrived at the medical school "with a body, warm, still bloody, and fully clothed." The death being suspicious, information was given to the authorities by the doctors involved. Alexander Perry was questioned, confessed and implicated Ross and another fellow, Albert Hawkins.[13] Perry was charged with suggesting the murder of Emily Brown "for the purpose of selling her body for dissection."[14] The jury charged Ross and Hawkins with inflicting wounds on her skull "and by incised wounds of the thorax, penetrating the heart." Of the three men tried, only Ross was convicted of first-degree murder and was hanged on September 9, 1887.[15]

The *Evening Star* concluded its report, stating that "the greatest excitement exists among the negroes in the thickly populated section in which the woman was murdered. Some of these people declared Perry had frequently boasted of the number of people he had assisted in disposing of. An old woman named Mary Nantze, who lives in the neighborhood[,] had been missing for a week, which fact added to the excitement."[16]

Undoubtedly, for many people this story, even in Washington where it was reported as well, added to their paranoia and confirmed their worst fears that body snatchers were murdering the living for dissection in medical schools.

The Arraignment and Trial of George Christian

The *Evening Star* reported that on December 13, 1873, George A. Christian, Charles Green, and Margaret Harrison took up dead bodies from burial grounds in Washington "for the purpose of disposing of them for gain, against the peace."

The Arraignment

[T]he judge fixed the amount [of bond] at $1,000 each, but after waiting sometime for their friends, about 4 o'clock the Marshal of the Police Court accompanied them to jail for a hearing. The woman seemed to be considerable affected, and on the way over there Christian remarked that she was innocent however guilty he might be. Charles Green, the colored man, was silent and seemed quite indifferent. The officers stated this morning that it is ascertained that the duty assigned this female was to attend all funerals as a mourner for the purpose of locating the graves and to take note of the general surroundings in order to facilitate the active partner in his night operations.

The paper noted the "Remarkable Diary" found on Christian and that it was a "Singular History of the Grave Robbing Business":

> In our report of this startling case on Saturday it was stated that the diary found on Christian contained a large number of entries, showing the wholesale extent to which he had carried on his business of robbing graves for the dissector schools[;] it seems by this diary and the letters accompanying it that Christian, under various aliases, was in correspondence with medical schools all over the country for the supply of cadavers or corpses, and that he had made very complete arrangements with parties in this city to post him and give personal aid, with a division of the proceeds of the business.[17]

The diary began on January 1, 1873, and the last entry published by the newspaper was December 8, 1873. Included with the newspaper's published account (some names were censored) were two letters and Christian's membership card in the Young Men's Christian Association. Unfortunately, the diary has been lost, and we only have available to us what was printed in the *Washington Evening Star* on December 15, 1873.

The district attorney charged Christian with robbing burial grounds of dead bodies and "disposing of them to medical colleges in different places throughout the country. Dr. George A. Otis recommended Christian's immediate dishonorable discharge from Government service. This was approved and Christian was out of two jobs."

The diary contained "incriminating evidence and was turned over to the Chief of Police and given to one of his Surgeons; it was censored, and portions were given out for publication in the city papers. Many names of those who had been out with Christian were, for good and sufficient reasons, omitted."[18]

The First Trial

On December 17, 1873, the *Evening Star* reported on the trial in the Police Court primarily of George Christian, accused of stealing the bodies of A.C. H. Webster from the Congressional Cemetery on October 29, 1873, and Thomas Fletcher from the Holmead cemetery on December 13, 1873. Christian's lawyer was planning to plead that the "acts were committed ...in the interests of science" but decided on not guilty. Christian's diary was key for the prosecutor. After some objection the diary was admitted as evidence and two officials from the Surgeon General's Office verified the diary was in Christian's handwriting. The prosecutor read from the diary October 29th, "Attended a funeral at Congressional cemetery to-day and brought the subject into Georgetown College to-night."

The next case concerning Thomas Fletcher was argued with eyewitness testimony from the officers involved as well as the sextant at the Holmead cemetery. The cases were remanded to the next day, when Christian was convicted and sentenced by the judge on December 18th to a one year in jail and a fine of $1,000. Margaret Harrison was not charged and Charles Green was returned to jail.[19]

George A. Christian's Diary

For our purposes I will give an account of Christian's general business activities and entries in his diary showing his involvement with the Washington medical schools (censored in the diary), his collaborators in the "ghastly business," and his shipment of corpses beyond Washington.[20]

The newspaper reported that "the diary which is in cool business form" begins with January 1, 1873, and the first entry relating to body snatching is as follows:

> January 3d.—1873 B. and C. went out and got two cadavers to-night.
> April 4th Dr. C and I went to the Washington Asylum Cemetery to-night and confiscated two sets of extremities and one head.
> Saturday 5th—There was quite a little excitement in this morning's market about our little adventure last night, many believing that another murder had been committed. No one suspected us.
> Sunday. April 8th—Went out to Washington asylum this morning, and went through the institution with Dailey, who has been appointed resident student.
> Tuesday, June 3d.—Called on Dr. _____ to see about getting some tickets to Tom Wright's execution. Did not succeed.
> Thursday, 5th—Received a pass from Dr. _____ for the execution.
> Friday, June 6th—Went to see Thos. Wright hung to-day. Everything went off smoothly, and he died by strangulation.
> June 29th.—Sunday.—Went out to the Washington asylum this morning to see Dailey. He showed me around the hospital, and I stayed to dinner with him. Rode home with Dr. Schleimer.

Christian's diary was censored by the press or at least before the details were given to the *Evening Star*. Generally, the names of many doctors and the medical schools where bodies were delivered for dissection were censored. However, there is enough information given to assess Christian's operation and who he was directly involved with. In these first lines from the diary, we see the importance of the Washington Asylum (also referred to as the almshouse) as a base of operations and the exploitation of the burying ground there.[21]

The Washington Asylum in the early 1870s was a combination of a poor house, a hospital, and a jail for criminals. As one writer who visited the Washington Asylum in 1870–1871 wrote, "We passed through a part of the building where, amongst old, toothless women, semi-imbecile girls—the relicts of error, the heirs of affliction—three babies of one mother were in [the] charge of a strong, rosy Irish nurse." In addition, "a few yards off, though out of hearing, were the thick forms of criminals, drunkards, wantons, and vagrants, seen through the iron bars of their wickets.... The association of the poor and the wicked affected us painfully." For the hospital portion he described its "syphilitic wards, where, in the awful contemplation of their daily, piecemeal decay, the silent victims were stretched all day upon their cots; amongst the idiotic and the crazed; into the apartments of the aged poor." As for the burying ground, "we stood at last amongst the graves of the Almshouse dead—those who have escaped the dissecting knife." Clearly not so![22]

Of the officials mentioned in these first few lines of the diary, Dr. David Schleimer is the most important for our purposes, as he appears throughout and seems to be George Christian's partner. Schleimer is one of a group of doctors who were all connected with the Georgetown medical school in the body-snatching business at the Washington Asylum. He is reported as a resident medical student at the Washington Asylum on February 1, 1873. He received his MD from Georgetown College on March 6, 1873, and his specialty was smallpox.[23]

Daily is likely B.E. Daily, who received his medical degree from Georgetown in 1874 and appears to have taken over as the resident medical student after Schleimer received his medical degree in early 1873.[24]

Doctor C, who is noted as being involved in body snatching, is most likely Moses Cooper, who in 1874 was a physician at the Washington Asylum and received his MD degree from Georgetown College in 1874.[25]

On Thomas Wright and his hanging, the following was reported in the *New York Times* on December 28, 1872. The "colored desperado" was arrested on December 25 and charged with the murder of Samuel Rogerski, "whose dead body was found in an alley horribly mangled." The *Chicago Daily Tribune* reported on June 6 that "Thomas Wright was hanged to-day in the jail-yard for the murder of Rogerski.... At 10 minutes past 12 the drop fell. Life was not extinct until a lapse of 17 minutes. His neck was not broken, the man being choked to death." (This confirms Christian's report of strangulation.)

There was great interest in Wright's execution, and the crowds explain why it was difficult to get a ticket. "There were about 500 persons in the jail-yard, and several thousand outside, many of them on the house-tops and other high points, where they could have a full view of the execution."[26] Christian did not indicate that he had tried to obtain Wright's body; however, Wright was suspicious that he might be the victim of body snatchers and earlier asked to see the sexton of the Mount Olivet cemetery (Catholic, founded in 1858). He informed the sexton that he would like his body placed in the vault and that "no doctors should get it, and being thus assured he expressed his thanks to him, as also to his friends for what they had done for him. He thought that the doctors might want his body to see how his neck cracked, which seemed to bother him a great deal."[27]

Beau Hickman's Body.

Sept. 2—Dr _____ and I went out prospecting this evening, and succeeded in getting (characters in cipher), referring evidently to the body of Beau Hickman. It was a lovely moonlight night, and everything went off smoothly.

Sept. 3rd—There was a great hue and cry in all the daily papers today about the grave of Beau Hickman being robbed last night. Have not seen any one who seemed to know who did it.

"Beau Hickman" as noted in the diary was more than a local celebrity. He had come to Washington as a young man with an inheritance that he promptly squandered. Over the years he became well known to visitors to Washington as well as statesmen and politicians, so much so that his death was reported in newspapers across the United States. He was basically an honest grifter whose personality and storytelling skills helped him secure an income. As a guide, he also earned money by taking visitors to the local gambling dens and brothels. Overall, he was viewed as peculiar, harmless, and entertaining.[28]

On his death, Hickman had no money. A local undertaker provided a plain coffin. Hickman's remains were taken to the burial ground attached to the Almshouse (the Washington Asylum's Potter's Field).[29]

According to Christian "everything went off smoothly" but, based on the following account, perhaps not as smoothly as he had bragged in his diary.

The following report concerning Hickman's body appeared in the *Alexandria Gazette* on September 4, 1873. Learning of Beau's death, Mr. Dorsey Clagett and John Langley wanted to give him a Christian burial and started "a subscription list" for that purpose. Funds were raised,

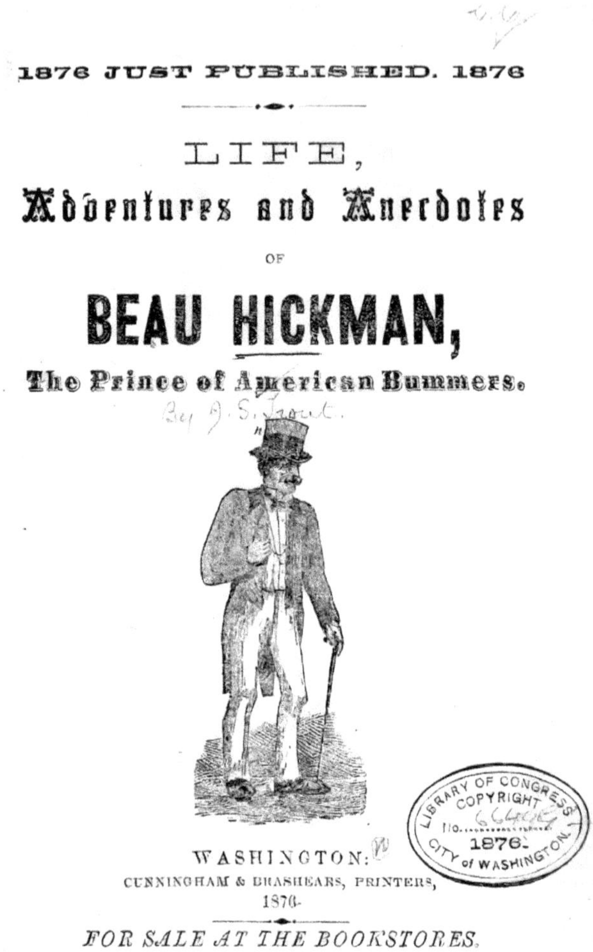
1876 JUST PUBLISHED. 1876

LIFE,

Adventures and Anecdotes

OF

BEAU HICKMAN,

The Prince of American Bummers.

WASHINGTON:

CUNNINGHAM & BRASHEARS, PRINTERS,

1876.

FOR SALE AT THE BOOKSTORES.

"Beau Hickman." James S. Trout, *The Life, Adventures and Anecdotes of Beau Hickman, the Prince of American Bummers*(1876) (Library of Congress).

> The services of an undertaker were secured, and about 2 o'clock yesterday afternoon, he proceeded to the Potter's field and was pointed out the grave of the late Beau Hickman by a colored man, who originally dug it.
>
> After a few spades full of earth had been thrown up a suit of clothes was unearthed, which was recognized by the first gravedigger as those belonging to the body of Hickman. Proceeding with the excavation the box containing the body was finally reached. The top was found to be shattered to pieces, while the sides hung together by mere splints. In this condition it was withdrawn from the grave, and on the removal of the lid the body presented a most horrid spectacle. The arms had been removed at the shoulder joints, the legs amputated at the hip joints and the head cut off, all of which had been carried away. The head had been skinged [skinned] and done by so skillful a hand as to leave the features of the face recognizable. The breast had also been opened and the heart removed, but so speedy was the departure of the perpetrators that they dropped it, and it was found about fifteen feet from the grave. Beside a grave near the one where the remains rested, was found a surgeon's knife, by which the operators performed their butchery, which was left behind in their hurried departure. The trunk and skin of the face of the deceased were replaced in another box and removed to the congressional vault [Congressional Cemetery vault] by the undertaker, where they will remain until interred. It is supposed that the resurrecting of the body was the work of medical students,

> but it is believed from the skilful manner in which the face was skinned that a professional surgeon had a hand in the job. The whole affair is deserving of the strongest censure from the entire community and those that would thus willfully and unchristianly descrate [*sic*] a body deserve and should be brought to punishment.[30]

In addition, the desecration of Beau Hickman's body raised fears among Black Washingtonians of the "resurrectionists ... and many dared not venture out after dark for fear of night doctors ... [who] ... would grab them before the undertaker had wrapped them in funeral robes."[31]

The report on the diary continued:

A RESURRECTION FIRM ESTABLISHED.

Sept. 10—Dr. Schlimer [*sic*] called at the house for me this afternoon, and I rode out to the asylum with him. We talked about resurrecting next winter, and partly promised to go in together.

Sept. 11—Called to see Dr. _____ at his office this morning in regard to furnishing material to his class for dissection. Dr. Schlimer called on me at the office to-day. We agreed to divide, giving him 8–15.

Sept. 12—Called to see Drs. _____ and _____ in regard to furnishing material for dissecting. They were both agreed.

Sept. 18—Called on Dr. _____ this morning, and he promised to let Dr. Schlimer, and I furnish his college with material this winter at $15 each—we to inject and remove it.

According to Christian, Dr. Schleimer was a partner and let his customers know that the doctor was a partner. Note that the names of the colleges are censored. We learn the local price of cadavers, and part of their agreement is to remove the bodies and/or cadaver parts from the dissecting rooms likely so that the customers would not get caught with ill-gotten remains.

THE DOCTOR'S RESURRECTION MONEY COMES TO GRIEF.

Friday, Sept. 19—Jay Cooke and Co. suspended yesterday, and I was unfortunate enough to have some money in their hands. Went up to see about it today but everything is closed, and no information can be had.

Sept 20—Went out to the asylum this afternoon and staid [*sic*] until after dark with Dr. Schlimer. There was a cadaver on hand, but we could not get it. Went down town in the evening.

Sunday 21—Went out to the Washington asylum early this morning and staid to dinner. Dr. Schlimer drove me around after dinner. We got a subject this evening.

Sept. 22—Staid at asylum last night with Dr. Schlimer and took breakfast there. Went to college this morning and injected our subject. Went out to the asylum in Dr. S. place to-night.

Sept. 30—Got a permit from the Board of Health to-day to bury the material from the dissecting room of college. Did not go to the asylum to-night.

Christian is referring to the Jay Cooke & Co. bank when it became overextended in the building of the Northern Pacific Railway and failed. The bank had its headquarters in Philadelphia and had a branch in Washington, D.C.

Christian seems to be a regular visitor to the asylum and may have even posed as a doctor: "Went out to the asylum in Dr. S. place to-night," undoubtedly sizing up inmates near death.

It is hard to believe that the Board of Health was not aware of something going on with Christian requesting permission to bury leftover material from the dissecting rooms.

Business Of Another Kind.

Oct 4th—Miss H called to see me professionally; this afternoon I gave her Tinct. Gentian, co. zi gtt der die.
Sunday, Oct. 4—Called to see Miss H, this morning, and found her doing as well as could be expected.
Oct. 7—Miss H came to spend a week with us this morning.
Oct.—Got excused from the office for four hours today. Was sent for to come home and attend Miss H. who was suddenly taken ill. She had a miscarriage of a female child at 11 p.m.
Oct. 15—Dr. Schlimer drove to the city this evening and took a subject to the _____ College. We got in just before the close of lecture but got up quietly without being seen.
Sunday, 26th—We got a subject at Holmead's Cemetery for _____ College to-night.
Oct. 29—Attended a funeral at the Congressional Cemetery this afternoon and brought the subject in to _____ College to-night. Called to see M to-day and found her doing well.

According to Suzanne Shultz, who looked at whether Christian was also an abortionist, due to the limited information given she could not completely confirm he was an abortionist.[32]

Holmead's (old name Western Cemetery) was one of the oldest burial grounds in the District of Columbia. In 1871 a health committee recommended that the graveyard should be closed.[33] The conditions there were so bad that people were buried in plots two and a half foot deep for fear of striking water (perhaps another reason why Holmead was popular with body snatchers). The legislature did not "heed the recommendation," and again in 1874 the District of Columbia Board of Health recommended that the cemetery "be condemned without delay as a nuisance injurious to health."[34] In 1884 excavations were begun to move bodies from Holmead Cemetery. Over three thousand bodies were ultimately removed to other rural cemeteries "to make room for residential development."[35]

The Congressional Cemetery was established in 1807 and got its name because "Senators and Representatives who died in Washington in the early 1800's … as well as other dignitaries" where buried there.[36] The Congressional Cemetery was not immune from body snatching. On October 29, Christian reported his visit to the cemetery. According to one account, a man named A.C. Webster, a prominent mason of the Washington Lodge, passed away. He was reported to be a fine specimen for dissection. George Christian was a member of the same lodge and attended the funeral and "accompanied the remains to the grave." That evening he and his fellow resurrectionist, Percy Brown, visited Webster's grave. The tomb was "re-opened, and Webster's body soon lay on the grass beside it." His clothes were removed except for the "masonic regalia," which was "thrown back into the coffin." As they were about to leave with his body a noise startled the two, and "they dropped the cadaver" and took off "running until they reached the Capitol steps." Talking it over, they decided the "securing of such a choice subject was worth the risk of returning." They went back and found Webster's corpse where they had dropped it. "Before daylight Webster's body had been dissected by five of his friends."[37]

Feels Sleepy After A Busy Night.

Oct. 30.—Was out until 3:30 a.m. last night on business for the College. Felt rather sleepy to day and had a slight chill this morning.
Nov. 2. Went out to the Asylum. Took a ride out to Glenwood Cemetery and the Soldiers home. Took a cadaver into _____.

Glenwood Cemetery was established in 1854 as a rural cemetery outside the city of Washington and was modeled after the Oak Hill Cemetery.[38] The Soldiers' Home

Cemetery was founded in 1861 and consisted of five hundred beautifully laid-out acres. By 1871 there were 5,488 interments.[39] Unfortunately, even these new cemeteries were easily exploited by Christian.

A Disappointment.

Nov. 3—Dr. Schlimer and I drove out to Harmony Cemetery this afternoon. Saw some subjects in the vault and went after them tonight but could not get into the place as it was locked. Hazen went with us.

Nov. 4th—Tried to get Hazen to go with us this evening but he would not do it. Dr. Schlimer took me down town to-night but would not go anywhere.

Nov. 5—Walked out to Piney Branch Hotel this afternoon but did not find what I went for.

Mr. B. and I went out to the asylum this evening with Dr. S. and brought in a subject for N.B

Harmony Cemetery (officially Columbian Harmony Cemetery) was the successor to the original Harmoneon Cemetery, a burial ground for free Blacks. Harmony was established in 1859 and from the early 1880s to 1920 was the "most active black cemetery in Washington."[40]

Hazen was likely Dr. David Henry Hazen, who graduated from the Georgetown College School of Medicine in 1873.[41] Again, we find another member of the body-snatching ring, a recent Georgetown medical school alumnus. It appears that of all the doctors involved, Schleimer was the most active body snatcher, as described in Christian's diary.

Not So Fortunate As To Meet Another Funeral.

Nov. 9th—Sunday, Dr Schlimer and I went out riding this afternoon, hoping to see a funeral, but were not so fortunate as to meet one. I waited two hours near Ebenezer Church but did not find anything.

Out Prospecting.

Nov. 10—We went out prospecting at Rock Creek Church cemetery this afternoon but found nothing. We went to Holmead's that evening and got a subject, which we took to _____ College. Got home before twelve.

November 11—We succeeded in getting a subject at Ebenezer cemetery to-night. Boardman went out with me as Dr. Schlimer could not leave the Asylum.

It is difficult to read parts of this diary when we perceive the cold, calculating eyes of Christian and his cohorts surveying funerals looking for potential victims while family and friends are in deep mourning saying goodbye to loved ones and expecting the interred to remain in their final resting place.

The Ebenezer Church that Christian mentions was a Black church in Washington, and any burials would likely have occurred in the Ebenezer burial ground.[42] The Rock Creek Church Cemetery he visited later in the day is in Washington, D.C., It was founded in 1719 and by mid–nineteenth century was "laid out in the fashionable picturesque rural cemetery manner."[43]

Based on what we know of Holmead's cemetery, it was not unusual that Christian obtained a body that evening. The Ebenezer burial grounds were established in 1838. The conditions at the Ebenezer cemetery were not much better than at Holmead. In 1874, the District of Columbia Board of Health wrote of the Ebenezer Cemetery that "they found it in bad sanitary condition, undrained, and with graves so near one another as to crowd the locality … [and] to cause the earth to become impregnated with decayed animal matter and fetid gases that will be a source of injury to the public health." The board recommended "further interments therein be prohibited."[44]

Boardman was likely Charles Vernon Boarman, MD, another graduate of the Georgetown College of Medicine. "In 1873 he was the demonstrator of anatomy at Georgetown." Given the Georgetown connection with many of the other physicians, mainly graduates in 1873 and 1874 connected with Christian, I believe it is likely that he was a member and a customer of this body-snatching ring.[45]

TWO SUBJECTS BOTH FEMALE.

November 12—Boardman went out with me again to-night and we got two subjects from the dead-house at the poor-house. Took them to _____ College. They were both females.

Apparently, Dr. Boardman (Boarman) was active in body snatching as well and had no qualms about obtaining bodies from the Washington Asylum. Since he was the demonstrator at the Georgetown medical school, we can surmise that the bodies were delivered there for his dissection demonstrations.[46]

ANOTHER FEMALE.

November 13—Staid at the Asylum last night so as to see Mike. Dr. Schlimer, Stephenson, and I went out to Holmead's cemetery and got female subject for _____ College. Got through at 8 pm.

Could Stephenson be James Stephenson, who was thirty-five years old in 1884, a Black laborer who was later caught along with the notorious grave robber Vigo Jansen Ross and charged with robbing graves? Stephenson would have been twenty-four years old in 1873. He claimed that he had never robbed graves before, but when he was questioned with his boss Jansen, Jansen said that he had never robbed graves either, and then the three culprits (the third person was Thomas Bowie, Black, age twenty-four) all laughed at that joke (see Chapter 10).

SETTLING ACCOUNTS.

Friday 14th—Called on Dr. Schlimer and set for all but five subjects.

November 15—I came home before 3 o'clock to-day and lay down. Dr. Schlimer called just before dark, but I did not feel able to go with him.

Sunday, 16th—This has been a beautiful day. I stayed in the house until 3:30 o'clock p.m., when Mr. B., Mrs. B., Saide and I took a walk. Went through the Congressional and Methodist cemeteries.

Monday, 17—I went to the alms house in the evening and tried to get Dr. Schlimer out on a night expedition, but he would not go.

The Congressional and Methodist cemeteries were across from each other.[47]

FOUND THINGS TOO WET.

Nov. 18—The rain of yesterday has turned things into a wet snow storm. Dr. Schlimer called for me and we went out tonight but found things too wet.

Nov. 19—I went out to the alms house to-day and stayed until evening, expecting to get a subject that was buried today. When we went down after dark, however, we found it not, on account of the darkness.

November 20—Schlimer (M.D.) went to the lodge to-night, and left me to get the subject myself, which I did, and delivered to college dissecting rooms.

November 21—Walked out to the alms house to-night, but our expectations were disappointed.

November 24—I went to the Washington asylum in the evening with Dr. S. after a subject. We got one in Potter's Field.

Nov. 25—Went out with Dr. Schlimer to get a subject, but found too much work to accomplish, and abandoned it, as one came in this evening to be interred to-morrow.

The names "alms house" and "Potter's Field" burial grounds are used interchangeably. From the diary, the asylum had become a major source for the grave robbers.

A Handy Appointment.

Nov. 26—Dr. Schlimer was today appointed physician to the poor in the 9th district. We got two subjects in Potters field to night.

Christian and Schleimer used the burial grounds like a warehouse in which they could easily retrieve the recently dead for their business. Christian probably believed that Schliemer's appointment would give the doctor more opportunities to observe the poor and recommend that those without family and at death's door be admitted to the poor house or the hospital to be buried in "Potter's Field" for later extraction.

Based on some of the reforms that came later at the Washington Asylum, officials and the public must have taken notice of what was happening at the asylum, as detailed in Christian's diary. Although none of the doctors or staff mentioned in his diary were prosecuted for their grave-robbing activities, in a report covering November 1, 1876, to November 1, 1877, there is a discussion of the many improvements made at the Washington Asylum. Besides new staffing and a new head, we learn that one of the reasons why Christian and Schleimer were able to act with impunity was the recordkeeping was lax. Even during this later more restrictive period, the number of Potter's Field burials was 549, and only 6 corpses were removed "by request of relatives or friends." Previously, not being able to produce a dead relative could simply be attributed to badly kept records; additionally, requests for buried inmates were minimal and hardly presented a problem for the staff.

Nevertheless, the new administration took recordkeeping seriously as well as the protection of the graves of the inmates from desecration. "The digging of the graves in the 'Potter's field' was done by inmates of the institution under the direction of the intendant, [and] an accurate record is kept by him of the number of each grave, together with the name and descriptive list of its occupant."[48] The "cemetery is guarded so as to prevent desecration."[49] Also, there was "no case of 'resurrection' or effort of body snatching ... reported" from November 1, 1876, through November 30, 1877.[50] Although some aspects of the reform and improvement of the Washington Asylum could be attributed to the actions revealed in Christian's diary, the diary and its contents are not specifically mentioned in the intendant's report.[51] Unfortunately, it seems that these reforms were short-lived, and once again Potter's Field would become a warehouse for the District's medical schools (see Chapter 10).

Dr. S. "Red Hot."

Nov. 27–Thanksgiving Day—Stayed at the Almshouse last night and saw all the patients this morning. Did not get through until 10 o'clock. Came in and found Dr. Schlimer "Red Hot."

I interpret Christian's term for Dr. Schleimer as "Red Hot" as meaning that he was upset with Christian visiting the hospital patients. According to a report on conditions in the Washington Asylum in 1873, the "buildings were sadly out of repair and overcrowded on both the prison and pauper department; the hospital was sunk in a hollow, hidden from the sun and air; the poor-house inhabited by a favored crowd, who had under pernicious practices which had grown up, been mutating for years between the poor and prison departments; in fine there was such an utter lack of system, that nothing but a radical change could affect needed reform."[52]

As noted previously, one visitor to the Washington Asylum in 1871 described the facility as a combination of criminals placed with the destitute and the insane with the merely sick in the same overcrowded facility.[53]

Because there was little physical division between the criminals, the poor, and the hospital patients and aged, who were alert to their surroundings; the groups could easily communicate with each other. Some residents of the asylum undoubtedly recognized Christian as a body snatcher, and word spread among the sick poor and the hospitalized that he was taking inventory for future acquisitions. This likely caused an uproar in the hospital that Dr. Schleimer had to quell. Christian's description of him being "Red Hot" suggests that Schleimer was not happy with Christian making the rounds the evening before.

A Mistake About The Body Of Henry Young.

Nov. 28, Friday—Attended the execution of Henry Young today and took Mr. B in with me. Dr. S. and I went to Ebenezer cemetery to get him tonight but found a woman instead.

Nov. 29—Received a letter from the University of Virginia and Michigan and answered them both; also wrote to Ossle asking him to try and get me an order for subjects in Cleveland.

Nov. 30—Dr. Schlimer and I got a subject for shipping to-night at Potter's field.

Monday, Dec. 1st—Shipped two subjects to Dr. Frothingham to-day. Sent them in whisky barrels by express to J.D. Quimby & Co. for him.[54] Dr. Schlimer and I went to the asylum but got nothing. He gave up the keys.

Dec 2—It rained a good deal last night. Dr. Schlimer, Dr. _____ and I went to Ebenezer to-night and found three new graves, but the ground was too wet to get them.

The reason Christian did not get the body of Henry Young was because his body was being shipped to Alexandria, Virginia, for burial, not to the Ebenezer burying grounds. According to the *Evening Star*, Henry Young, a Black man, had robbed and murdered a Virginia drover named Frank Hahn. After his trial while awaiting execution, Young was visited by several clerics; one of the most prominent was Reverend Daniel Draper, minister of the Union Bethel African Methodist Episcopal Church. Reverend Draper also spoke at Henry's execution. Perhaps Christian thought that Henry Young had arranged to be buried in the Ebenezer burying grounds (the church's cemetery), because Draper was involved in his last days. However, after Henry was hanged, he was lowered into a "plain stained coffin" with "black rosettes." The lid was secured, and the coffin was taken "in charge by J.W. Plant, the undertaker [I wonder if he took a ribbing for his name?] and carried to the wharf for Alexandria."[55]

For the out-of-state shipping of bodies, Christian refers to the University of Virginia, Michigan, and Cleveland, Ohio. The demand for corpses was especially high in two of these states. In Virginia the legislature refused to "sanction the dissection of executed murderers, so it was impossible to dissect legally." Bodies were secretly obtained locally or shipped in from out of state and dissected privately.

Michigan had a total of sixteen medical schools. In 1866 the University of Michigan had 525 students enrolled in its medical courses, "which made it the largest extant at the time in American anatomical classes." There were not enough local cadavers to meet the needs of the school. Bodies had to be shipped in barrels from outside the state.

In the state of Ohio, there were forty-two medical schools vying for cadavers. One of the largest suppliers was the grave robber William Cunningham, or "Old Cunny." He was active between 1855 and 1871. Even Old Cunny shipped bodies across state lines.[56] Once Old Cunny was gone in 1871, the demand for cadavers only increased. There were others such as Dr. Charles O. Morton, body snatcher in Ohio, who also shipped bodies across state lines.[57] For Christian, this was an opportunity he could not ignore.

CATO TO GET 2.00 A SUBJECT.

Nov. 3 [*sic*, probably should be Dec. 3]—Got Cato, our janitor, to go out resurrecting with me to-night. We went to Ebenezer cemetery but did not succeed in getting anything. We promised to pay him 2.00 a subject, to come out of Dr. S's share.

A POOR NIGHT'S WORK.

Dec. 4th—Went to Holmead's and Young Men's Cemeteries[58] this p.m. Did not find anything at either. Hospital Steward, Hilton was sent over to help me today.

Christian involved other staff members of the asylum in his grave-robbing activities. The pay for Cato was roughly equivalent to a little more than a full day's wages. In 1873 an average daily wage for an unskilled worker at ten hours per day was $1.81.[59] However, statistics do not indicate what these rates were in Washington, D.C., and what the rates were for Black employees. Nevertheless, this was probably an attractive figure for Cato for only a few hours of work. Also, we do not know what Cato and Hilton were told to bring them into this activity.

BUSINESS DULL AGAIN.

Dec. 5—Wrote to Dr. Davis this morning, promising to send him two subjects tomorrow, went to Holmead's and Young Men's Cemeteries this evening, but did not succeed in getting anything.

Dec 6—Went out to the Alms House this afternoon. Did not find Cooper there. Cato and I went out to Ebenezer this evening and got a subject which we put in barrel ready to ship.

Dec. 7th—I went out to the Alms House this morning and saw Cooper. Found Bennie at the house when I came back. We went out riding together I got a subject at Holmead's myself.

Monday, Dec. 8—Sent two subjects to Virginia this morning, and wrote a letter to Dr. Davis in regard to them. Cato and I went out to Mount Zion tonight, and got a subject for N.B.

Dr. Davis was John Staige Davis of Charlottesville, Virginia. He was a "demonstrator of anatomy at the University of Virginia" from 1845 to 1849. He was later a professor of anatomy at the University of Virginia until his death in 1885.[60] Christian wrote that he sent him two subjects on December 8.

The Young Men's Baptist or Mount Pleasant Plains Cemetery, a Black burial ground, was founded in 1857.[61]

Christian does not indicate where the body from Ebenezer was shipped, but it seems likely it was one of those shipped to Dr. Davis as was the body from Holmead, as they were sent out the following day, and he wrote a letter to Davis regarding his shipment.

Back to business, Christian and Cato collected a body from Mount Zion, a Black cemetery. This was Christian's last entry, as he was arrested a few days later.

The following letters addressed to Christian under one of his aliases are curious and shed some light into the way the transportation of cadavers was managed at the University of Virginia.

TRANSPORTATION
Dec. 2, 1873.

Dear S.E. French, Dear Sir:

The last mail brought your letter. Please send me at once two subjects of merchantable quality and securely barreled. I have had infinite trouble in consequence of a bloody liquid escaping from one of the barrels last winter.

Send them by freight to Dr. J.S. Davis, University of Virginia and notify me by mail that you have sent them.

Yours truly, J.S. Davis

P.S. if the arrangement works well l will get from you chiefly.

Dr. Davis's involvement in the cadaver trade went back to the 1840s. He worked with a "covert team of people who harvested [primarily slave] cadavers for medical research, transporting bodies from Richmond to Charlottesville where they were sold to the faculty." His letters show that the trade in bodies was a "highly organized" and "fully functioning business." Because of teaching methodology, he required "twenty-five cadavers per year" to allow each student an individual dissection. In the letter, he required "good subjects, properly shipped." Following the Civil War, southern physicians turned to harvesting the corpses of former slaves and free Blacks in local cemeteries by closely monitoring "black funerals because they had to act within four days" to ensure a specific travel time before decomposition of the corpse began.[62]

Davis may have turned to Christian for an additional supply of cadavers. It is unlikely that Christian would have been his only supplier.

Ann Arbor, Mich.,Dec. 4, 1873

Dr. S.E. French, 303 East Capital St. Washington, D.C.

Dear sir:

Boxes have come or rather barrels. Do not send barrels: they always get the heads knocked in and excites suspicion if they do not as the subjects shake about so. The best way to pack is in a box three feet by two, or near that dimension, the subject having legs and thighs flexed and head resting on the chest sawdust packed about to prevent odor and subject from shaking about in the box. Two can be put in a single box a little larger than the one I describe. You may keep on sending until I am done work at $25.00 for the good ones. We sell for forty to the students all injected and I have to get mv pay for keeping the room and all incidental expenses. The express averages about 7 dollars a subject, so, you see the price you mention could not be afforded. Your money will be sent promptly on the receipt of goods, and you may send me just as fast as you can between now and January 1st.

In haste, Yours Truly,

G.E. Frothingham.

In this letter details are given for shipping cadavers to Ann Arbor, Michigan, probably for a dissecting room at the University of Michigan. The buyer gives specific instructions on the best way to ship the bodies to prevent odors and details his attendant costs and profit. Likely if two bodies were shipped in one box, the buyer would realize a greater profit.

An Active Young Christian.

The prisoner had upon him at the time of his arrest a certificate of membership in the Young Men's Christian Association though, of course, that association had not the slightest reason to suspect the nature of the "active" night work he was engaged in.

The following is a copy of the ticket of membership: "This ticket certifies George A. Christian is a member of the Young Men's Christian Association of Washington, D.C., for the year commencing."

The sarcasm in this report concerning Christian's membership in the Y.M.C.A. is self-explanatory.

George Christian's appeal on February 9, 1874:

> This morning in the Criminal Court. Judge Cartter. George A. [when later pardoned he gave his middle initial as H.] Christian, who it will be recollected was arrested in December last, on the charge of desecrating a grave and removing a dead body [that of Thomas Fletcher from Holmead's burial ground] was tried, convicted, and sentenced December 18th by the Police Court to one year in jail and to pay a fine of 1,000, was called up for sentence, having been found guilty a few weeks ago in this court, to which he had appealed. Judge Cartter [after hearing Christian's answer that he had nothing to say why sentence should not be pronounced], said that the court had come to the conclusion to remit the fine imposed below upon the information that it would operate as a punishment to Christian's family and the court did not propose to add to the affliction of the family. He would therefore remit the fine. This case was not that of a student of science in the pursuit of intelligence for the purpose of advancing qualifications. If it was such a one much could be said in his behalf. The living were interested in the knowledge of the structure of the human body and this knowledge could only be obtained by the examination of the dead. But in this case the sensibilities of the living have been wounded. your case is without apology; you pursued this business, according to your book, and have brought grief to the living. There is nothing in the case to induce the court to remit the imprisonment. He would, therefore. impose the sentence, one year in jail, less the time already served under the sentence below. Charles Green, the colored man arrested with Christian at the same time under the same charge, was jailed under the impression that he had been instructed by counsel to enter a plea, but he answered to the information that he was not guilty of taking the body; was not in the employ of Christian, but in the employ of Dr. Schlelmer to attend to his horse. &c. He was therefore sent back to jail.[63]

Although the public was against grave robbing and saw Christian's conviction as justified, nevertheless Christian had support in high places in Washington. On September 24, 1874, President Ulysses S. Grant issued a pardon for George H. Christian, who was convicted in February of "removing dead bodies for gain" and sentenced to one year in prison, "strongly recommended by many of the most prominent members of the medical profession in this City, including the faculties of the 'Georgetown' and 'Columbian' medical schools, the editors of the leading Washington papers and many other citizens of the District of Columbia, as well as by Senator John Sherman, and a large number of the Ohio Representatives in Congress."[64]

The two schools that benefited most from Christian's activities came forth under the protection of the medical community in Washington, D.C. Perhaps the schools were concerned that Christian might implicate them even more in his activities, but more likely he was being held in prison and was an example to others who might have taken over his business that they too could be imprisoned. By procuring him a pardon and having him leave Washington, the pressure was off the schools and their potential suppliers.

As for why Senator John Sherman and other Ohio representatives were there, it would have made sense for several reasons. President Grant was a son of Ohio. Ohio had a long history of violent riots against medical schools and suppliers that the mob thought were using bodies gotten illegally from local graveyards. The Western College of Homeopathic

Medicine witnessed a violent attack in February 1852 when a rumor spread that the remains of a young girl were found in a cesspool in one of the college buildings. A Mr. Johnson believed that it might be his daughter who had been stolen from her grave. Over two hundred people formed a mob and attacked the building, destroying equipment and valuable collections and finally lighting the building on fire. The mob decided to attack the home of an anatomy professor as well, and the riot was finally quelled by the state authorities.[65]

Shortly afterward in June 1852 on Walnut Hills Road near Cincinnati, another riot broke out when a small shanty was discovered to have "disconnected skeletons," "bodies in barrels," and "corpses with their clothes on." A mob formed and rioted and tried to lynch the men responsible. The authorities prevented the lynching. It was later proven in court that the bodies were legally obtained and that the men were preparing the bodies for medical purposes.[66]

For the Ohio medical schools, it was paramount to obtain bodies legally—this meant from out of state and not locally—and not give the mob an excuse to attack the medical schools. For example, the Homeopathic College in Cincinnati hired Edward C. Wetherell as its anatomy teacher in 1853 because he could furnish plenty of "dissecting material for the students from the city of New York." However, he soon retired in 1858 and died that year from cholera.[67]

Nevertheless, there was still a dearth of cadavers for the medical schools, and people such as Christian who supplied from out of state were a necessity for the schools to have enough cadavers on hand. We also saw the earlier example of Old Cunny operating in Ohio and shipping bodies out of state. As late as 1878 Old Cunny's widow was arrested with five other persons in Cincinnati for "selling the body of a black girl...."[68]

However, to conclude this beyond Christian's pardon, in 1878 "a body snatching episode of paramount significance, occurred in the state of Ohio." On May 26, 1878, John Scott Harrison, U.S. senator passed. He was the son of William H. Harrison, who served as president for one month in 1841, and the father of Benjamin Harrison, who became president in 1888. After John S. Harrison was put in his grave, his son and a cousin heard rumors that a friend's body had been stolen and taken to Cincinnati. "In their investigation, they canvassed the Medical College of Ohio (University of Cincinnati), without finding any evidence of the subject they were looking for and were about to abandon the project. At that moment, a body was raised up into the dissecting-room by means of a hoist. Its head and shoulders were covered with a cloth. When the hood was removed, both young men recognized it as being the body of John Scott Harrison."

The deceased's son, Benjamin, "the newspapers of the city and, in fact, the whole nation contributed their share in arousing the emotions of the populace."[69]

In Ohio, in 1879 body snatching "became a penitentiary offense with a heavy fine." The law passed in 1879 was amended in 1880, and on February 19, 1881, "all unclaimed bodies which had to be buried at the expense of the town became legally available for anatomical dissection."[70]

Until the law of 1881 there was a lack of bodies for the Ohio medical schools. It made sense for the Ohio legislators to support Christian's pardon, because cadavers shipped in by men such as Christian (attempting to take advantage of the market in Cincinnati, already a "distribution center" for corpses imported into Ohio), would provide the cadavers to meet most of the needs of the medical schools. Although they could not meet all the needs, there still was a local market, and it would depress this market and keep the price of cadavers down.[71]

Oddly enough, I could find no public mention of Christian's pardon in the District of Columbia papers. It seemed to have been discreetly buried in Grant's presidential papers at the time.

Nevertheless, no new anatomy law was immediately passed in Washington, and therefore the demand for illegal cadavers did not cease. Soon George Christian was replaced by Vigo Jansen Ross in Washington, nicknamed the "King of Resurrectionists."

10

The Heyday of Body Snatching in the Nation's Capital

Vigo Jansen (Ross), "King of the Resurrectionists"

The conflict between the medical faculty and other elites who supported the need for bodies to improve medical education and those who deplored the theft of bodies from the burial grounds can be seen in the treatment by the courts of those accused of body snatching and convicted. For example, in the case of the well-known body snatcher Vigo Jansen, he was repeatedly arrested. The demand for cadavers was so high in Baltimore that "he departed from the prudent line of stealing only the bodies of the poor and carried on his depredations in a cemetery for the better class."

In "Washington, he stole the body of a criminal who had been hanged and sold it to a medical school: the next night he stole it again to sell it to another ... [and] ... was caught with his booty in a hack. After serving his sentence he ... lectured on body snatching in one of the smaller theatres, giving practical illustrations with a sham corpse."[1]

According to newspaper reports, Jansen presented this lecture at the Theatre Comique on May 18, 1884. The interest in body snatching was not as popular as he anticipated. The *Evening Star* critic was not impressed, headlining his column "The Ghoul at Work." He wrote that Vigo Jansen, the "king of resurrectionists," delivered a lecture "on his chosen profession at the *Theatre Comique* last night and drew an audience of about sixty persons, the major portion of which consisted of newspaper men, policemen and attaches of the theatre. The rest consisted principally of visiting bicyclers. The total absence of colored people was noticeable, but not very wonderful."

Jansen was introduced by Dr. Selden W. Crowe, himself an alleged body snatcher, having stolen the body of a man named A.T. Stewart. On the stage in the rear was a "natural looking grave, consisting of a mound of earth carefully sodded with green turf and decked with white flowers."

Jansen, "a short, stout man, with a heavy dark moustache and goatee ... [was] attired in a dress suit ... [and] walked across the stage in a nervous manner twice before he said a word and would evidently have sooner faced a graveyard than his small audience of eager listeners." As soon as he began to speak, the audience began to shout "louder, louder," finally inducing him to go into an "harangue, in which he attempted to prove that the ghoulish business was not disreputable but was a human necessity." He gave examples of how his business benefited humanity, leading to doctors trained on these corpses providing thousands of beneficial surgeries over their lifetime of practice.

He charged the surgeon general of the army as "being the biggest resurrectionist of all" and then stated that in his experience that "he had been shot at and hunted by dogs just as if he was the worst criminal in the community."

After this the curtain went down, and Jansen changed into different clothes, including a "brigandish-looking hat and a long coat with a high collar, and when the curtain went-up he presented quite the appearance he desired." He announced that he would demonstrate how to "dig up" a body from the ground.[2]

Dr. Crowe assisted Jansen, posing as a laborer "on the job and, came sneaking on with a spade in his hand. Jansen picked out the head of the grave and felt the turf to find out whether the grave was a fresh one" and tiptoed around and "marked off about two feet at the head of the grave to be dug up." When this was done, he reached down and removed some boards, and by the united efforts of the two, the alleged "stiff" was drawn out, "covered with a white shroud, his head and bare legs showing."

> A colored boy who had been enticed in, when he saw this, bolted for the door at break-neck speed. In getting a fresh hold on the "stiff," Jansen got his hands under the arms of the corpse, which tickled the negro who represented the "stiff" and caused him to laugh and work his legs. He finally stiffened his form, and the two resurrectionists carried him off the stage, as Jansen said, in a sepulchral tone: "Well, just put it over there behind the fence." The grave was filled, and the sod and flowers were replaced, and the curtain went down on the ghastly exhibition.[3]

The reviewer for the *Evening Critic* was not finished with his criticism of the performance and in another column the same day wrote, "It is a pity there is no law which would have permitted the authorities to have stopped the disgraceful exhibition of Jansen at the *Comique* last night. Grave robbing is a crime which should send its perpetrators to the penitentiary, instead of to the lecture platform."[4]

Clearly, his attempt onstage was not successful.[5] In October 1884 Jansen "renewed his ghastly business in the District." He and his party with their "plunder" were taken prisoner while trying to enter a cemetery.[6] According to the *Evening Critic*, while in jail Jansen asked a reporter if Dr. A.C. Adams was up in court. When told he was not, the reporter wanted to know why Jansen asked for this man. Vigo Jansen replied, "He is the demonstrator of anatomy at the National Medical College [also called the Columbia College Medical Department] … the college for which I am furnishing subjects." He also informed the reporter that he was going to fight the charge, as there was no law against grave robbing in Washington, D.C., and that he was employed by the faculty, who provided him with counsel. "It's a shame to arrest me for this," he continued. "There is no law against it, and the last time I was convicted they had to go back 187 years for a decision in England. Those colleges have got to have subjects. What does a dead body amount to," he said, contemptuously, "when it can be used for the advancement of science?" "He said that if Dr. Adams had been sent for last night he would have been released."

To give some idea of the rest of his confederates, a reporter asked Jansen's two Black assistants, James Stephenson, thirty-five, laborer, and Thomas Bowie, twenty-four, oyster-shucker, "How long have you been in this business?" Stephenson replied, "Only las' night, boss. I wouldn't done if I hadn't been drunk. I wouldn't done it no how, if he hadn't told me a lie. He comes to me an' says, I want to git a stiff." He said he was afraid at first, but Jansen said, "They can't do nothin' with you, 'cause I've got a permit to dig 'am up.' But when the police come, he didn't show them the permit he showed mo."

Bowie refused to talk. Stephenson said he had never been engaged in this business before. "Neither was I," said Jansen, with a dry smile. "Then they all laughed in chorus."[7]

For all Jansen's bravado and connections, he was "sentenced to jail for eleven months and twenty-nine days." The tools of the trade, "ropes, picks, spades and hooks[,] were confiscated by the police."[8]

The newspaper report identified Jansen, thirty-five, as a well-known grave robber in Washington and Baltimore as a "notorious depopulator of graveyards" who had given the "disgraceful lecture at the *Theater Comique*." Jansen was so infamous that the captain of police, Charles R. Vernon, was informed that Jansen was planning to rob the Black Young Men's Burying Grounds and was spotted "attending funerals and lying concealed on the vault watching the places of interment." "The police had information he planned to pay the place a professional visit that night and they were on the lookout."[9]

The medical community was actively collaborating with Jansen and his cohorts. It became obvious that Jansen was not only well known and easily identified by the public but also was naming doctors and medical schools in defense of his profession and as part of his legal defense. The medical schools did not want to be openly identified with this immoral and ghastly profession but had to support it to obtain their cadavers. The publicity was too much, and the solution for the medical schools was to make "up a purse to induce him to leave, as, during his presence, the police were so active that what may be termed the quiet and respectable pursuit of the business was impossible."[10]

Vigo Jansen Ross later committed suicide in New York City on November 3, 1887. According to the report, "letters found on his person show he was driven to the deed by starvation."[11]

Body Snatching After Jansen: Tolerated but Not Acceptable

I will argue here that with Jansen's admission of the involvement of the medical colleges' illegal use of subjects in their dissecting rooms as well as the various U.S. medical services admitting to the same, the authorities in the District of Columbia realized that without a body-snatching law or a "penal code" allowing the use of criminal bodies (all criminal dead were required by statute to be buried), a solution had to be found to obtain subjects for the medical schools. The answer was to look away from the digging up of bodies in the "Potter's Field." Besides a certain amount of cupidity on the part of the medical schools to remain in business and the demonstrated improvements in medicine, there were the religious and social changes in the attitude toward the poor, especially the idea for the charity given to them in life, they owed society a debt in death. However, to tolerate the exploitation of the bodies of the poor, the resurrectionists were not to stray into the other respectable Washington cemeteries, and if they did and they were caught, they would be prosecuted because the public demanded it.[12]

Even with this "understanding," most of the cemeteries in Washington were still being frequented by body snatchers, as "there is probably no other city in the Union where the proportion to its size, [and] grave robbing is carried on so extensively as it is in the Capital of the Nation. The crime is fostered by men of science and winked at by the authorities." Occasional "efforts have been made … to suppress it," but these efforts were generally unsuccessful.

The superintendents of the cemeteries in Washington when interviewed about this issue were naturally circumspect, especially those representing cemeteries with Washington elites buried in them. Examples include, the Glenwood Cemetery containing members of old Washington families; the superintendent admitted only that there were two grave robberies nearly four years previously. The Prospect Hill cemetery contained the bodies of wealthy citizens of German descent. The superintendent did not admit to any grave robberies but noted that he recently saw a "fellow prowling in the dark looking for a grave recently filled in on that day." He sent his dogs after the resurrectionist, who when he "saw what was coming ... made quick tracks for the fence" and escaped. The Oak Hill Cemetery contains the bodies of many distinguished Washingtonians. Its superintendent noted that it was the only cemetery "that has not been desecrated by body snatchers because it is the only cemetery in the United States where bricking in of the grave is obligatory." No doubt the statements made by these superintendents were to instill trust in their lot holders. However, the article quoting the superintendents concluded that "to equip their dissecting rooms the colleges have, therefore bought annually 100 bodies stolen from graves belonging to the lot owners in cemeteries where the well to do and wealthy bury their dead."

Nearly all the Washington cemeteries had some security but still fell prey to the resurrectionists when the demand for "subjects" increased. One cemetery, the Asylum's Potter's Field, had no security. It was "known by the colleges, by the authorities and by the resurrectionists as Scientific Ground." For example, during the twenty-five years prior to 1892, on average there were buried 400 persons per year. Daniel Tyndall, a clerk in the Washington Asylum, estimated that "few of the 10,000 bodies once buried in Potter's Field are now there." When asked what had become of all those bodies the reply was that "the resurrectionists and medical colleges of Washington can tell."

As for why there were so many paupers in Washington and, by implication, why they were not missed when the graves were emptied, the explanation offered was that Washington is a "cosmopolitan city" and unique because "all sorts of ... Senators, Congressmen, diplomats, and government officials ... cling to Washington when their days of usefulness are over. Many men of former greatness are today picked up in the gutters. They beg drinks and pennies where once they bestowed charity and hospitality with a lavish hand. To-morrow they may be in the almshouse, the day after to-morrow they may be in the Potter's Field, and on the third day they will most surely be on the dissecting table of a Washington medical college."

Black cemeteries also offered security, but to the anatomists and resurrections the value of a Black body was equal in value to a white body, so the exploitation of Black cemeteries was as lucrative to the resurrectionists as any elite, fashionable, or public cemetery and just as dangerous. For example, on December 12, 1892, the watchmen at the "colored" Harmony Cemetery had a full battle "with half dozen resurrectionists." The resurrectionists were digging up a grave and were surprised by three watchmen. The resurrectionists fired their pistols, and the watchmen returned their fire. "The ghouls retreated from the grave and escaped." One resurrectionist was wounded but managed to escape, leaving a trail of blood behind. The authorities at the Harmony cemetery claimed that they only knew what graves had been robbed if they discovered the "ghouls at their work." They were of the opinion that a "general re-opening of the graves in the cemetery would probably reveal hundreds of empty coffins."

The medical colleges for their further protection added a layer of deniability. Both the National Medical College and Georgetown's medical school received their subjects in the middle of the night, dropped off and received by the janitors at the two schools with no questions asked. At the National Medical College, the procedure was completely anonymous. At Georgetown the janitor alone received the cadavers and took them to the dissecting room. The aim was to protect the demonstrators, doctors, and students, who in this way had no knowledge of who the subjects were, where they came from, or who delivered them.[13]

The Body-Snatching Case of Dr. W.W. Beall, 1892–1893

An example of the issues I have noted is illustrated in the following body-snatching case of Dr. W.W. Beall, accused of snatching the bodies of Mrs. Alvina "Venie" Cheek and Mary E. Hawkins on the evening of December 20, 1889, from the Congressional Cemetery and Potter's Field, respectively.

The case was reported in the *Evening Star* on December 23, 1889, and began with the following admission about Potter's Field: "The law against the desecration of graves by body snatchers is openly violated in this District night after night, but prosecutions for the ghastly work are few. Potter's Field is generally chosen as their scene of operations because they can go there at any time after dark and drive off with their plunder undisturbed."[14]

It was first reported at the jail located near Potter's Field that the guards and prisoners admitted to seeing a buggy on Friday night stopping near the cemetery, a buggy they had seen on numerous nights. Everyone knew they were waiting for an opportunity to "go down to the burial place of the poor and to carry of[f] their ghastly burden." Further, on Friday night the "guards were certain that there were cadavers in the vehicle, but they did not imagine that any burial place other than potter's field had been visited."

After stealing the two bodies, the grave robbers made their way toward town when an officer approached the buggy. He heard the driver talking and recognized the voice of Dr. Beall, having known him for many years. The officer followed and then approached the buggy. The two men in front of the buggy ran away, and the driver attempted to flee with the buggy, later jumping out of the buggy and running off. The empty buggy held two female cadavers, "one white and the other colored, and they were taken to the morgue and the buggy turned in to the property clerk."[15]

Because it was thought that both cadavers had come from Potter's Field, the officers were told that "no effort was made to have them identified." Body-snatching rumors spread quickly, and "hearing that dead relatives have been removed … inquiries to that effect were being made at the cemeteries." The rumor must have gotten out that one of the bodies was that of a white woman, because that Saturday afternoon a young man arrived at the morgue and "asked permission to see the body of the white woman, saying that his sister had been buried in the Congressional Cemetery a few days ago." Obviously, there were suspicions that bodies from other cemeteries had been taken. One rumor circulating even involved the recovery of a corpse from a medical college: "a body was recently taken from another cemetery and traced to a medical college. The work of the resurrectionists was discovered and the body returned to the grave before the dissecting knife had been used upon it."[16]

After viewing the body, the young man thought it was that of his sister, but when a station clerk "telephoned the East Washington station he was informed that the bodies had been removed from Potter's Field." He told the young man of this, but he was still troubled by what he had seen and left in an "uncertain frame of mind."

Meanwhile, Officer Oliver, who earlier had seen the white woman's body, was not convinced that her corpse had come from Potter's Field. He "thought that there was a look of refinement about her that is not often seen about persons who occupy graves in the pauper cemetery, and he was not satisfied with the investigation that had been made." He looked more closely at the body and noticed in the "undergarment" that was wrapped about it the name "B. Cheek." When he checked further with the health office, a record showing her address, cause of death, and burial site was discovered. The body was that of Mrs. Alvina Cheek of No. 1015 South Carolina Avenue southeast; she had died on December 11 of the ravages of phthisis (tuberculosis) and was buried in the Congressional Cemetery the previous Tuesday.

The piece of clothing with her name on it was taken from her corpse and "brought to the house and there it was learned that the name had been written on Mrs. Cheek's undergarment. Meanwhile, Mr. Cross, the superintendent of the Congressional Cemetery inspected the grave site and said that the grave was 'all right and had not been |disturbed.'" The theft of Alvina Cheek's body was confirmed when the grave was reopened on December 22, and "in the broken coffin was found the body of the child that had been buried in the grave with its mother."

However, when her husband reached the morgue, he recognized the body of his late wife "lying on the board ready to be, placed in the ice box." Mrs. Cheek "had been sick for some time and had gradually wasted away until there was hardly any flesh left on her form. Her remains, with the body of her infant, which was only a few days old, were interred" in the Congressional Cemetery "on a knoll overlooking the Anacostia River and not far from a gate which opens into the rear end of the work house grounds." Opening the grave would have been relatively easy for an experienced resurrectionist, as the soil had not been fortified, and her body would have been easily removed with a grappling hook, and afterward the grave was "refilled and the flowers on it placed where they had been left by the bereaved husband." The body was said to have been "taken through the gate or over the fence and stripped of clothing." From there "it was carried through to potter's field" and there kept until the body of Mary E. Hawkins was "lifted" from the poor house burying ground.

Officer Oliver had made a thorough investigation of the buggy in which was found the bodies of the two women as well as the grave clothes taken from the body of Mrs. Cheek. He also discovered a heavy iron hook attached to a long rope that had been used in lifting the two bodies from their graves.

Related to the case, a strange event occurred on the morning of December 22. Dr. A.C. Adams, the demonstrator at the National College of Medicine and the doctor Vigo Jansen asked for when he was arrested, put in a claim for the horse and buggy in which the two bodies were found. Adams swore under oath that it was his property. "When the doctor went to the sixth precinct station to get the horse and buggy, he met Mr. Thomas B. Cheek there." "Mr. Cheek was greatly incensed at what had taken place." He questioned the doctor sharply, but the latter said he did not own the team. The police lieutenant told them not to have any trouble there, and the doctor drove off with the buggy. Later that day Mrs. Cheek's remains were placed in a casket, taken to the cemetery, and placed in the receiving vault, where they were to remain for some days (to be made unsuitable for dissection).

On December 23, Mr. Cheek went to the police court and swore a warrant out against Dr. Arthur C. Adams, charging him with the desecration of his wife's grave.

According to the newspaper report, neither the officials in the morgue or elsewhere nor the police in general were willing to do anything to identify the two female bodies. They would have been buried anonymously in the poor house cemetery, only to be dug up for the dissecting table or even sold secretly to one of the medical colleges, no questions asked. The identification of Mrs. Cheek was thanks to one policeman who suspected that one of the women was not taken from Potter's Field and followed through on his own to discover her identity and prove that her body had been stolen from the Congressional Cemetery, obviously an important distinction in official Washington.

Meanwhile, because of events concerning the seizure of the horse and buggy with the two female bodies left behind in the carriage, probably unknown to Mr. Cheek at the time, the police did not think that the perpetrator of the crime was Dr. Adams but instead was another physician.

The Trial of Dr. W.W. Beall for Robbing the Graves of Mrs. Alvina Cheek in the Congressional Cemetery and Mary E. Hawkins in Potter's Field on December 20, 1889

On the evening of December 20, 1889, Dr. W.W. Beall left his home with two confederates and made his way in his horse and buggy with the tools of his trade, including a customized grappling hook, to obtain a body in the Congressional Cemetery and another in Potter's Field. The Congressional Cemetery was established as the Washington Parish Burial Ground in 1807, but soon after Congress "took control of the cemetery," and all members of Congress interred in other cemeteries were moved there. It also served as a cemetery for other prominent Washingtonians. Alvina Cheek's body was removed first from the Congressional Cemetery, and then Beall and company went to Potter's Field and dug up the body of the "colored" woman, Mary E. Hawkins, and placed her next to Mrs. Cheek's body in Beall's buggy. The account continued describing the circumstances of the capture of the buggy and its contents as I related earlier.[17]

Dr. Beall's trial took place on January 6, 1890, in the police court. One newspaper opined about Dr. Beall's trial that "Dr. W.W. Beall's grave robbery excited a sensation in this city."[18] The prosecution began by having the bodies of the two women identified. The driver of the work house ambulance identified Mary Hawkins, and the undertaker involved in Mrs. Cheek's funeral identified her body. Mr. Cheek, the husband, was called to the stand as a witness. He was greatly affected by the events and "nearly broke down as he piteously told of opening the grave and finding the little baby thrown back in the grave on its head."[19]

Additional information on Beall's capture was added. A second officer testified to finding a steel hook in the buggy, the stock-in-trade of a body snatcher. Another witness, A.B. Anderson, a blacksmith, "testified to making such a hook for Dr. Beall ..., although he could not be sure, that it was the one found in the buggy." Another witness testified to selling Dr. Beall the steel to make the hook.

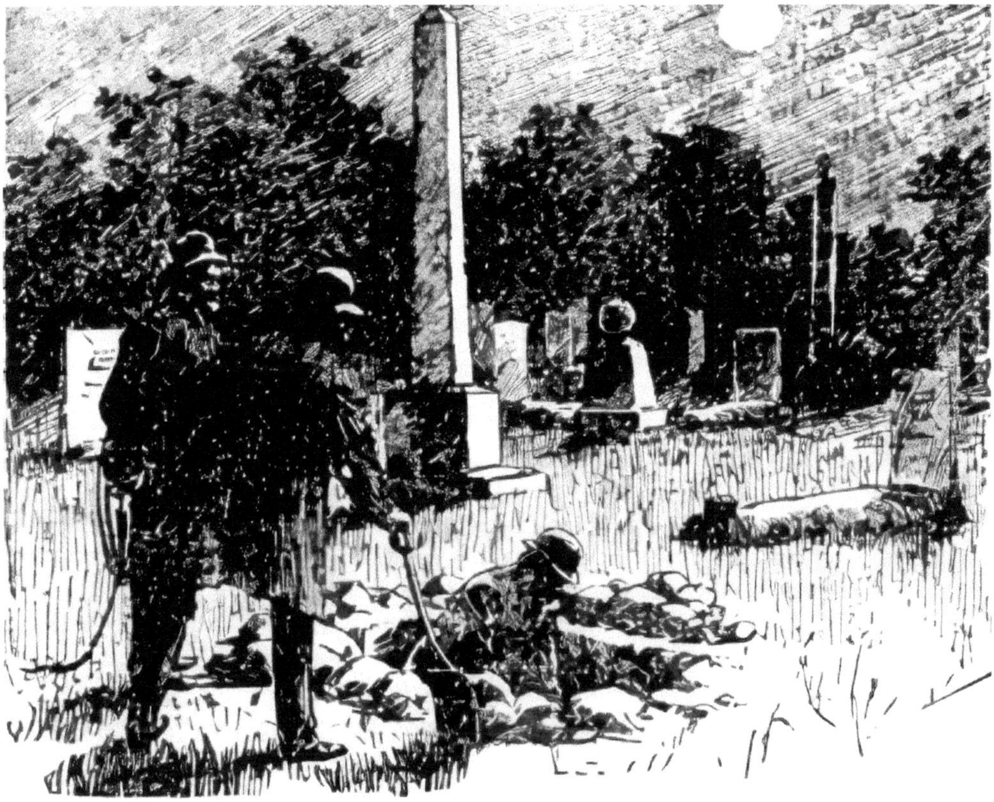

"Body Snatchers at Their Ghoulish Work." ***Crawford Avalanche*****, Grayling, Michigan, December 30, 1897, 3 (Library of Congress).**

Testimony was given stating that Dr. Beall was seen "walking away from the scene of the capture of the buggy by the officer." Another witness positively identified Dr. Beall as the owner of the buggy. Detective Raff told of the "chase and escape of Dr. Beall at the Washington Grove." The last witness praised the doctor, but his admiration in this case was misplaced, and he said that "the doctor was a hard worker at his trade, making an average of three trips a week to the grave yard after subjects."

During the questioning the disposition of the buggy was raised. The prosecution thought it strange that Dr. A.C. Adams, who Mr. Cheek originally thought was the body snatcher, had come to recover the horse and buggy. The prosecutor wanted to know if it was at Beall's request and if, as the demonstrator at the National College of Medicine, he knew where the college obtained its subjects. He replied that he recovered the buggy at Dr. Beall's request and "he did not know" how the subjects were obtained.[20] The prosecution rested its case.

The Beall trial was resumed on January 8, 1890. There was great public interest in the case. It was "an unusual thing for the court to hold an evening session, and quite a crowd of people attracted by this fact and by interest in the case itself, gathered by gas light in the court room." The only "evidence heard was for the defense." Dr. Beall's main witnesses were unsavory characters. First was R.J. Ewing, a younger man who lived with the doctor. He testified that Dr. Beall was at home the night the robberies occurred except for "twenty minutes when he was called out to see a patient. George Marlow, a negro, testified that on the same night he summoned Dr. Beall to attend his wife, and that the doctor was with the woman between 9 and 10 o'clock, the time at which the police found Dr. Beall's buggy containing the two bodies." Marlow's wife confirmed the testimony, and the defense rested.

The prosecutor rebutted the testimony, arguing that Ewing was Dr. Beall's "assistant in robbing the graves and urged that neither of the other witnesses were trustworthy, owing to their contradictory statements made on cross examination." In addition, "Marlow had already served two terms in the penitentiary."

Judge Miller summarized the case, saying that it was a misdemeanor, it was strange that Dr. Beall did not take the stand himself, and it was unusual that the doctor recovered his buggy in such a roundabout way.

Interestingly, unlike the attitude of the authorities who had no interest in either identifying or protecting the bodies from Potter's Field, perhaps because the thefts of the two women's bodies were tried together and the judge wanted to show that the law was serious about this crime, he said that the "defense was not sufficient to explain" the amount of "circumstantial evidence against Dr. Beall." He imposed a fine of $200 and imprisonment for ninety days in each case for "desecrating the grave of Mrs. Cheek and that of the colored woman." The total fine was $400 and six months in prison. A "motion for a new trial was immediately made by Dr. Beall's counsel."[21]

Dr. Beall's case was finally heard in the criminal court on June 6, 10, and 11, 1890. The prosecution and defense presented their witnesses. The defense produced a new witness who claimed that he saw Dr. Beall's "horse and buggy going through Lincoln Park on the night of December 20, with two colored men in it."

Dr. Beall took the stand in his own defense. He "got very much mixed up during the cross examination.... His explanation as to why he visited Potter's Field so often was looked upon as being very weak, as was also his excuse for not going to headquarters and claiming his horse and buggy." A witness in rebuttal testified to "having seen Dr. Beall visit Potter's Field and mark certain graves." Dr. Beall concluded his time on the stand by denying "all knowledge of the grave robberies, and accounting for all of his time on the night of the robbery. On the next morning ... [he said he] ... found his buggy gone from his stable."[22]

The case went to the jury on the afternoon of June 11. The jury was out for over five hours and was not "able to agree, [and] the judge discharged them."[23] "Soon after the doctor felt it healthy to leave town." He took up a new practice in Baltimore.[24]

The public was willing to tolerate the removal of the bodies of paupers from Potter's Field as long as it was out of sight and out of mind but could not accept a body snatcher living in their midst, a known "ghoul" of Washington's other cemeteries. Even if the jury could not render a verdict, it seems that the public did.

Post-Beall Washington

With the self-exile of Dr. Beall from his body-snatching activities in Washington, grave robbing continued unabated in D.C.. According to an exposé titled "Ghouls at Their Work" printed in the New York newspaper the *Morning Advertiser* on January 16, 1893, since Jansen's conviction (as Beall was not convicted) it had been a "number of years now since grave robbing has been punished in the District of Columbia."

It flourishes now "as Medical science demands more subjects now than ever before." Georgetown College School of Medicine, Howard Medical School, and Columbian College Medical Department also called the National Medical College (which was the medical department of Columbian College since its founding)[25] were named, and all three medical schools required more "subjects ... from graveyard resurrectionists."[26]

The chief resurrectionist was a "colored man named Marlow and he worked out of a barracks in the west part of town." After interviewing several superintendents of Washington cemeteries, the paper learned "that a well-known practicing physician in Washington" was at the head of Marlow and his "gang of ghouls." The doctor apparently enjoyed "the protection of the police."

The paper reported that the "body snatchers outfit in Washington consisted of a wagon, a spade, a crowbar and a grappling hook." The wagon was common enough so as not to arouse suspicion after midnight; it can "carry the body of a full-grown man without doubling it up." It is covered in a "dingy white canvas." There is just enough space for the body snatchers "to sit one over the head and feet of their dead passenger." The giveaway of their trade is the "hook." The spade and crowbar are common enough, but the hook is specialized to their trade and is "lowered into the coffin when the head of the subject is exposed, and by a dexterous jerk the hook is fastened to the jaw and the body pulled from the coffin."

Interestingly, as we saw earlier, George Marlow and his wife were the chief witnesses for the defense in the Beall trial. The description of the wagon and tools of the trade was similar to the buggy and tools named in the Beall trial as well. Although the article claimed that Marlow had police protection, strangely there were some policemen who recognized the wagon and what he and his cohorts were up to. On November 23, 1893, the *Evening Star* reported the arrest "at an early hour Saturday morning of the three negroes in a wagon on the Brentwood Road." The "arrest caused some comments in police circles.... [I]t was supposed by some of the officers that the men were probably the burglars who have been visiting all sections of the District.... When they appeared in the Police Court on Saturday their counsel ... demanded a jury trial and the case went over." The judge "saw the arsenal taken from the prisoners, the large sack and rope ladder and then fixed the bond at 1,500." The men "were unable to give bail and they were thereupon committed to jail."

One of the prisoners was George Marlow, Sr., "an ex-convict." Because they "were arrested ... near Columbia Harmony cemetery, the first impression made on the officers was that the men were resurrectionists, and they are still of that opinion. The appearance of the burglars in East Washington Saturday night while the negroes were in jail dispelled the idea that they were the burglars, while the interest taken in the men by physicians caused the officers to believe that they were violators of sepulcher."

However, while the three men were in jail Saturday night, "resurrectionists were at work in Mount Zion cemetery, a colored burying ground in the suburbs of Georgetown. The cemetery was visited sometime during the night and there in sight of several dwelling houses the men did their ghastly work and took from the grave the body of Spencer Mitchell, a colored man, who departed this life earlier in the week." Mitchell, a driver, "had been injured by a horse." Taken to the hospital, he died a few days later. An autopsy was performed on his body.

After his burial, "the sexton of the cemetery ... [saw] ... that Mitchel's grave had been disturbed and following footprints from the grave he soon saw blood stains on the ground." The trail of blood stains led first to his discovery of "portions of the entrails of the dead man" and finally "he found the body that had been stripped of its clothing and dragged … far from the grave." The police surmised that "a physician saw the body and did not want it because of the post mortem examination having been made."

No doubt as these two events occurred while the accused men were in jail, that evening the men were promptly released the next day, much to the disappointment of Marlow's neighbors who had been anxious to get the original case tried, as they were "desirous of getting rid of Marlow as a neighbor."[27]

What we do learn from the report is that the police on the beat were willing to arrest suspected body snatchers even though it was known that the police were compromised at the highest levels on this issue.[28] In addition, the police were patrolling all cemeteries including the Black burying grounds. It also seemed that "the interest" taken in Marlow and his men "by physicians caused the officers to believe that they were violators of sepulcher." Finally, the obvious state of Mr. Mitchell's grave, the trail of "blood stains," and his desecrated body were highly unusual. Also, as the article suggests, if a doctor was there to judge the quality of the grossly mishandled corpse, he was taking a tremendous chance that he might be caught and ruined.

Perhaps one of the most brazen examples of the work of the resurrection men and their collaboration with the medical colleges and authorities viewed by the public was the following incident.

On October 29, 1892, hundreds of members of the public saw a "demonstration that a robbery of graves and the traffic of human bodies was being carried on with extraordinary audacity." The "fashionable Fredonia Hotel" overlooked a public alley next to a private courtyard belonging to Columbian's National Medical College. On that day looking from the "upper windows of the hotel the guests saw two nude bodies lying in the narrow court." As described by the reporter, "the waiters, bellboys, and chambermaids thronged into the alley and peered through the cracks in the fence. Passersby's seeing the curious crowd, stopped, and looked in their turn," including children. "Straining necks were at all the upper windows of the Fredonia Hotel." What the crowd saw were the naked dead bodies of a forty-year-old "Negro" man and a twenty-five-year-old "mulatto" woman.

While all this activity was going on, the owner of a nearby horse stable telephoned the dean of the faculty of the National Medical College, Dr. Albert King, who in turn called Dr. William P. Carr, the National Medical College demonstrator in anatomy. Meanwhile, a policeman in street clothes saw the bodies and went to "call a patrol wagon." Dr. Carr rushed over to the college and picked up the bodies each in turn, within the full view of the spectators, and "dragged them … down a flight of stairs to the cellar." There he injected them with "preserving fluid." They were taken "to the dissecting room … and cut with scalpels, so that they became 'subjects' and the property of the college." When the policeman returned with the patrol wagon, he searched the college and the grounds "but could find no trace of what he had seen." The "discovery and Dr. Carr's ready action occurred between 8 and 9 o'clock in the morning."

The cause of this embarrassment and commotion was because the body snatchers had "arrived with their burden about 3 o'clock in the morning. They drove their cart down the public alley to the 'stable' adjoining the college north." This annex to the college was not a stable but was used exclusively "for the reception of 'subjects,' and opens directly into the rear of the college." The body snatchers had a key to unlock the "stable" and place their cargo inside "without notifying anyone connected with the college." That morning "the resurrectionists broke the key in the lock and couldn't open the door." The "subjects were a special order." They could not travel around town with them, as it was too dangerous, "so they tossed the dead people over the fence."[29]

The Washington, D.C., Medical Community "Comes Clean"

Shortly after Vigo Jansen was paid to leave town, the Washington medical community began to lobby for an anatomy bill. While the daily operations of trafficking with the resurrectionists continued, no doubt the college administrators wanted to relieve themselves of the odious burden of dealing with these men. But as we will see, they had become dependent on them for a variety of reasons, and an anatomy bill that at first may have held out promise later caused the colleges to have second thoughts.

However, the success of an anatomical bill in Pennsylvania a little more than a year earlier had been national news in spite of the involvement of the medical establishment in Philadelphia in a major body-snatching scandal. Dr. William F. Forbes, the author of the Armstrong Act (an anatomical act) of 1867 in Pennsylvania and demonstrator at Jefferson Medical College in Philadelphia, had been implicated in a major body-snatching episode involving the Black Lebanon Cemetery in Philadelphia. The Washington newspapers had carried the news on this scandal. The *Evening Star* reported that "the colored people, who mainly use the cemetery, are very much worked up over the matter." The prisoners came into court by a back door to avoid the furor of the mob.[30]

The situation was tense, and luckily for the medical community in Philadelphia, the issue was resolved to their satisfaction through the amendment of the Armstrong Act, resulting in the Pennsylvania Anatomy Act of 1883, providing more subjects by the enforced compliance of officials who dealt with unclaimed bodies across the state and reducing the traffic in human bodies. (See Chapter 11 for a full account of this episode.)

Also, articles such as those that appeared in the *Alexandria Gazette* in support of Dr. Forbes advocated an anatomy act for Washington, D.C., to provide subjects to the medical schools and prevent robbing the graves of respectable people.[31] The medical community and their supporters likely believed that it was an opportune time to craft an anatomical law that would finally meet their needs.

The Struggle to Craft a District of Columbia Anatomy Bill

The first anatomy bill of 1886 for the District of Columbia was passed by Congress. It was taken "virtually verbatim" from "an act to provide for the protection of the study of anatomy in the State of Maryland" and approved by the Maryland legislature on March 30, 1882. The District of Columbia anatomy bill was vetoed by President Grover Cleveland on April 26, 1886. President Cleveland vetoed the bill because the law was not sufficiently definite in "designating the authorities responsible for the disposition of the bodies of the unknown and pauper dead."[32]

A second bill was proposed in 1888 to overcome Cleveland's veto and called "for the promotion of anatomical science and to prevent the desecration of the graves in the District of Columbia." Its supporters were "distinguished gentlemen of the medical profession residing in the city of Washington." These gentlemen from the medical schools and government officials in their letters of support admitted to the illegal use of cadavers in their activities.

For example, the dean of the faculty of the National Medical College, Dr. Albert F. A. King, wrote that in the "District of Columbia during the past sixty years or more (the oldest medical school [National Medical College]) is now in its sixty-eighth session, the bodies used for dissection have been surreptitiously obtained, often enough at the risk of life and limb, as well as liberty. The police and judicial authorities are fully cognizant of this method[,] the former often visit our dissecting rooms at their pleasure and could if, they chose, arrest every one of us."[33] Of course, the authorities arrested the body snatchers but not the doctors or those in the dissecting rooms.

It was not until Jansen's arrest that schools were named in the newspapers. Not only had Jansen named the National Medical College and various doctors working there, but he had also earlier during his onstage appearance "charged the Surgeon-General of the Army with being the biggest resurrectionist in the country."[34] It was likely that no one attending his performance believed him.

Yet, in the accompanying report supporting the third attempt at an 1890 bill, the following statements in letters (written in March 1888) and an army memorandum confirmed his charge. Not only was the surgeon general of the army involved, but the surgeon general of the navy was involved too. As for the navy, during the 1870s the surgeon general confirmed using stolen bodies in the navy's Medical Corps examinations.

> Not only do medical colleges require material for dissection, but the Government of the United States actually commands those persons desirous of entering the Medical Corps of the U.S. Army, and U.S. Navy shall as a prerequisite therefore, "perform surgical operations upon the cadaver."
>
> In some instances, such operations were performed by candidates for admission to the Medical Corps of the U.S. Navy in the dissecting rooms of our colleges and upon the dead surreptitiously obtained.[35]

Dr. Albert F. A. King wrote that the only means of doctors dissecting bodies for anatomical training in the District of Columbia "is by illegal methods of operating upon cadavers surreptitiously obtained," although anatomy is required "according to an act Congress approved in 1838." The "District of Columbia affords no legal method by which the means of obtaining such anatomical knowledge can be secured."[36]

The surgeon general of the navy, F.M. Gunnell, wrote on March 22, 1888, that "candidates for admission to the Medical Corps of the U.S. Navy" were required to dissect and operate on a cadaver. Currently, he wrote, examinations are held in Philadelphia, but "the examinations were held in Washington, D.C., from 1871 to 1879, and anatomical material was obtained from the medical department of the Columbian University, and the operations performed in the anatomical rooms of that institution."

The surgeon general of the Marine Hospital, John B. Hamilton, wrote on March 22, 1888, that "the examining boards meeting in this city have been much embarrassed for the want of anatomical material; that portion of the examination requiring the performance of surgical operations on cadavers has been waived because of the scarcity of bodies."[37]

In 1888, a Michigan congressman argued in the House of Representatives in support of the bill that "as regent of the University of Michigan, having included with it the largest medical college in the United States, we had to meet and solve, so far as we could, this question. We found that in that part of the State of Michigan near to our medical college something analogous to a reign of terror prevailed amongst people who were called upon to bury their dead; that there was a feeling that no grave was sacred, and there was no assurance the dead would rest where they had been laid. We found frequently the friends and relatives of the deceased discovering the removal of the remains and following them to the dissecting-room and reclaiming them."

He also added that "the State of Michigan enacted a law very similar to, almost identical with, the bill now [under consideration] … [;] the effect of the law, that grave desecration in the State of Michigan since the enactment of that law has almost entirely ceased, and that complaint of the law has ceased on every hand. People now lay the bodies of their relatives and friends in the grave with the most absolute assurance they will repose where they are laid."

Notwithstanding the support for the bill, there was a lively debate in the House of Representatives on March 27, 1888, over "which bodies should and should not be dissected." Some representatives in the House argued that the proposed bill was a war on the poor, especially those who died in the almshouse, a jail, an asylum, or a hospital. The representatives argued that given the conditions in which some people died, they had no idea what would happen to their bodies, and some would be in no condition to make their last wishes known. Only for those buried at public expense was a "harsh penalty for the character of their lives, [and] they shall after death be laid upon the dissecting table and cut to pieces."[38]

The House members also debated the plight of the poor being at the mercy of the resurrectionists if the law was not passed. Some of the proposed amendments to protect the poor inmates in these institutions included "notifying relatives of the deceased and maintaining the accountability of officials and medical schools involved in conveying the dead bodies to medical schools." (As we saw previously, the bodies of the poor in the asylum cemetery served as the illegal "Scientific Ground" for the colleges.) The bill's supporters listed the sixteen states with anatomy laws highlighting bodies to be dissected as defined in their laws to resolve this issue. Its supporters concluded that most of the states named selected "bodies for dissection in the manner provided in the District of Columbia."[39]

As to the bill, King et al. posed the question "can subjects be provided for dissection without offense to public sentiment." He argued from the economic view that "colleges would not go to the expense of purchasing material at the high prices paid resurrectionists, when they could obtain them at less cost, and in a legal manner." Also, from a sort of "boosterism" and the old truism of protecting the sepulchers, "shall the capital city of the country, the very center of science, art, education etc., lag behind the neighboring states in the humane proceeding of legally protecting the graves of people from the resurrectionists."[40] And finally, providing the "proper education of a physician of Washington and the surgeons in our Army and Navy, which the United States Government actually commands, shall operate on and dissect the bodies of the dead."[41]

King also stated that "the authorities accept the need for dissection [and] they know our methods prevail in other cities everywhere anatomy is taught," and when "suitable legislation is passed" there is a "legitimate provision for bodies." The argument concluded with the old but useful truism that this will "put an end to the disreputable business of resurrecting bodies of respectable persons from cemeteries."[42]

The second anatomical bill was not passed in 1890. A third bill was introduced in 1892 after a plan developed by the Washington medical colleges "to throw the odium attached to body snatching off themselves." The bill was introduced on February 1, 1892, by Mr. John J. Hemphill of South Carolina, chairman of the House Committee on the District of Columbia. It was a bill for "the promotion of anatomical science and to prevent the desecration of graves in the District of Columbia."[43] The bill would have established a procedure for the delivery of cadavers of those who were to be buried at public expense from hospitals, prisons, almshouses, jails, morgues, and asylums within the District of Columbia to the authorized agents of D.C.'s medical colleges. The bodies were to be proportionately distributed by the number of students in each college. Exemptions were provided for those who previously asked for burial and the requests for their bodies from relatives, friends, strangers and travelers to be buried. To ensure identification, the names of the deceased were to be published in a daily paper in the city of Washington before they could be sent to a medical college. After use the body was "to be decently buried."

However, the most troublesome part of the bill for the medical colleges was the severe punishment for those who engaged in the trade:

> Whosoever shall use such body or bodies for any purpose other than that aforesaid, or shall remove the same beyond the limits of the District of Columbia, and whosoever shall sell or buy such body or bodies, or in any way traffic in the same or who shall disturb or remove bodies from places in which they have been buried, shall be deemed guilty of a misdemeanor, and shall on conviction be imprisoned for a term not less than two or more than three years, at hard labor, in the jail of said District.

The bill received a second reading in the House and was referred to the Subcommittee on the Judiciary; however, no further action was taken on the proposed bill, as no one "was pushing it." The commissioner of the District of Columbia, G.W. Douglass, chairman, notified the House committee on February 26, 1893, that they were "not prepared to make a report." According to a newspaper report, the bill was "pigeonholed," and the "medical Colleges in whose interest it was alleged to have been drafted, do not want it passed."

The delay was due to second thoughts by the medical establishment in Washington. The schools realized that "grave robbery in Washington would go to the wall." The "colleges feel they cannot exist without the aid of the grave robbers." The reasons were "counting out the pauper dead under fifteen years" and those requesting a proper burial, and the colleges "could not get more than 150 bodies a year." They would still need 150 bodies and require the resurrectionists. However, the law would cut off the "ready material" of the resurrectionists because Congress threatened them with a three-year imprisonment at hard labor that would force them to find other employment or "raise the tariff on the subjects to an exorbitant rate." According to the newspaper, the medical schools "had a great deal to lose by the passage of this bill."[44]

Although there were other attempts to introduce an anatomical bill in Congress for the District of Columbia, it was not until April 29, 1902, that the U.S. Congress finally passed "An Act for the promotion of anatomical sciences, and to prevent the desecration of graves in the District of Columbia." The law included an anatomical board for the control and distribution of dead human bodies that consisted of "a district health officer, two members from each medical school, one from the post graduate school and one from the medical school of the army and navy." Those who died unclaimed within the District of Columbia had to be "apportioned to the medical institutions according to the number of students enrolled each year."[45]

Nevertheless, there were still extensive restrictions included in the new law. For example, the board had the power to appoint and remove officers and had to keep detailed records of transactions and facts regarding the "receipt and distribution of bodies" and allow any board member and the district attorney of D.C. access to these records. All officials encountering dead bodies had to give written notice to the board, and requests made by the deceased for burial or cremation or by friends and relatives had to be honored.

Notices to relatives were required, and the board was mandated to list the names of the dead in Washington newspapers once a week. All bodies had to be used in the District of Columbia. However, the punishment was mitigated for breaking the law. Anyone who trafficked a body outside Washington or conveyed a body from a grave or vault (without a permit) would be punished with not more than a $200 fine or up to a year in the workhouse. Any official or individual who transgressed this law would be tried in the police court and could expect a similar sentence. No doubt the difference in the punishment from a possible three-year prison term at hard labor as proposed in the 1892 bill to one year in the workhouse was obviously a compromise to maintain the availability of some resurrectionists and to obtain buy-in from the colleges.[46]

In summary, during the 1880s and well into the late 1890s the city government of Washington, D.C., and the federal authorities actively supported the body-snatching activities of the Washington medical schools. As noted previously, the dean of the National Medical College had already admitted in 1888 in a letter sent to Congress that the "police and judicial authorities are fully cognizant of this method ... [and the police] ... often visit our dissecting rooms at their pleasure—and could if they chose arrest every one of us."[47]

The colleges had free rein over Potter's Field, even calling it the "Scientific Ground" while using a procedure to ensure deniability and anonymity to protect themselves if bodies were obtained from other cemeteries.

Due to the nature of D.C.'s footprint, the medical schools and authorities realized that to obtain sufficient subjects the resurrectionists needed to be retained and tolerated, and this explains why the D.C. anatomical law passed by Congress in 1902 substantially reduced the punishment for trafficking in dead bodies from the 1892 proposed anatomical law.

Unfortunately, it is sad to admit that the period from the early 1880s to the late 1890s was the heyday of body snatching in Washington, D.C., and Washington likely led the nation in this crime.[48] As a New York City newspaper reported, in the District of Columbia "the violation of sepulture is almost as common as house robberies in New York City."[49]

As for the anatomical law being sold to the public in Washington eliminating the trafficking of dead bodies, Dr. Llewellin Eliot was not so sanguine. He wrote in regard to body snatching in 1916 that "I do not believe any law will ever stop body snatching, what Sir Astley Cooper said before a committee of the House of Commons: 'There is no person, let his situation in life be what it may, whom, if I were disposed to dissect, I could not obtain.'"[50] Dr. Eliot, having experienced body snatching and the tortured passing of the anatomy law in Washington, D.C., was right to be pessimistic about its entirely ending the practice there.

11

Observations on the Victimization of Blacks, the Poor, and Immigrants

Recently much has been written about Blacks and their role in the history of the progress of medical science, especially their "powerlessness" in the face of the need for cadavers for dissection due to the rise in the number of medical schools in the United States in the nineteenth century. Like the poor and immigrants, the newly freed Blacks found themselves on the low end of the social hierarchy for the living and the dead. The pinnacle of the dead was the "respectable white citizens interred in churchyards."[1]

We have seen examples of this in earlier chapters, especially in Washington, D.C., where grave robbers exploited the private "colored" cemeteries and "colored" sections of public cemeteries for years with little resistance, and later whites and Blacks who ended up in the Potter's Field burying ground would end up on the dissecting tables of D.C.'s medical colleges. Many of the reports of body snatching in the Washington newspapers had as their victims Blacks.[2]

Body snatching was a lucrative endeavor, made more so when less investment was required. Throughout the nineteenth century the "resurrection men" avoided being "exposed to the wrath of an organized religious community," confronting "watchers," or having excessively difficult access to the grave by robbing the graves of indigents and Blacks as "ideal victims of the anatomists."[3]

The following examples illustrate the egregious exploitation of Blacks in the body-snatching activities in the Northeast from the late eighteenth to the end of the nineteenth century.

The Case of Anthony Frederick and His Wife Jenny

I begin with the interesting body-snatching case of Anthony Frederick, a free Black man, and his wife Jenny. Based on the document from the trial, there is no doubt that the judge harbored a deep antipathy toward Frederick, but what is even more intriguing was his unusual support at this time for the idea of body snatching, especially for medical education. Unfortunately for Frederick he could not have chosen a more biased judge to come before with his claim. After reading this case, as the reader will see, the judge is named in a well-known medical document, one of only two that has survived from this period that helps to explain much of what is found in the record of this case.[4]

In 1782 in Boston, Anthony Frederick brought the following writ, as summarized by Israel Keith, a judge of the Massachusetts Court of Common Pleas. "As Mr. H.

[Frederick's lawyer] in aggravation of ye injury supposed to done by Doctor [Benjamin] Curtis,[5] to Anthony Frederick, representing it not only as an impiety and unmerciful attack upon the feelings, the Honor and reputation of said Anthony, but even as an outrage upon the Dead: and as there is great reason to believe there was some dead creature brought into a room under Doctor Curtis' roof, and there dissected."[6]

Keith was unsympathetic and admitted up front that he was on "the other side of the question." And as we will see, there is more to be gleaned from his response than a judge irritated by a free Black man bringing charges against a doctor both white and an elite member of the community.[7] "I will suppose for the sake of argument that Jenny the wife of Anthony Frederick was dug up, brought to Doctor Curtis' house and there dissected. Now if this is a crime it must arise from all or one of these three reasons. Because it was an impiety, a violation of the rights of the individual or a breach of the Laws of Society…" said Keith. "That it is not an impiety or disobedience to any divine law is most evident, because it is no where said that thou shalt not dig up or dissect a dead negro…." He explained why it was not a case of impiety. "Is it not equally impious to disturb the bones, which have lain fifty years, as those which have lain but one? The Deity has given no commands concerning it—The world has done as it pleased—in Egypt they embalmed, in Rome they burned … and thousands are very carelessly tumbled into the sea. In fact, it is no matter what becomes of the body. It is but a broken cage."

As for it being a "violation of the rights of the dead, this is absurd; for a dead body has no rights or property. It has no capacity to feel or power to revenge an injury…. The hope of a future state of existence first taught men to bury the dead with decency, and the vulgar idea that the same particles of matter were necessary to the resurrection has invested them with all their imaginary rights…. But since S. Paul and Mr. Locke[8] have been read in the World these false ideas are wearing off by degrees and dissections—and the making of skeletons has become the common practice in all the countries where the Arts and Sciences flourish."

Keith made his case for dissection:

> Are not the malefactors which are hanged at Tiburn [Tyburn, England] given to the surgeons; and are not strangers everywhere dug up and dissected,—And how great an advantage this has been the world is beyond the power of language to express for if surgeons cannot form their practice in some measure from the dead, they must do it upon the living at the hazard of life. The propriety of this measure is so much felt here at present that though dissections have been performed in this town [Boston] for two or three years past without secrecy, yet no one complained till Anthony Frederick.[9]

Not content with this argument, Keith goes further and brings in the death of doctor and general Joseph Warren, the elder brother of Dr. John Warren. John and several other medical students who formed the Spunker Club studied under Dr. Joseph Warren at Harvard. It has been suggested that Dr. Joseph Warren may also have participated in the Spunker Club.[10] Joseph Warren died at the Battle of Bunker Hill in Charlestown, Massachusetts, in March 1775. His body was buried by the British on nearby Breeds Hill. Keith continued:

> Could not the immortal Dr. Warren have slept as quietly. Would not he have been more uneasy at the blowing tempest or the rattling hail under the clods of Charlestown than in Boston? It was the pride in human nature that caused his removal.

The public wanted to honor Joseph Warren by finding his body and removing it to the "Old Granary cemetery in Boston."[11] But to do this Joseph Warren's body had to be identified among the many dead. Just prior to the battle Paul Revere had made two artificial teeth for Joseph. Keith wrote that both the colonialists and the enemy were "crowded into one common vault" (buried on the battlefield); "must the bodies of these poor men who dwelt happily … be disturbed … after lying a year in the bosom of the earth! and all for the sake of one man! Even their teeth were examined! Nevertheless, this disturbing of the dead has never … been called an injury. Doctor Warren was raised and brought over to Boston in triumph."[12]

Judge Keith said that even the recently dead were disturbed, and I would add that there is no doubt their bodies and skulls were manhandled looking for the two artificial teeth that Paul Revere had fashioned for General Joseph Warren that would identify his body.

After lecturing Frederick and his lawyer on the many possibilities as to why a body might rightly be disturbed in the grave, Keith turned to the task at hand. He began by insulting Frederick and his late wife. Earlier he had said, "suppose for the sake of argument" the body was Jenny's. Now saying Jenny was "no stranger or malefactor, but the wife of Anthony, and though she has suffered no injury, yet the feelings of an affectionate husband have. The writ says … it caused … Anthony great pain and distress of mind. Could I really believe this I would pity him.… But where are the scales, where is the balance that shall way [*sic*] the feelings of Anthony Frederick?" Keith addressed Frederick:

> Have you not repeatedly affirmed that Jenny was a whor [*sic*], a slut, and a drunkard, and that you was [*sic*] glad she was dead! Did not you tell me in my office with a laugh that Doctor Curtis had got his pay for tending Jenny while alive by converting her into his own use when dead? Are these the feelings that are valued at a thousand pounds? I have seen a horse that would feel more for his great grandfather![13]

Keith finally addressed the third issue, the law itself. Accordingly, he wrote that there was no law that gave Frederick "a right or property in the body of Jenny of a longer duration, than that expressed in the marriage covenant—'until death does them part.'" Although one historian has noted that Keith reduced the former couple to the "status of strangers,"[14] it was unfortunately the way common law was understood and not unique to Keith in determining the case before him.[15]

Judge Keith concluded that all Frederick could bring against Dr. Curtis was a "simple action of trespass." Even on this issue Frederick had not offered proof that the dissected "negro" in Dr. Curtis's house was Jenny. Keith knew on this charge that there was also no common or statutory law in Massachusetts to award the husband damages, "and what do our Statutes say upon the subject? Nothing! They are as silent as the Negro that is dissected."[16] He unnecessarily heaped insult and injury at Frederick by insulting his late wife and at Frederick by exposing what he had likely said in confidence to the judge. No doubt that he asked for $1,000 in compensation (a substantial sum in 1782) added to what Keith probably thought was Frederick's effrontery.

Why was Judge Keith so familiar with arguments in support of the doctors' and surgeons' need for cadavers as well as arguments countering religious and philosophical objections? This knowledge was likely acquired by his having spent two years attending Dr. John Warren's lectures on anatomy. It also explains Keith's familiarity with General Joseph Warren's reinterment and rabid antipathy to Frederick's case.

As evidence, Keith received what exists today as only one of two examples of the original and historically important certificate given out by Dr. John Warren and printed by the engraver Paul Revere.[17] Written on the certificate is the following: "These may certify that *Israel Keith Esq.* has diligently attended an entire course of my Anatomical Lectures & Demonstrations; together with Physiological & Surgical observations at the dissecting Theatre in the American Hospital, BOSTON: whereby he has had an opportunity of acquiring an accurate knowledge in the structure of the human body. John Warren F.M.S. [Fellow. Medical. Society?] BOSTON March 28th, 1782."[18]

The Frederick Anthony case is a rare and early example of the position of the way in which a free Black man found himself entangled in the courts in Boston over the obvious stealing of his wife's corpse for dissection purposes and a judge who, unfortunately for the Anthony Frederick case, appeared to have been a hyper-partisan supporter of medical views likely limited to a few elites at this time.[19]

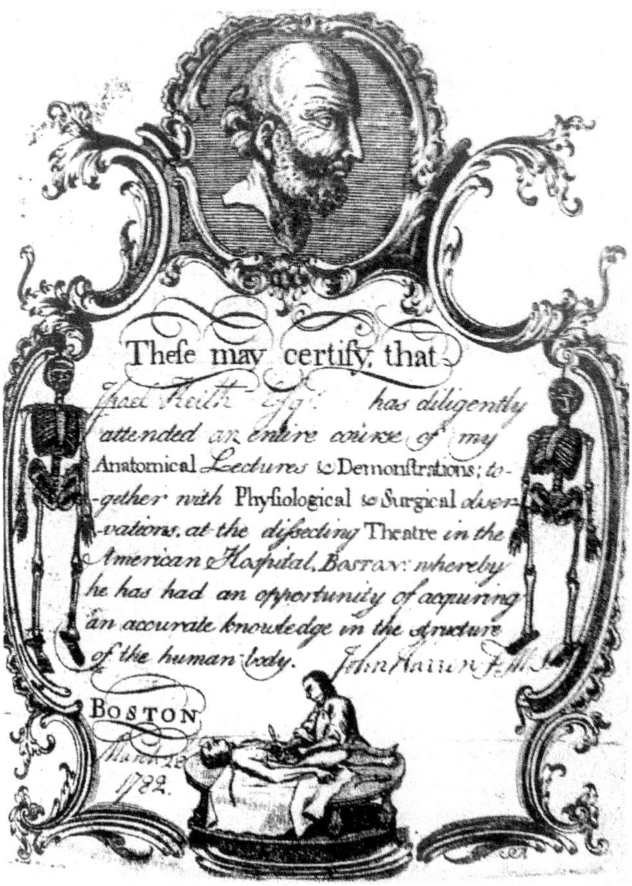

Judge Israel Keith's "Certificate of Attendance at Dr. John Warren's course of anatomical lectures." Harrington, Thomas F. *The Harvard Medical School a History, Narrative and Documentary.* New York: Lewis Publishing, 1905, v. 1, 84. (courtesy of the John Hay Whitney Medical Library, Yale University).

Black Bodies in New England

Later in Massachusetts on February 20, 1810, John Warren and Aaron Dexter presented a "Memorial and Petition for the Removal of the Med. Lec. To Boston." They argued "for moving the Harvard Medical School from the University's home in Cambridge ... to Boston." As one historian wrote, from there the medical school "could avail itself of cadavers of the poor black and white denizens of the almshouse."[20] The medical school moved to Boston a year later. The Harvard medical students appeared to prefer the Almshouse cemetery.

Initially, students at Harvard Medical School had sufficient bodies to undertake their studies. But as medical schools proliferated in New England, the competition for subjects became intense. "Students from the developing schools were sent to Boston to procure subjects which they did in a careless and sloppy manner. The public thus aroused by blatant grave robbing set grave watchers in the burial yards."[21] John Warren of the Harvard Medical School was forced to send to New York for anatomical specimens. It is almost certain that many of these cadavers purchased from New York were Blacks, as the primary "victims chosen by the grave robbers were those interred in pauper's graves or the Negro burial grounds, chiefly because large numbers were buried together, frequently without coffins, making procurement of cadavers infinitely easier."[22]

Black Body Parts Noted in the Dartmouth Dissection Laboratory

Although slavery had been on the decline in New England, Dartmouth College in New Hampshire had been "one of the largest slaveholders" in the New Hampshire "colony and later the state, and its officers buried enslaved and free black laborers in the college cemetery."[23] In 1810 Ezekiel Cushing, a Dartmouth medical student, wrote to his sister that "I have this moment returned from the dissecting room, where there are at present the remains of fifteen of our fellow creatures in every stage of decay, and of all ages, sexes and colours," indicating that the dissecting room contained "negro" specimens.[24]

In 1811 the Dartmouth medical school obtained its own building. The basement was soon filled with "human and non-human bones." Craig S. Wilder surmises that many of the skeletons in the basement of the new medical school were "likely those of enslaved and free black people" who, like Cushing's specimens, undoubtedly had been originally buried in the Dartmouth cemetery.[25]

Generally, few medical colleges in New England acquired anatomical subjects from "remote areas" before the advent of railroads. Most of the country medical schools, such as those in Vermont and New Hampshire, claimed to acquire subjects from large cities, but most were locally sourced. In large cities they claimed that bodies were acquired from remote areas. "It is likely that nearly all cadavers used in each medical school in New England before the Civil War were disinterred in the immediate neighborhood." The receiving of cadavers from long distances was only possible after "the railroads became common and especially after the Civil War, when bodies of southern Negros were used in northern medical colleges. Bodies were shipped in barrels labeled as some commodity."

> A gentleman now deceased, who was a demonstrator and later a Professor of Anatomy in a medical college in New England, told me a few years ago that during several years in the eighties and nineties he had an arrangement under which he received twice in each session a shipment of twelve bodies of southern Negroes. They came in barrels marked "turpentine" and [were] consigned to a local hardware store that dealt in painting materials. The receipt of two large shipments of turpentine in the season of the year when little painting was done created no suspicion as to the real contents of the barrels.[26]

The Story of the Negroes Burying Ground in the City of New York

In the city of New York in the late 1780s, approximately 15 percent of its population was Black, consisting of slaves and free blacks. Free Blacks who were not poor and slaves "were buried in the Negroes Burying Grounds, a segregated section of the potter's field, which was adjacent to the Almshouse." Both private doctors and Columbia College's medical school obtained many of their cadavers from the Negroes Burying Grounds.[27] On February 14, 1787, the recently freed Blacks and slaves petitioned the city's common council.[28] They complained that "it hath lately been the constant Practice of a Number of Young Gentlemen in this City who call themselves Students of Physick, to repair to the Burying Ground assigned for the use of your Petitioners, and under cover of the Night, and in the most wanton Sallies of Excess, to dig up the Bodies of the deceased friends & relatives of your Petitioners, carry them away, and without respect to Age or Sex, mangle their flesh out of a wanton Curiosity and then expose it to Beasts & Birds."[29] The petitioners recognized the value of "consulting dead subjects for the benefit of Mankind" but only asked the board to adopt traditional measures and limit dissection to "people convicted of capital crimes," the original source of subjects for dissection.[30] Unfortunately, the petition was unsigned and was not endorsed by the city clerk and did not appear in the minutes.[31] Later on February 16, 1788, a "letter of protest" appeared in the *New York Daily Advertiser* stating "few blacks are buried whose bodies are permitted to remain in the grave." Complaints followed that female bodies not taken due to "alarm" were being devoured by swine, and human flesh was found "along the docks, sewed up in bags."[32]

The Black community could not marshal the resources to protect and secure their dead, and the plundering of the Negroes Burying Ground continued.[33]

Throughout the nineteenth century, Black people were especially sensitive to both body snatching and dissection from a religious and moral point of view. They, as others, believed in "a literal corporal rising from the grave."[34] Dissection "represented a gross assault upon the integrity and identity of the body and upon the repose of the soul."[35] For Black people the wound was deeper; following the Civil War, being recently freed, they saw the inability to protect their cemeteries and dead as "emblematic of their failure to gain equal rights."[36]

In addition, free Blacks knew that dissection was also a method "to punish rebellious slaves."[37] One notorious example was the treatment of the body of Nat Turner, a slave who had led a revolt in Virginia in 1831. Following his execution, his body was likely dissected. Virginia whites saw bodily mutilation as a "sign of their contempt and an additional humiliation to the person executed," a common fate of rebellious slaves.[38]

The Nation's Capital

The reader is advised to see chapters 9 and 10 in this book for many examples of the exploitation of Black cemeteries to provide subjects for Washington's medical schools and the attempt to export illegally obtained Black bodies out of the district for use in medical schools in other states.[39]

For example, we have the newspaper reports of the notorious Washington grave robber George Christian's diary published in the *Washington Evening Star* on December 15, 1873, as evidence that most of the burying grounds he visited were either for Blacks or in the "colored" sections of public cemeteries.[40]

Another but somewhat contradictory fear was the stories about "night doctors" started after the Civil War by southern whites trying to prevent Blacks from migrating to northern industrial centers. "Among the most effective rumors deliberately circulated by southern whites concerned the kidnapping and murdering of urban African Americans for anatomical dissection."[41] The rumors where so effective that even whites feared the "night doctors,"[42] although there was no evidence that people were being murdered to supply the dissecting tables of American medical schools, especially those in Washington, D.C., until as previously discussed the "burking" of Emily Brown.[43]

To conclude, even Black soldiers who served in the Civil War were not exempt for a final service to the medical profession. As a result of the "death rate from disease, malnutrition, and dehydration," a preponderance of Black cadavers "became the subjects for autopsies" by the military surgeons. In a study titled *The Negro as a Soldier* (1868), 405 autopsies were performed, and of these 381 were on Black corpses and 24 on white corpses.[44]

The Lebanon Cemetery Scandal of December 1882

Perhaps of all the misfortune and treatment of Blacks regarding the exploitation of their bodies stolen from cemeteries and burying grounds for dissection, one of the most egregious was the theft of bodies for at least eleven years from the Black burial ground the Lebanon Cemetery in Philadelphia, Pennsylvania, that culminated in the arrest and trial of a band of "resurrectionists" in December 1882. Yet in the end, the effective resistance of the Black community that threatened to riot and close the renowned Jefferson Medical College in Philadelphia led to a reformed anatomy law in the state of Pennsylvania that later served as a model anatomy law for other states. The events and the law had national implications and influenced later events in Washington, D.C., as noted in Chapter 10.[45]

In 1867 a liberal anatomy act had been passed by the Pennsylvania legislature called the Armstrong Act. It only applied to Philadelphia and Allegheny Counties. There were not enough legal bodies available for the medical schools in Philadelphia. It was suspected by some journalists and a few "Negro leaders" that "resurrectionists" had been visiting the Lebanon Cemetery for the past fifteen years to obtain cadavers for dissection.[46]

Suspicions leading to the Lebanon Cemetery scandal were aroused the previous March when a Jefferson Medical College student sitting in Dooner's restaurant in Philadelphia asked about a recently deceased popular Black waiter named Canon Wicks. Mr. Dooner told him the waiter had been dead for at least a week. The student remarked, "I saw him only two days ago."[47]

Mr. Dooner visited Mr. Louis N. Megargee, city editor of the *Philadelphia Press*, who had let his body-snatching suspicions be known and told him of his odd conversation with the medical student. Megargee decided to observe activities at the Jefferson Medical School. He became suspicious of several men and "obtained complete information on the men's occupations and haunts." Megargee and his colleagues, posing as doctors, began mixing with the suspected resurrectionists. The men were "watched in the act of carting bodies away from the [Lebanon] cemetery, and in the act of transferring them from the express wagon to the very room in the Jefferson Medical where the subjects are prepared for dissection."

They had "discovered an organized gang of dealers in dead bodies." They learned that there was a citywide conspiracy of "doctors, graveyard superintendents, and undertakers who were involved in the ghoulish business." However, as warm weather was approaching, the confrontation had to be put off. Operations were suspended in the summer and would resume at Jefferson Medical "with the cold weather, and the renewed demand for subjects for the dissecting knife." Once the cold weather set in, they began preparing for a "confrontation" with the resurrectionists.[48]

On the evening of December 4, 1882, three men were moving stolen bodies from the Lebanon Cemetery to the "receiving vaults of the Jefferson Medical School." The three men were stopped at 11 p.m. and arrested at gunpoint by Mr. Megargee, four reporters, and a recently hired Pinkerton Agency detective named William Henderson. The men arrested included Levi Chew (Black), Frank McNamee, and Henry Pillet. Robert Chew, brother of Levi Chew, the cemetery superintendent, was arrested later that evening, and Andrew Mullen, a mail carrier, was arrested the next morning. McNamee was an express man. His wagons advertised his name on both sides. Mullen, or "Yank," was employed by McNamee to carry mail in his wagons, and Pillet, or "Dutch," also was an employee of McNamee's. Levi Chew was a laborer.[49]

The wagon carrying the bodies and the men were taken to Eberle's stables, where the men were held under arrest. The wagon and horse were returned to McNamee's stables, and the six cadavers were returned to the morgue, where "all but one of the bodies was identified." According to further reports, even at that early hour "a large crowd gathered around the Morgue[;] ... some individuals were apprehensive that the bodies stolen might be those of friends."

The prisoners' hearing was to be held at 4:00 p.m. that day. The news spread like "wildfire[,] ... creating tremendous excitement among the colored population." The accused entered through the back entrance to the building. Once the crowd realized who, they were there were shouts of "Who's got a rope?" and "Bring a rope." "Passing from lip to lip ... [there was] a disposition to lynch the prisoners." Others reported a more demonstrative Black crowd; "the crowd made another rush, and men and women attacked the captives, who shrank and cowered before them."[50]

After the accused were questioned, Megargee described the events of their capture, and how three men were later taken to the Pinkerton Agency. And most importantly, he implicated Jefferson Medical College by telling the magistrate that McNamee had keys to the Jefferson Medical College doors. Megargee also described the arrest of Robert Chew that evening. Chew said that "he had been at the cemetery eleven years, and bodies had been taken away for eleven years by his brother, by Solomon Butcher [his brother-in-law], John Mayer, and McNamee: sometimes bodies left in the receiving vault over night were removed, and the empty coffins buried." Some of the bodies were buried in shallow graves of only three feet so the gang members could easily dig them up later (especially in an area called the "homestead" in the cemetery). Coffins without bodies were buried containing stones and bricks along with the clothing of the dead.[51] Records showed that in two months fifty-five bodies were buried in one grave.[52]

Each prisoner had bail set at $5,000 for a further hearing. The streets were filled "solidly from wall to wall" with "an enraged crowd, and while no serious trouble was apprehended, it was thought desirable to avoid so far as possible any chance of a misunderstanding between the crowd and the officers."

The prisoners were kept in a back room until the crowd outside receded. "Word was sent to the Central Station, and [with] ten reserves coming up as an escort a procession was formed, and the march to the jail began." However, the crowd quickly "collected again as the prisoners were led along, and followed them hooting and making uncomplimentary remarks, but as far as is known, no demonstration of violence."

On the afternoon of December 6, 1882, at an emergency meeting that was called to address the body snatching scandal at the Lebanon Cemetery, the trustees of the Cemetery dismissed Robert Chew from his position as superintendent of the cemetery. The subject of prosecuting the trustees of the Jefferson Medical College was "broached," but no definite action was taken. A resolution to "employ counsel to prosecute the criminals who despoiled the graves" was passed.

The graves of eight people in the cemetery were opened. "In the grave where Josephine White was supposed to be buried, the bodies of Elizabeth and John Gibbons were found. The body of Louise Morris, aged 103 and Leah Lynn's body who was buried December 29, 1880, was missing. In their place where two bodies should have been, was found a coffin with nothing inside."[53]

The president of the Board of Trustees, Guy M. Burton, an undertaker, explained the body-snatching procedure. Bodies were taken by "resurrectionists" from the "homestead" portion of the cemetery, where bodies were buried "scarcely more than three feet in depth." Bodies in the middle of the cemetery were removed under the direction of the superintendent and brought to homestead, "where they were placed under a few inches of earth, ready to be taken away by McNamee." The graves were then covered up. The trustees offered help to every lot holder who wished to examine a grave. They also resolved to ask the police chief to place an officer near the cemetery to preserve order.

This request was necessary because the excitement created by the "disclosure of the wholesale body snatching at the Lebanon Cemetery for the use of medical students of anatomy at the Jefferson Medical College" did not subside. No doubt the testimony uncovering the "ghoulish" practices of the body snatchers engendered one shock after another. Excitement reached a fever pitch. The *Philadelphia Inquirer* reported that "yesterday the colored people having relatives buried in the cemetery flocked to the grounds. As the morning wore on at least 2000 colored people congregated within the enclosure[,] many provided with shovels and picks with which to dig up the coffins of the departed."

However, only those with permits from the Board of Health could disinter their deceased family and friends buried there. Those who did not have a permit were refused permission.[54] *The Philadelphia Inquirer* reported for December 7 that "no diminution was observed ... in the crowd of colored people, which ever since the exposure of the resurrectionists, has been thronging Lebanon Cemetery from mid-day to nightfall. If anything, these numbers acceded those of the day before[;] ... a squad of policemen was dispatched to the scene." Likely to quell the digging in the cemetery, the Board of Health cautioned that there would be no more permits issued because of the possible exposure to bodies of persons who had died of smallpox, diphtheria, or other contagions.[55]

The "Indignation Meeting"

A meeting was called at "Liberty Hall" on December 7 to protest the profanation of the cemetery. The meeting occurred in a large "densely packed" hall, composed primarily of "colored men and women." Before the meeting began the more "excitable" members of the audience made vigorous denunciations of the superintendent of the cemetery, Robert Chew, and the "Trustees and faculty of the Jefferson Medical College." Members of the audience who had "deceased friends and relatives interred in the ravaged burial grounds were moved to tears in their doubts concerning the safety of their bodies."

The chairman of the meeting was Major James H. Teagle, who sat on the dais with several others including clergy. He said that "it was one of the worst wrongs ever perpetrated on the colored people." Several speakers followed, united in expressing their "sympathy" for those who had suffered this "calamity" and exhorting the audience to prosecute those responsible for the "outrage."

At this time, a resolution was adopted thanking the members of the press who had been "concerned in the arrest of the grave robbers." Several other addresses followed the passing of the resolution. The mood was somber and quiet until the jailer at the Seventeenth District police station, H. Price Williams, rose to speak. He first spoke of the episode that had brought them together and then turned his ire on the Lebanon Cemetery Board of Trustees, claiming they were "unworthy of the trust reposed in them." The audience exploded in "angry mutterings" and shouts of "indignation." He stated of the "fifty-five bodies buried in one grave in the space of six weeks that the cause of their removal had been going on for nine years past" and accused the Board of Trustees as the brains behind this activity, declaring that "every member of the board of trustees ought to be behind bars."[56] He then challenged the integrity of the president of the Board of Trustees, Guy M. Burton, and claimed that as an undertaker his actions conflicted with his duties as a "responsible official of the Negro cemetery's governing board."

When Burton rose to reply, some audience members moved forward with "revolvers in their hands." Police officials had to restore order. Other speakers came forward to describe the "horrible nature" of the crime of December 5, and while one speaker urged no violence "until every effort of the law had been exhausted, this speaker did suggest the lynch law as a last resort."

When a minister spoke and demanded "that twenty years of body snatching at the Lebanon Cemetery be avenged," there was immediate "boisterous applause." A second minister charged the faculty of Jefferson Medical College with "culpability on the principle of the receiver being as guilty as the thief."

With order restored the meeting concluded, with the Black audience "reflecting its outrage" by offering two resolutions. The first concerned the "disgraceful robbing of the graves in the Lebanon Cemetery by a class of human fiends," and the second was an expression of appreciation for "Megargee and his colleagues for the 'arrest and imprisonment of the body snatchers.'"[57]

The Trial

The trial of the grave robbers was held on December 15, 1882. Six bills of indictment were drawn up "charging them with violating the right of sepulture," in removing six bodies from the Lebanon Cemetery.

A jury was selected that consisted of eleven white men and one Black man, Charles H. Davis, the foreman. Just prior to the trial Mr. McNamee and Mr. Pillet changed their pleas from not guilty to guilty.

Prior to the beginning of the trial of Robert and Levi Chew, who pleaded not guilty, an affidavit was presented to the court by the district attorney on behalf of a trustee of the Lebanon Cemetery "charging Dr. Forbes, Benham and Lohman of the Jefferson

Medical College, with conspiring with the defendants to violate the right of sepulture, also to disturb the cemetery, and he asked for a warrant to be issued for the arrest of those persons."[58]

The direct involvement of the Jefferson Medical College in this body-snatching scheme had been earlier confirmed in the first reports concerning McNamee having the keys to the building. On December 6, 1882, the day Robert Chew was dismissed, a former janitor had come forward with more explosive information connecting the college with the body snatchers. He revealed that "he had helped receive subjects brought to the college by the prisoner." His duties had been to put them in "pickling vats" to help Dr. William S. Forbes, anatomy demonstrator at Jefferson, to "inject them" and to hoist the "stiffs" out of the vats into the "dissecting room." He said he could not bear the "stench" and quit. He was told not to reveal anything about "his duties at the college."[59]

As a result of the district attorney's request, the court issued a warrant for the doctors. Forbes and Lohman were brought into court that day and were released on bail.

Witnesses were called against Robert and Levi Chew. They included Megargee, his four colleagues, and Detective Henderson. Afterward the "Commonwealth rested their case."

Robert Chew claimed total innocence. He said that he was confused when Megargee came to his home to confront him and that he told him "he was afraid of ghosts and that was the reason he didn't assist in snatching bodies." His brother Levi said that he came to the cemetery "purely by accident" and that when he told his brother he had a "small pox patient he was simply joking." (Earlier it was determined that the password for obtaining bodies was that they had a smallpox case.)

The case went to the jury, "who without leaving the box, rendered a verdict of guilty." The Black foreman of the jury remarked in a soft voice, "Is there no law to hang them?"[60]

In some respects, the community had gotten some justice with the guilty verdict of the body snatchers, but the trustees knew that the community wanted some punishment rendered to the cause itself, the Jefferson Medical College trustees, and the faculty. Punishing them was the only way to prevent the future exploitation of the bodies of their family and friends buried in the Lebanon Cemetery. McNamee admitted that his business had been ruined with the publicity and the guilty verdict at the trial. Speaking on his own behalf, he tied the body snatchers directly to Jefferson Medical College.

McNamee admitted that Dr. Benham had gotten him started in the business three years earlier by hauling legal cadavers. McNamee was introduced to Dr. Lohman, at Jefferson Medical College, by Benham, who took him down to the burying ground to obtain corpses. Lohman cheated McNamee of the money he was owed. McNamee began dealing directly with Dr. Forbes, cutting out the middleman. Forbes said that anything McNamee had to do for the college "he would get me to do it, and then I would be paid." Levi Chew would inform McNamee when bodies were available, and he would go to Dr. Forbes and say, "We will have some bodies coming tonight." Forbes would "give him the keys and tell somebody at the college to stay up and receive the bodies. Dr. Forbes knew where we got the bodies from; as he told me about it before I knew anything about them."

At one point McNamee had asked Dr. Forbes if he could get in trouble for hauling these bodies from the cemetery. Dr. Forbes said, "You can't have anything done to you; you do nothing but the hauling." Later he told McNamee that there were two judges connected with the college, and "I wouldn't, and they wouldn't do you any wrong." McNamee also claimed that he never went to any other cemetery.

Pillet stated that he only worked for McNamee and did not know he was doing anything wrong. Sentencing was deferred for the guilty. As stated earlier, the two physicians from Jefferson Medical College appeared, and bail was set. The court then adjourned. Dr. Benham was from out of state and did not appear.[61] The four found guilty had their sentences delayed "until Forbes was brought to trial."

On December 18, 1882, Dr. Forbes was indicted on eight counts that included "conspiring with McNamee and others to despoil the graves at the Lebanon Cemetery" and "violating the right of sepulture, by removing bodies from the grave." The prosecution brought McNamee from the "prison to be used as a witness before the grand jury."[62]

Rumors were rife that the district attorney was attempting to rush Dr. Forbes's trial while passions were inflamed. According to the *Philadelphia Inquirer*, prominent members of the elite reform Committee of One Hundred in Philadelphia rose to his defense, questioning if this was appropriate and protesting that a delay would offer a better opportunity for a fair trial.[63] "They argued [that[Dr. Forbes position could not seek exposure in so grave a matter for no proportionate object and that whatever he had said to McNamee had reference solely to legitimate sources of supply to the college." It was also argued that McNamee had threatened Forbes "if he did not get counsel for him." And it would be "contrary to the traditions of the court to base any trial actions on the unsupported testimony of a convicted prisoner and one who, it is said cannot be believed upon oath."

Sentences for the four men were handed down on March 29, 1883, following the conclusion of the trial of Dr. Forbes on March 17, 1883 (see below). Robert Chew, because he was the superintendent of the Lebanon Cemetery, was the most culpable. He received two years in prison. His brother Levi Chew, who had access to the cemetery and worked there, was also culpable and received eighteen months. Frank McNamee and Henry Pillet, as "strangers in their relations to the cemetery[,] have been guilty of no breach of trust and Pillet having no part in the planning of the crime least guilty of all." McNamee received eight months in prison, and Pillet received four months in prison.[64]

Jefferson Medical College Responds to the Accusations

The morning following the reports that the Lebanon Cemetery had suffered the grave robberies, a gaggle of newsboys appeared in front of Jefferson Medical College "loaded down with copies of the *Press*" crying out "arrest the body snatchers," "startling disclosure," and "violated graves." Other cries prominently mentioned Jefferson Medical College. A crowd of two hundred students and newsboys quickly formed. The students' remarks showed that they did not take it seriously: "we know nothing of this" and "I'm glad we don't have to furnish the stiffs." The professors looked very serious. When Dr. Forbes appeared at the school, people could see that he "was as white as a sheet."[65]

Following the hearing on December 5 when testimony established that McNamee had keys to the college doors, the college administration argued that "the case was entirely exceptional, and that the authorities would have acted with great promptness in suppressing the offense, had they known of its existence, and bringing the guilty parties to justice." They claimed that "nearly all the bodies brought for dissecting were obtained by means known positively to be legitimate, and that the man employed to bring them to the institution was supposed to be trustworthy."

In defense of the college one doctor claimed that when "irregular offers were made to furnish subjects they were rejected; the regular agent was furnished with keys to bring in bodies because he was believed to obtain them legally." Also, they had figures on the subjects, and these "would vindicate the college with authorities."

Dr. Forbes, the demonstrator of anatomy, said "that man has hauled unclaimed bodies for us from the prison and the House of Correction, for which service he was paid, and the keys entrusted to him."[66]

Following the "Indignation" meeting on December 6, one doctor was reported to have said that there was likely to be trouble at the college because of the "reception of the stolen bodies from the Lebanon Cemetery." This would go straight to the Board of Trustees because they had chosen the current "demonstrator of anatomy," Dr. Forbes. The demonstrator is "required to give bonds that the dead bodies shall be procured ... from such sources as the hospital, almshouse, prison, and morgues. When they have been unclaimed by their friends." The "recent disclosures ... prove that more care must have been exercised formerly than at the present in obtaining bodies for dissection."[67]

The physician proved prescient when on December 15 Dr. Forbes was indicted by a grand jury on the testimony of McNamee.[68]

Meanwhile, the dean of the college got the local authorities to guard the college against any assaults.[69] While the dean was having the school guarded, Professor and Dr. William H. Pancoast of the college invited a distinguished alumnus, William J. McKnight, state senator, doctor, and convicted body snatcher in his youth.

As a youth, McKnight had been studying medicine with the local doctors in Brookville, Pennsylvania, in 1857. One of the doctors, Dr. Simons, had ambitions to become a surgeon and was eager to dissect a recently deceased Black man named Henry Southerland. Due to a series of misadventures, the body prepared for dissection was discovered in an icehouse. Murder was at first suspected and inflamed the town. The *General News Press* reported the story in the following manner. "The body was laid on ice, with a board under the shoulders and head, the legs and arms spread out, the entrails taken out and the skin taken off, evidently in a position for the purpose of dissection." Twelve men were called to the scene to function as a jury, and after examining the site they concluded that the body had been removed from a local graveyard and that they believed it was "the body of Henry Southerland, a colored, being buried several days previously."

According to McKnight, the townspeople were unhappy with the doctors involved, and David Barclay, a congressman, was preparing to prosecute the men involved. McKnight's brother, a young lawyer, had heard rumors of the intended prosecution and convinced him to turn himself in to the authorities. McKnight subsequently appeared before Squire Smith and was charged "under the act of 1849, to protect graveyards." He pleaded guilty and was fined twenty-five dollars and court costs. His brother had convinced him to go to court to avoid "double jeopardy" in the event Barclay's case went forward and Barclay tried to implicate McKnight in having played a more serious role in the "resurrection" rather than only having acted as a lookout.[70]

It was McKnight who would successfully advise Dr. Pancoast on what to do to save Jefferson Medical College. During dinner on December 10 the question arose as to "what effect 'this scandal would have on the college.'" Dr. Pancoast exclaimed, "The College is ruined." McKnight replied that this was an opportune time "to secure legal dissection for Pennsylvania." Naturally, the other guests disagreed with him. He said it should be presented as an "act to prevent the traffic in human bodies and to prevent the desecration of grave yards." Dr. Pancoast saw the merit in this approach and asked him to meet with the dean of the college the next day. The meeting was unfruitful and had elicited a "violent confrontation." McKnight told Dr. Pancoast that "if you get the Philadelphia Anatomical Association to draft a suitable law, and send it to State Senator Reyburn, of that city, I will support it through the Senate."[71]

Dr. Pancoast attempted to calm the deans and the medical staff at Jefferson Medical College as well as other medical people in Philadelphia. A member of the Philadelphia Anatomical Association, Dr. Pancoast asked them to consider McKnight's counsel for a new anatomical act. Initially, with the indictment of the grave robbers and their proposed trial in mid–December, he undoubtedly thought this would make his task easier. However, with McNamee's confession in open court and the indictment of Dr. Forbes, it seemed that Jefferson Medical College had been put in a "precarious" position. This also raised the question of Philadelphia's future role in medical education and its ability to compete with New York, Boston, and other places with more progressive anatomical laws.[72]

The Trial of Dr. William S. Forbes

The next hurdle for the college was the upcoming trial of Dr. Forbes, scheduled for March 16, 1883. According to the obviously sympathetic approach of the *Philadelphia Inquirer* to Dr. Forbes, his prosecution was begun under "great and unreasoning public clamor."[73] Dr. Forbes was charged with engaging in a "conspiracy with Frank McNamee and others to rob the graves of the Lebanon Cemetery." The judge's summary to the jury was that even though the bodies were illegally obtained by McNamee and the two Chews, Dr. Forbes must be judged on whether he is a "party to a conspiracy either by original agreement or subsequent assent" to take corpses from the Lebanon Cemetery. It was only on this basis and this alone that "the charge must stand or fall."

Other issues such as the value of anatomy to society, although discussed in the trial, had nothing to do with the case, as jurors were to decide "not what the law should be but what it is." Two key issues supported by others in their testimony were that the supply of bodies from local institutions was inadequate—"bodies are frequently obtained from other sources," generally unclaimed bodies and only from suppliers they knew—and that Dr. Forbes was not in charge of the anatomy room; it was Dr. Hawson who received supplies for the facility. Dr. Forbes had only met McNamee once and had never heard of the Lebanon Cemetery until the news of the body-snatching episode was published.

The judge addressed the jurors before their deliberations and emphasized the character of McNamee and Forbes. The judge also reminded the jurors that McNamee had been convicted of a crime and that the "law looks upon the testimony of an accomplice with grave doubt. Uncorroborated by other testimony, direct or circumstantial[,] it is not in law sufficient to convict." Dr. Forbes was presented as a man of great character and probity and, unlike McNamee, had nothing to gain.[74]

Forbes's supporters thought that the matter would be quickly settled and that the jury would return immediately. However, it was not until the following day that the verdict of not guilty was rendered. The courtroom erupted in a thunderous ovation.[75] The only concern by his supporters was that Forbes had to go through the trial in the first place. His final words during an interview after the trial where that he had not known "of any such place as the Lebanon Cemetery."

According to the *Philadelphia Inquirer*, there was no "proof produced worthy of a moments consideration," and "he should never have been indicted. The public were not satisfied with the conviction and punishment of the robbers of graves." The article continued by placing the blame on the Jefferson Medical College, as "the real defendant" was not Dr. Forbes but rather the college itself because it was the college that was "responsible for the course of study pursued in the Anatomical department." Dr. Forbes's only responsibility was to "receive the material for that department without questioning the source."

The article concluded with the need to provide material for the study of anatomy and urged legislation to avoid this problem in the future.[76]

The crusading newspaper the *Press* wrote "that when Dr. Forbes's professional and collegiate associates assert that the acquittal clears him ... of any complicity with or knowledge of the bodysnatchers, they impose a tremendous strain on the evidence which it will not bear."[77]

A Modified Anatomy Act

Before the acquittal of Dr. Forbes and shortly after the trials of the men who had robbed the Lebanon Cemetery, Dr. Pancoast, on the faculty of Jefferson Medical College and a member of the Anatomists Association, at a meeting of the association on December 28, 1882, "induced" it to frame and forward a new state anatomy act and send it along to a friendly senator in the state legislature. Following a series of meetings and drafts in January and February 1883, on February 9, 1883, a committee within the association was appointed to send the petition to the legislature. The petition was titled "An Act for the Promotion of Medical Science for the Distribution and Use of Unclaimed Human Bodies for Scientific Purposes ... and to Prevent Unauthorized Uses and Traffic in Human Bodies."

Importantly for our purposes, the petition spoke to the concerns of the entire community but especially the Black community, whose ire had been raised by the long-term exploitation of Black burial grounds such as the Lebanon Cemetery. At the forefront of the petition, besides increasing facilities for medical education in Pennsylvania it included "and in preventing desecration of burial grounds."[78]

On February 28 the act was offered to the senators in the Pennsylvania legislature. McKnight, who had actively participated in this proposal and had promised to move it forward with all dispatch, saw to it that it was presented the next day to the senators. There was a contentious debate, with senators from outlying counties arguing that the proposed act was "discrimination against the poor unfortunate person who has no relative claimant." Others argued over the "sharp class distinction" that the government was proposing. Some thought that the idea of dissection was "disgusting ... especially because the commonwealth's most miserable class of citizens was expected to supply the subjects" and wondered whether our poorest would "be devoted to science, to investigation, and study."[79]

The historian Horace Montgomery noted in this case that the arguments against the proposed act "betray the late 19th century resistance to enlightened methods in medical education." Certainly elites, who were aware of new ideas from Charles Lyell and Charles Darwin undermining the hold of religion on nineteenth-century thought and the impact of Jeremy Bentham and Herbert Spencer on the individual's role in society, especially the latter two, seemed encouraged by the idea that for a poor person who had failed in life, when taken care of by society, there was a debt owed and that the debt in death was to be paid on the dissecting table for the greater good for the living.[80]

As noted previously, the arguments against this law did not stem from benighted ignorance but did have validity. The fear of being dissected harked back to the debasement of the criminal body after death as a further punishment for a crime. The concern for the poor as noted in the repeal of the Connecticut Act of 1833 was based on the fear that anyone could end up destitute if circumstances worked against them. Among many religious people, the resurrection of the body was still considered a reality.[81]

As for the improvement in medical education, it had certainly begun but not wholly on the dissecting table, and in fact gross anatomy was being replaced by physiology, microbiology, and evolutionary theory as well as a host of newly developing subfields.[82]

Other overt political aspects of the argument were the accusations that the Philadelphia senators were only ever interested in their own city and that they argued for the removal of the section in the proposed act that "the corpses of the poor of the interior of the State shall be dragged to Philadelphia ... if they say the necessities of medical education require it."[83]

Senators John E. Reyburn, who oversaw the bill, and William McKnight responded to their colleagues' arguments. Reyburn replied that "the true test of humanity of medical education was the competence of the State's physicians" and was likely more important to allay the fears of the Blacks and others throughout the state to "assure a second result of ending such desecration of graves as recently occurred in Philadelphia." Finally, unless the act was passed, Philadelphia would see a decline in its medical schools through a lack of cadavers in relation to cities such as New York, with more liberal state anatomy laws.[84]

Finally, McKnight argued in support of the act. He addressed the "essentials of medical education as well as the polemics of the opposition." Further, "Humanity ... should first be shown to the living," for it was they "we must legislate for ... not the dead."[85]

The bill was passed in the Pennsylvania Senate by a vote of 26–7 on March 7, 1883, and sent to the lower house.[86]

There is no doubt that the revolt over the desecration of graves in the Lebanon Cemetery had been a motivating factor for rapidly moving the act forward to prevent another episode. The senators were debating this act in early March prior to the trial of Dr. Forbes. As Forbes later wrote, public indignation over this had not died down from his "day of arrest to the end of the trial, [and] certain newspapers of this city during the entire period, with the most determined rancor, continued to arouse the public to a great pitch of excitement."[87]

Visiting the Dissecting Rooms and the Pickling Vats of Philadelphia's Medical Colleges

While the doctors and legislators had been active following the arrest and conviction of the Lebanon Cemetery body snatchers, there remained the trial of Dr. Forbes. If he was convicted, it was believed that this would have a chilling effect on the future of medical education in Philadelphia.

With the acquittal of Dr. Forbes their fears were diminished, and on March 28, 1883, representatives of the Pennsylvania House legislative committee working on the modified anatomy act were given a tour of the Philadelphia medical colleges that included Jefferson Medical College, the University of Pennsylvania, Hahnemann College, and the Philadelphia Dental College. The report gives us an unusual view of the medical colleges' work rooms and incidentally suggests the racial makeup of most cadavers used in these institutions.

The first college visited by the committee was Jefferson Medical College. The committee witnessed a young man "whittling a bone from a dried and partially dissected colored cadaver." There were thirty-nine tables in the room, and four held cadavers. When the covering on one body was pulled back, the trunk was splayed open, and a strong odor permeated the area. Representative William Bryson of Columbia "succumbed" and had to leave the room.

Dr. Forbes met the committee in the receiving room and took the members to view "five large square wooden tanks[;] … one of these was opened and five bodies, black and white, were exposed." Meanwhile, Dr. Forbes explained how the cadavers were preserved through their "pickling process." He also pointed out that there were fifteen bodies in the tank, which represented the current "stock of subjects on hand in the college. The winter session [was] … at an end." One assistant on hand said that "175 bodies had been through the tanks" during the prior session.[88]

What was not said was that most of the bodies were undoubtedly "colored" and that many were likely from the Lebanon Cemetery. Mr. McNamee was the main supplier to Jefferson College. As one witness, Henry Allen, "testified, in 1881 and 1882 he had been employed by Dr. Forbes at the Jefferson College to preserve bodies and to take care of the dissecting room." He claimed that McNamee had brought bodies to the Jefferson College "about once or twice a week; he often brought three or more bodies; they were generally colored people, although, there were one or two exceptions."[89]

Dr. Forbes "pointed with pride to the general cleanliness of the room." Considering his indictment and acquittal, he probably thought it would be a good idea to remind the committee that he ran a quality operation and said that "he was glad to show the representatives that this department of the college was conducted as properly and with as much regard to privacy as possible."

The legislators moved on to the remaining schools, taking the longest time at the University of Pennsylvania. Most of their time was "spent in the dissecting room and but a few moments in the pickling vaults." The dissecting room was a marvel for its time, said to be the "best arranged, lighted, and ventilated … with fifty-five tables." That day there were three subjects arranged on the tables, and a fourth cadaver "supplied by the coroner" was being worked on.

The chairman of the committee, Thomas McReynolds, called his members together at the conclusion of the tour and asked the doctors about their thoughts on the "bill now pending in the Legislature providing for the supply of medical colleges with legitimate subjects." The physicians replied that the committee should understand that medical students came from the entire state, and as a result they believed that the 1867 law should be applied statewide and that unless an "adequate supply of legitimate subjects would be provided the supremacy of Philadelphia as a metropolis of medical education would be lost."[90]

The committee was true to its word, and the House passed the bill "with a minor amendment back to the Senate on June 4, 1883. Governor Robert Pattison signed the Act on June 13, 1883."[91]

Importantly, the act prominently proclaimed that it was intended to not only further the medical sciences but also prevent trafficking in human bodies. It was titled "An Act for the Promotion of Medical Science by the Distribution and Use of Unclaimed Bodies ... and Prevent the Unauthorized Uses and Traffic in Human Bodies."

The act contained eight sections and applied to the entire state and, most importantly for the first time in any American anatomical act, required compliance. The first section established a board for "the distribution and delivery of dead bodies." In the second, officials were required to notify the board of all bodies to be buried at public expense except those with kin who requested interment and travelers who died suddenly. The third section required that the board was to receive bodies and distribute them. The fourth section states that the board "may employ a carrier or carriers for the conveyance of said bodies." The fifth section stated that medical persons had to be bonded before they could receive any corpse. The sixth section stipulated that the board would regulate the price of bodies and that the cost would be "paid by those receiving the bodies." The seventh section stated that anyone who neglected their duties "enjoined upon them by this provision of this act" would be fined not less than one hundred dollars or more than five hundred dollars. And the eighth section stipulated that all acts inconsistent with the act would be repealed.[92]

Besides the medical needs that would be met by this act, there was the social uproar and the potential danger to the continued success of the medical community in Philadelphia. On the practical side, the physicians and colleges were sensitive to the potential threat from the Black community if the acquisition of illegally obtained Black corpses continued. It was hoped that this new law would suppress the unlawful theft of cadavers, eliminate the need for colleges to deal with the loathsome "resurrectionists," and ensure that physicians and the colleges of Philadelphia would never have to experience both the threats of violence they had just witnessed and the legal assault that might have come to the schools if Dr. Forbes had been found guilty.

The Pennsylvanian Anatomy Act of 1883 established a model for anatomical acts in other states.[93] By 1896 the American Association for the Advancement of Science wrote of the Pennsylvania Act that "of the anatomical laws which are in force in this country the committee is of the opinion that the law of the State of Pennsylvania is best." For their purposes, not only was it best for the promotion of medical science, but it also mitigated "the desecration of the resting place of the dead."[94]

In 1905 a professor of surgery at Jefferson Medical College, Dr. William Keen, commenting on the Pennsylvania Anatomy Act, also called it the "best in the United States" and spoke not to desecration of the dead but instead to the hurt to the living and their indignation that helped engender the act, "which provisions carefully prevent wounding the sensibilities of the community."[95]

Clearly one of the reasons for the genesis of the anatomy act of 1883 was the indignation and threats by the Black community of Philadelphia. No doubt the credit given to Dr. William Forbes as the father of the anatomy act of 1867 that formed the basis for the anatomy act of 1883 is deserved, and even the actions of the doctor Senator William J. McKnight for helping to pass the act were merited. From the late eighteenth century to most of the nineteenth century, Black grave yards, burial grounds, and bodies were exploited with ineffective resistance. With the wholesale body-snatching episode at Lebanon Cemetery, for the first time Black resistance had forced the medical and political elites of Philadelphia to pass a law to stop this outrageous practice. The act limited the wholesale theft of the dead and appeared to provide sufficient bodies for the medical community of Philadelphia. The irony is that the Black community in Philadelphia received little or no recognition for the important part they played in helping to bring the loathsome traffic of unbridled body snatching to an end in Pennsylvania through passage of what the scientific and medical authorities of the time considered one of the "best" anatomical laws in the United States.

Immigrants and Poor Whites

Black people "were not the only victims of the widening gap between the legal supply of cadavers and the demands of medical schools. Body snatchers preyed most frequently on the dead of impoverished and powerless whites. White paupers crowded the country's almshouses, particularly outside of the South. In death they filled most of the graves in potter's fields."[96] Even though some states created "legal channels" for obtaining executed criminals, the numbers were "pitifully inadequate." For example, between 1800 and 1830 "Massachusetts executed less than 40 persons," a totally inadequate number for the anatomists of Massachusetts.[97] While the Connecticut Anatomy Act of 1824 was also proven inadequate to meet the needs of the anatomists and physicians,[98] it seemed that the least objectionable way to obtain cadavers without "provoking public outrage" was to "steal the dead of groups who could offer little resistance and whose distress did not arouse the rest of the community." Besides Blacks, the other groups were immigrants and poor whites.[99]

Interestingly, in his oft-referenced article, John B. Blake wrote that the failure of even "liberal anatomy acts" passed after the American Civil War essentially "subordinated the supply of cadavers to the prejudice of institutional directors."[100] This was even evident in the earlier anatomy laws passed in Massachusetts and Connecticut.

For example, in 1850 Dr. John C. Warren of the Harvard Medical School, commenting on the Massachusetts Anatomy Act of 1831, concluded that the obstruction to obtaining cadavers was due to the superintendent of the House of Industry, who opposed the law. The superintendent died in 1847, and Warren maintained that now "an ample supply was obtained for the Medical School particularly in consequence of the influx of Irish paupers, and the great mortality among them."[101] However, in 1855 Dr. George Hayward somewhat ghoulishly wrote that "the supply has not been perhaps as great as could be wished: but, with the increase in population and pauperism, this objection will pass away." Even as late as 1881, Edward M. Hartwell wrote that the bodies of the dead in Massachusetts are "valuable material at the bottom of the graves.... The anatomists wish that an administrative law could be passed so that all the appropriate bodies in the entire State, as well as Boston, should be delivered to them at their dissecting room."[102]

As we saw earlier, the failure of authorities responsible for the poor to support the Connecticut Anatomy Act of 1833 permitting the cadavers of the poor to be made available for dissection led to the rescinding of that portion of the act in 1834. Legal acts for obtaining bodies of the poor for dissection continued to lack the support of many officials in various states in which they were passed even as late as the early twentieth century. For example, a state hospital disposed of its dead in "quicklime so they could not be used for dissection." The hospital was only half a mile from a northern school by necessity, but importing cadavers from Tennesee. This showed the "lack of cooperation between different state institutions."[103]

As a result of the lack of cadavers for dissection, an increasing number of medical schools, physicians, and demonstrators turned to the illegal acquisition of the bodies of immigrants and poor whites. In the larger cities (such as Chicago), bodies would be procured "illicitly from three sources of supply. First, potter's fields; second, other cemeteries, (necessitating dangerous recklessness), and third bribery, directly or indirectly, almshouses and prisons before burial."[104] In addition to these, mental institutions and morgues were also utilized.[105] Public burying grounds, almshouses, and potter's fields were exploited the most by body snatchers. For example, in 1879 about five thousand cadavers were dissected each year in the United States; "at least a majority are illegally obtained, many of them by actual purchase."[106]

As noted previously, outside the South, native whites and immigrants made up most residents of almshouses. Of these a "disproportionate number of immigrants ended up in the illicit cadaver traffic." One-eighth of the population in 1880 was foreign born, but immigrants accounted for 34.6 percent of the enumerated almshouse population that year, while native whites represented 56.8 percent and Blacks 8.9 percent.[107] In 1913 a survey of fifty-five colleges asked them where they received the main supply of their subjects, and most named almshouses as their main supply. Other colleges gave tuberculosis hospitals as another primary source of cadavers.[108] Tuberculosis mortality rates were especially high among Blacks and poor whites, killing "150,000 people annually at the turn of the century."[109] By 1910, nearly "half the paupers in almshouses outside the Southern states were foreign born, mainly Irish and German."[110]

As Humphrey wrote, the passage of "a liberal anatomy act did not necessarily eliminate body snatching." State laws were not effective because, as we saw earlier, even in the nation's capital (although Washington, D.C., did not have an anatomy law and supplied bodies to other states), "illicit traffic in cadavers was a far flung, interstate business" that was difficult to police and to prohibit. Nevertheless, the anatomy laws passed in other states to prohibit body snatching served a purpose. The legalization expanded the supply of bodies "and by limiting dissections to unclaimed bodies, substantially reduced the amount of personal suffering caused by the seizure and dissection of recently deceased relatives and friends." On the other hand, legalization continued the attitude of "the days when judges condemned a criminal to dissection after execution."[111]

There is evidence of the fear of this stigma and its persistence throughout the nineteenth century documented earlier in the century by the father of Joseph Smith, Jr. (future founder of the Mormon faith), Joseph Smith, in Palmyra New York, in 1824. Even though he was said to be on the verge of losing his property, when a rumor spread that his son Alvin's body had been stolen and dissected, Smith still was able to find the money to advertise "in six consecutive issues of the *Wayne Sentinel*" the following:

> NOTICE TO THE PUBLIC: Whereas reports have been industriously put in circulation, that my son, Alvin; had been removed from the place of interment and dissected, which reports, every person possessed of human sensibility must know, are peculiarly calculated to harrow up the mind of a parent and deeply wound the feelings of relations; therefore, for the purpose of ascertaining the truth

of such reports, I, with some of my neighbors, this morning repaired to the grave, and removing the earth, found the body which had not been disturbed....

This method is taken for the purpose of satisfying the minds of those who may have heard these reports, and of informing those who have put them in circulation, that it is earnestly requested that they would desist; therefrom; and that it is believed by some, that they have been circulated more by a desire to injure the reputation of certain persons than by a philanthropy for the peace and welfare of myself and friends.

Joseph Smith sr.
September 25, 1824[112]

The rumor turned out to be false. Joseph felt the need to advertise this fact because the real fear was that if Alvin had been exhumed and dissected, it would have carried a "stigma" suggesting his family "as people who were unable to protect their dead, whose dead deserved no protection." As the nineteenth century progressed, the concern with respectability was not just among the middle classes but also those who aspired from the lower classes. The need to continue to differentiate themselves with respect to their dead from "indigents, criminals, blacks, and Indians" was paramount.[113]

Even by the early twentieth century, the same fear of a pauper's burial persisted. As one writer reported, "the poor ... naturally have a horror of a pauper burial in the light of the apathy and indifference of those who subject the bodies of the dead poor to humiliating indignities,"[114] including the stigma of dissection and the "humiliation imposed on social outcasts."[115]

The historian D.C. Humphrey was correct when he concluded that the new anatomy laws "confined dissections to a voiceless, widely scorned segment of society.... Legalization did expand the supply of cadavers and, by limiting dissections to unclaimed bodies, substantially reduced the amount of personal suffering caused by the seizure and dissection of recently deceased relatives and friends. But legalization also perpetuated an attitude that had not changed much since the days when judges condemned criminals to dissection after execution: dissection remained a humiliation imposed on social outcasts."[116]

Conclusion

Body Snatching and Rumors Leading to a Breach of Trust and Comity in Two New England Towns

Two examples of a breach of trust and comity in a small community and its consequences can be seen in the New England towns of Ipswich and Manchester, Massachusetts. In Ipswich, the traditional social and political leadership of the public's "betters" in what was still a highly structured society was severely damaged by the town's betrayal by its doctor, Thomas Sewall. Not only was he the trusted town doctor, but he had also married into the upper class in the town. A few months after the discovery of the missing bodies, at least one elite, the town minister, Reverend Crowell, seemed to do his best to calm the situation, condemn the perpetrator, and restore some comity to the town. The consequences of Sewall's actions following his trial and guilty verdict led to his exile from the town and no doubt a distrust and stain on this leading town family for generations.

A similar crisis of confidence occurred in the neighboring town of Manchester when the town minister, both an elite and someone understood to be preparing the souls of the faithful for the next life, became involved in what was presumed to be a possible body-snatching scandal. This was the result of an inartful letter sent to Dr. Sewall by his former brother-in-law, Dr. Rueben Mussey, professor of anatomy and surgery at the Dartmouth College Medical School. Mussey wrote that the town minister, Reverend Thurston, had made promises to attract a young doctor to the town, stating the doctor would be able to obtain bodies in the town for dissection. The information and ensuing actions of the minister tore the town and church apart, eventually leading to mistrust in the authority of the church. To resolve the issues, an outside ecclesiastical council was convened. An investigation into this specific charge and related charges was deemed so damaging possibly to all clergy that it might lead to a crisis in confidence throughout New England. The council refused to consider the charges and decided on a lesser charge, agreeing that the comity of the church in Manchester was beyond repair, and the council recommended that Thurston receive an honorable dismissal. He was forced to leave Manchester. However, for those who opposed Thurston, they believed that the honorable dismissal was unwarranted and reflected poorly on the ministers who approved this decision and no doubt created mistrust on the spiritual worthiness of these clergymen.

Attacks on the Medical Schools in New England

All the attacks in the New England medical schools were not spontaneous but instead were based on a breach of community norms. Citizens were terrorized by the ongoing body snatching, either real or suspected, from their burying grounds. The authorities whom they expected to provide some protection for them and their dead failed to do so. The citizens believed that they had a moral right to address their grievances by taking the following actions: threatening doctors and their students, marching on the medical buildings and dissecting laboratories, damaging them, and threatening to destroy or tear them down.

The memory of these crimes long endured in the communities affected. Many newspapers that reported on these crimes were not entirely sympathetic with these episodes and actively criticized them, while others called for various solutions to prevent these actions that included improving the sepulture laws by incorporating the anatomical needs of the medical profession.

The Heroic Age of Medicine

The heroic age of medicine during the heyday of body snatching was anything but heroic. There were few reported improvements in medicine to make the argument to the laity that benefits were accruing from the dissecting laboratories.

The public attitude toward the medical profession and medical students as late as the 1880s is strikingly illustrated in "A Poem of the Hubbardton Raid Read in the Congregational Church Hubbardton May 12, 1880," where the medical students and doctors are defamed as lazy, mercenary, and quacks. This was believed by the public at the time of the Hubbardton Raid in 1830 and would begin to change following the American Civil War but more so toward the end of the nineteenth century.

The "quality of medical care remained low" throughout most of the nineteenth century, "although it did become more standardized due to the popularity of medical school training." The ability to diagnose illnesses was "unsystematic and superficial." The treatment of serious illnesses was "characterized by bloodletting, purgative doses of calomel, emetics, and blisters, all disguised to reduce the patient's fever, inflammation, and related symptoms."[1] As one doctor noted at the time, "all bled, all gave emetics, all purged, all starved their patients. They were real Sangrados [quacks] mowing down alike the infant, the youth, the adult, and the old man."[2]

In the area of surgery where there should have been expected improvements (after all, why the justification to the public for cadavers?), because of the practice of dissection there was little improvement found. As late as 1842 the daily duties of the surgeon were still little different than those of centuries past: "bleeding, cupping, leeching and enemata and other injections, the stomach pump; bandaging[;] … the construction of ligatures; sutures and dressings." In addition, there was the treatment of "certain wounds and deformities; fractures, luxation's, [dislocations] with the construction of splints." Without anesthetics and "ignorance of the causes of infection," operations were dangerous and painful.[3]

During the American Civil War it became obvious that there were critical deficiencies in medicine and surgery. Following the war, a "definite and concerted action began to improve the program of medical education.… Emphasis was placed on needed improvement in certain subjects. Two of these were practical anatomy and operative surgery on the cadaver."[4] Ironically, this required more corpses, creating a renewed interest in improving the anatomy laws. Meanwhile, to meet the new demand before improvements could be made in the anatomy laws, there developed a brisk trade in cadavers throughout the country, as in Washington, D.C., following the Civil War.

As for overall improvements in general medicine and surgery, this can be attributed to the speculations of Louis Pasteur on the "germ theory of disease" and its application by James Lister in 1864 using carbolic acid to kill germs, making surgical procedures that previously led to deadly infections less dangerous.

Evolution of Anatomy Laws and the Legal Expansion of the Subject Pool

Initially, the need for cadavers in medical schools was limited because students did not do human dissections. Historically, in England doctors did not operate on patients; this was left to barber-surgeons sometimes under the direction of a physician. Early "surgeons depended on speed, brute strength and optimism." In colonial America besides doctors, surgery was also performed by lawyers, tavern keepers, tailors, and even cobblers.[5]

John Jones, an American surgeon and the author of the first surgical textbook in the American colonies, advised potential surgeons on two related matters to improve their profession and raise their status. Besides attending anatomical lectures, the student should perform "frequent dissections of dead bodies with his own hands" and be "acquainted with the branches of medicine which are requisite for an accomplished physician."[6]

By 1823, there were eight medical schools in New England. Now, with the influence of Parisian medicine, students were required to not only observe the dissection of a cadaver in the amphitheater but also do human dissections. The problem was that there was no change in the anatomy laws that would have more easily supplied subjects for dissection. There were only two options: either turn to grave robbing or give up on the teaching of anatomy with student dissection as a requirement.[7]

Body snatching and the New England states' anatomy laws are inextricably linked. The laws over time were an attempt to discourage body snatching by providing sufficient subjects for the medical schools to prevent the stealing of cadavers from burying grounds and cemeteries for dissection.

At the beginning of the national period, the states had continued to follow English common law. In Massachusetts, the first laws were imposed not to aid the cause of anatomy but instead to further punish the criminal. For example, in Massachusetts, first murderers and then duelists were candidates for dissection. The New York law following the "Doctor's Riot in 1788" for the first time extended those who could be dissected to those put to death for burglary and arson.

The Connecticut Anatomy Law of 1824 may have been influenced by the New York law because the former extended dissection to any prisoner who died in the state prison at Newgate. However, this law was not effective and did not meet the needs of the anatomists. For anatomists it was, however, a step in the right direction. Although no action was taken, there was discussion (perhaps for the first time in an American legislature) in the Connecticut House of Representatives about expanding the pool of subjects to include the poor. This early attempt failed because throughout a good part of the nineteenth century, the citizenry saw "dissection [as] an ignominy and anyone whose body was dissected suffered posthumous disgrace and was thereby allocated to the same class as murderers."

The next phase in the passage of anatomy laws in New England was a result of the William Burke and William Hare scandal in Scotland. The public became aware "that grave robbing was more frequent than they suspected." While the newspapers carried the stories, the medical societies and legislators became involved in this issue. In Massachusetts in the past, physicians trying to interest legislators in anatomy legislation were ignored because of the "well known popular aversion to dissection." In February 1829 the Massachusetts Medical Society proposed an anatomy bill to a legislative committee, but the committee would not put the bill forward without "the support of public opinion." A committee from the Massachusetts Medical Society "sought to educate the public"; a pamphlet was prepared "in support of the proposed law, [and] 10,000 copies were sent throughout the state." The bill was introduced in May 1830 and finally passed on January 31, 1831, as "An Act More Effectively to Legalize the Study of Anatomy in Certain Cases." It was the "first effective anatomical act in the English-speaking world" and preceded the "Anatomy Act of the English Parliament" by fifteen months.

The law required civil officials to surrender any body that was to be buried at public expense (with some exceptions) for dissection, "going beyond the former limitation to the bodies of major criminals."[8] In other words, "a certain description of paupers are [*sic*] appropriated to this object."[9] The law had many limitations that nullified its intended purpose and, as we saw earlier, primarily pertained to Boston, with a rich immigrant population to draw on for subjects.

The Massachusetts law directly influenced the Connecticut Anatomy Law of 1833, a law in conflict with Connecticut's poor law system. Besides an insignificant immigration pool to draw from as in Boston, the changing political situation, a deteriorating economy, and resistant public opinion from the beginning all contributed to the law's repeal in 1834.

An anatomical law like the Massachusetts law was passed in 1834 in New Hampshire. It was repealed in 1842. A proposed anatomical law in Vermont in 1835 was never passed.

The American Medical Association was organized in 1847, and for all the work of its committees, papers read, and proposals, it had little effect on reforming the anatomy laws.[10]

There were numerous factors that prevented the acceptance of reforming the anatomy laws in not only the New England states but other states as well. One of the most significant before the Civil War was the religious or spiritual resistance found in most people of the prewar era. When Dr. Crowell argued in his sermon in Ipswich, Massachusetts, against grave robbing and the horrors of dissection, it was a template for later arguments for a good part of the nineteenth century if not beyond. The seemingly strange inability by the public and their legislators to embrace what today would seem a commonsense argument for providing subjects for the dissecting rooms and the ongoing resistance to the reform of the anatomy laws stemmed from the innate religious beliefs of Protestant antebellum America. These beliefs would later be challenged by the carnage of the Civil War, and the resulting attitude shift, combined with postwar intellectual and scientific medical developments, led to a fourth stage of anatomy laws introduced in most states, including those of New England.

The historian Mark S. Schantz has convincingly argued that prior to the Civil War, most Protestants took an "anthropocentric view of heaven" and "saw existence beyond the grave in … material terms. Resurrected persons would live on not in spirit but in full possession of perfected bodies." Although there were a multitude of arguments over the nature of how this occurred, in the end for most believers' inconsistencies were set aside, and "antebellum Americans tended to strongly favor materialistic ideas about the resurrection body."[11] The arguments of the anatomists and those trying to pass legislation in most of the states to acquire more cadavers would have been hard-pressed to overcome this now deep-rooted religious objection to destroying the physical body of anyone and interfering in God's plan for their resurrection.

These ideas as they related to dissection can be illustrated in an article written before the Civil War by Henry Raymond, later cofounder of the *New York Times*. Prior to this he was the editor of *Harper's New Monthly Magazine*. In April 1854 he wrote an editorial titled "The Sacredness of the Human Body." A good portion of the article discusses religion and dissection. He wrote that even in death for the body, "there is still remaining something of the former selfhood." For him, the "necessities of medical science have been overstated. Even when want is conceded, the benefits may be purchased too dear. Best that the causes of some bodily diseases remain concealed, that the knowledge of them be obtained at the sacrifice of some of the best feelings of the soul."

Raymond argued that the number of subjects needed in the medical schools is absurdly high and that the "number of graves disturbed, and human bodies desecrated every year, must be reckoned in the thousands." His solution was anatomical representation, as he saw no need for students to perform dissections when illustrations and models were available.

Raymond found the core problem to be an "increasing indifference to the grave[,] and its sacred contents must produce a state of mind at war ... with the most solemn revelations in Scripture." From the religious view, Christ's most important work "was the redemption of the body as well as of the soul." Further, citing Corinthians 15:14–20, if "the dead rise not, then is Christ not risen and if Christ be not risen, then our faith is in vain." Raymond wrote, "The air of the dissecting room is unfavorable" to this belief, "not that the superficial scalpel of the surgeon could even penetrate the psychological and physiological mystery" but that the "tangible associations are hostile to the Scriptural view."[12]

> It is true the dissecting of the Lecturer, and the after combustion of the janitor, do more than hasten a process which is going more slowly in the earth; every body [*sic*] understands that as well as those who would permit it as their profoundest argument; but, as far as associations and feelings are concerned the difference is immense.

As for the question of whether it is the same corruptible body that will be raised, "it is enough it be the same body[;] ... what is sown in mortality will be raised in immortality," and his example was the body of Christ. The body in the grave, Raymond wrote, rests secluded in "divine guardianship of silent waiting for the great day of deliverance from the dominion of death and Hades; with the other we connect ...the ideas of ignominy, of vile abuse of irreverence, of irreligion." For Raymond, the Christian grave is "as a sacred chamber that contains a hidden treasure" and not, as we have seen earlier, a body referred to as wasted material at the bottom of the grave.

Raymond contrasts the religious view of the body "as the once loved temple of the human spirit" lying in serene repose with the corpse in the dissecting room. "Thus, lying mangled, debased, deformed, made the subject of unfeeling remark by some cold materializing lecturer and ruder hands of the hardened and it may be [a] licentious student."

Finally, Raymond turns to the legislators who would be responsible for the anatomy laws supplying the medical schools with their subjects. "It is the general demoralizing effect at which we have hinted, that should make legislators pause before they give facilities to practices which may involve such momentous consequences."

As for the poor, Raymond expresses the viewpoint that their life is hard enough, so why should their friends have to contend with their dead friend's "ignominious descent to the grave [and] ... be all the more painfully sensitive to the thought of violence to their remains"?

For his conclusion, Raymond returns to an earlier period: let the medical profession have its subjects but "the fewest as possible."[13]

As for how to treat the poor, Mrs. Sarah Gould in her influential book *The Guardian Angels: Or Friends in Heaven* (1857), instead of focusing on the impact of dissection on the friends of the poor, exalts the religious to feed and bless the poor and thus receive a "glorious reward."[14]

With viewpoints such as this likely among religious people, with the sacredness of the body in the corpse there remains "something of its selfhood," and indeed the same body "will be raised again." It is no wonder that there was great hostility toward reforming the anatomy laws, because doing could be seen by the religious as a society complicit in a threat to the basic Christian belief of the bodily resurrection.

Raymond articulated many of the core beliefs of the understanding of the body, its scaredness and the reasons for its treatment after death before the Civil War. To the religious, dissection of the body and the insistence on exploiting the poor for the use of their bodies in the medical schools were anathema.

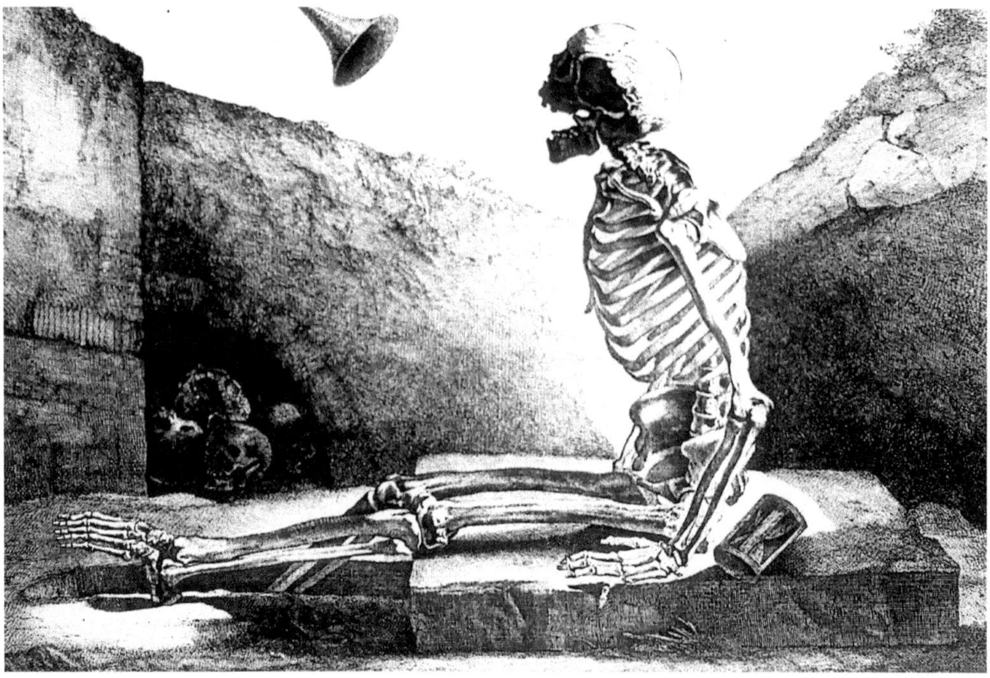

The resurrection as imagined by the artist on Judgment Day. Note the trumpet. The Latin inscription translates as "Arise from the dead and come to judgment." Jacques Gamelin, *Nouveau Recueil d'Osteologie et de Myologie*, Vol. 1, plate [7], 1779 (National Library of Medicine).

The Effect of the Civil War

Even though there was still resistance to anatomy law reform after the Civil War, the medical profession and society during the war had recognized the shortcomings of surgery and medicine in general. The deaths of 620,000 American soldiers, sons, fathers, and brothers as well as numerous civilians had traumatized American society and had consequences that would transform America's future and bring changes to the medical profession.[15]

The experience of the war in which even civilians saw themselves, thanks to Mathew Brady's photographs, led them to be "transfixed by the paradoxically lifelike renderings of the slain of Antietam" and the "prominence of bodies [that] overwhelmingly depicted their destruction and deformation[,] ... raising the question of how they [were] related to the persons who had once inhabited" those bodies. Obviously, these images were in stark contrast to the romanticized view of Raymond's article on the sacredness of the human body. For the soldiers it went even further, because "In the aftermath of battle survivors often shoveled corpses into pits as they would dispose of animals...."[16]

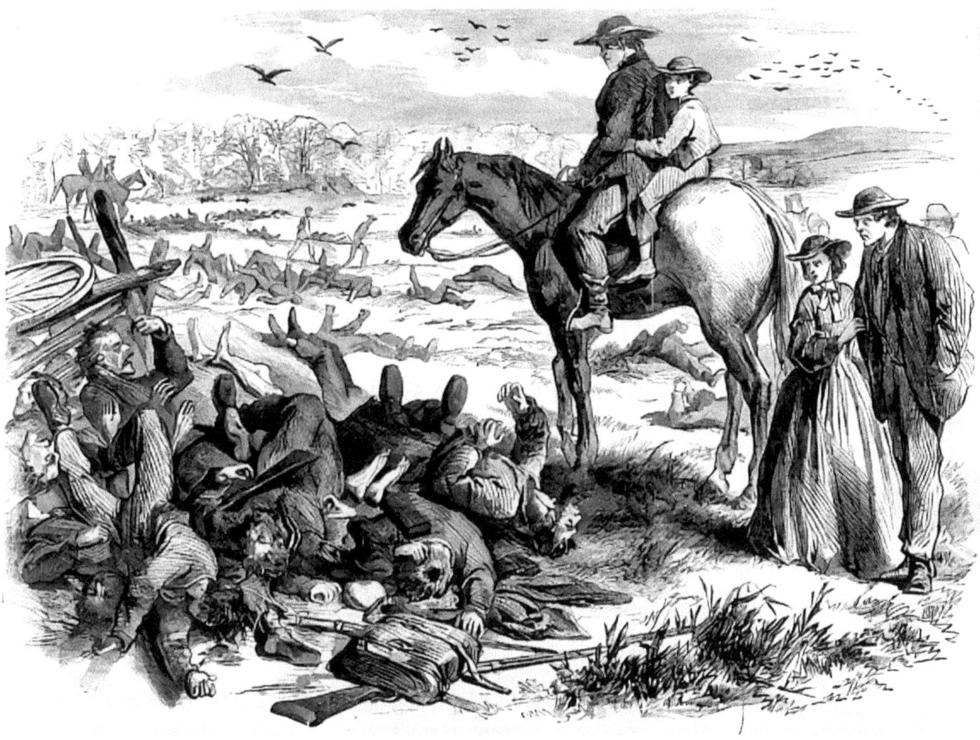

Civilians and soldiers confronting a pile of dead bodies along with bodies strewn on the field of battle. "Maryland and Pennsylvania farmers visiting the battlefield of Antietam while the National troops were burying the dead and carrying off the wounded." ***Frank Leslie's Illustrated Newspaper*****, October 18, 1862 (Library of Congress).**

Post-Civil War Society

After the war the prewar certainty of the body in the grave had been shattered. How many bodies were missing and never returned? The description of the mangled and deformed bodies in the dissecting rooms still had some impact but was likely lessened after witnessing the carnage on the battlefield. The certainty of religious views concerning the body and the assurance of religion teachings were being questioned by the experience of the war and new scientific research questioning other basic tenets of religion.[17]

Religious views among the upper- and middle-class Protestants had changed substantially following the Civil War. There was a new focus on improving "social conditions in the city, the saving of souls," and, more prominently, "the status of the spirit in the next life, [as] the corpse itself had become useless to religious instruction."[18] The Protestant mainstream religions had abandoned the corpse and stripped it of any "lingering sacrality, liminality or traces of power."[19] Christian authorities sacrificed their sanctification of the corpse to a "national [e.g., cemeteries dedicated to the war dead and the national outpouring of the funeral of President Abraham Lincoln], economic [i.e., the commodification of the dead through the rise of the funeral industry in Gilded Age America], and the medical interest in the dead [knowledge from the dissection of bodies now found a larger basis of support in society especially among Northern Protestants]."[20]

With improvements in living conditions and medical treatments for the upper and middle classes, the "omnipresence of death was mitigated."[21] This is not to say that there was a total acceptance of dissection and the anatomy laws. Still "resistance to the 'bodily profanation' ... of the corpse remained firm in the popular imagination of certain groups that more often than not provided the medical profession with the cadavers for study: the working poor, immigrants, and blacks."[22]

With the religious emphasis on the spirit rather than the body, the family death experience in postbellum America was being transferred to funeral directors as part of a new "commodification of death." Now the corpse was integrated into a "complex network" of commercial activity and was "represented as a potentially valuable object" for which the family purchased services (e.g., embalming) and "merchandise that reflected the approval of the deceased while alive."[23] Now, the family not only made a large financial investment in the funeral but was also expected to have the deceased in a professionally managed cemetery with a board of directors, and by the early 1870s some cemeteries began to offer perpetual care service.[24]

Funeral directors and cemetery managers moved their focus from the deceased to the survivors.[25] The expectation or trade-off for these professionally managed services was that the body would remain in peaceful repose in its new surroundings.[26]

Interestingly, in 1883 following the Lebanon Cemetery scandal, we have some evidence of these ideas being articulated. For example, "in 1883, the *Philadelphia Inquirer* praised the state's funeral directors for their 'steadily advancing appreciation of the aesthetics of modern society.' Those who appreciated art and aesthetics, particularly the pictorial ideal of park cemeteries, also appreciated the improved appearances of funeral service."[27]

These news ideas of cemetery management had not been lost on some of the lot holders of the Lebanon Cemetery. In December of 1882, they organized "to run board members against the Board of Managers of the Lebanon Cemetery ... after the outrage perpetrated upon the dead in the Lebanon burial ground." Their goals were to improve the lots, protect the general interest of the cemetery, and "aid the Board of Managers in collecting an annual tax on each lot and make it 'obligatory.'"[28] Unfortunately, when the election was held there were "large numbers of proxies," and in the end the old board was elected. One can see that there was an attempt by some of the more progressive lot holders to right the wrongs of the past and introduce modern cemetery management even if it was aspirational in what had previously been a neglected Black cemetery.

Post–Civil War society saw a "growing legitimacy of scientific thinking in nearly all aspects of social life, including public health and anatomical studies" in helping "to define the meaning of the corpse." Consumer culture combined with a professional class "re-established the value of the lifeless body for grieving survivors." Both "trends ultimately re-enforced the power of experts who took charge of the remains and began to manage their location in society."[29]

These factors all played a role in the next development of the anatomy laws. The fact that many of these new laws supported by public opinion suggested a trade-off, to prevent the illegal removal of the curated dead (whose bodies had value in the new funereal system) and to maintain the professional integrity of the funeral business where eternal repose of the body was promised, the business of body snatching had to be prevented or at least lessened. Public opinion began to side with the medical community. The unclaimed dead bodies of the poor would serve a useful purpose in the education of doctors, and sufficient corpses would be available to prevent or mitigate the now "valued corpse" perhaps embalmed and lying in permanent repose in the grave and provide comfort to families, as the new anatomy laws intended and the funereal experts promised.

However, this did not happen immediately, and there would be a series of local and national body-snatching scandals after the Civil War to mitigate this chapter in American medical history.

The Development of the Postbellum American Anatomy Laws

After the Civil War, a new phase in anatomy laws was instituted. Many of these laws were like the Massachusetts law. They were, however, criticized for being "discretionary and not mandatory." It was impossible to maintain a steady stream of subjects, because when officials were replaced the new officials were not always willing to provide cadavers. Bribery was also a problem. Similar laws were expanded to fourteen other states, many before 1880.[30]

Nevertheless, by the late nineteenth century wholesale body snatching and trafficking in bodies had in general been reduced but not eliminated, especially in the special case of Washington, D.C.[31] In another example, the Maryland Anatomy Act did not enforce compliance, so in 1893 when the Johns Hopkins Medical Department opened, "only 49 subjects came through the legally prescribed channels." The "deficit was made up by body snatching." Bodies had mysteriously appeared in the basement.[32]

Earlier due to state laws, access to cadavers was limited to convicted murderers. Doctors and students had no choice but to obtain bodies illegally. The wholesale plunder had been justified in the eyes of the medical profession for three reasons: State laws required dissection of humans as a prerequisite for medical licensing, this experience was critical for providing practice for physicians to avoid malpractice suits, and dissection would improve the ability of the physician to prolong the life and/or reduce the suffering of the living.

Throughout the period of the evolution of anatomy laws and the wholesale stealing of cadavers, the medical profession and its allies quickly realized that robbing cemeteries and burial grounds led to rioting and threats to local medical schools, especially when the bodies of respectable whites were stolen. Later the medical schools would use the unclaimed or buried bodies of the poor, immigrants, and Blacks, which they obtained illegally from almshouses, prisons, insane asylums, hospitals, and unprotected burial grounds, as these were less likely to cause outrage and rioting.

As for the predations of Black burial grounds, following the Civil War conditions had changed, and the wholesale robbing of Black burying grounds for bodies to supply the dissecting tables in the Northeast would finally be successfully challenged in the streets and in court. This challenge would lead to anatomy laws in various states that as part of their title would include ending the resurrecting of bodies from cemeteries. When the Lebanon Cemetery body-snatching episode and Dr. William Forbes's trial threatened the future preeminence of Philadelphia's medical establishment, these episodes led to a modified anatomy act in Pennsylvania that discouraged the wholesale robbing of cemeteries and burying grounds.

The solution to this ongoing conflict was to appease the respectable citizens by promoting anatomy laws that discouraged the wholesale looting of bodies from cemeteries and burying grounds by passing anatomy laws that discouraged resurrection men and implemented a state organization to legally obtain the unclaimed bodies of the poor and immigrants from the almshouses, prisons, insane asylums, and hospitals (places that had been illegally exploited earlier but whose bodies were now legally available). The argument, like the earlier contention, was that if the bodies in the graveyards were stolen and no one knew, there was no harm done. These unclaimed poor and immigrants would not be missed either. With improvements in medicine following the Civil War, there was now a common understanding that the poor and the unclaimed owed something to the state for the charity extended to them while alive and, thanks to McKnight in Philadelphia, that politicians should be "legislating for the living ... not the dead." It made sense that these unclaimed bodies of the poor should serve a purpose in death for the future well-being of the living.

Importantly, most of the new state anatomy laws passed following the Civil War had one drawback: the lack of compulsory enforcement to supply bodies. The Pennsylvania Anatomy Act of 1883 established this principle and a board to enforce it statewide, which undoubtedly explains why the Pennsylvania act was named the "best" anatomy law in 1896 by the American Association for the Advancement of Science. The award was given by the Committee for the Collection and Preservation of Anatomical Material.[33]

Ironically, the anatomy laws in New England (as well as the anatomy laws of other states after the Civil War) throughout most of the nineteenth century have been criticized because they were not compulsory in delivering bodies to the medical schools. This failure has, I believe, overshadowed the success of the physicians and elites over time to incorporate delivering the poor to the dissecting table. When adding the poor to the anatomist's pool of subjects was first suggested in the first quarter of the nineteenth century, the idea was roundly criticized.

In fact, only Massachusetts and New York had anatomy laws on the books prior to the Civil War that included the poor as prospects for dissection. Massachusetts managed to incorporate this measure in its anatomy law of 1831, but it was so limited that its effects were not felt outside of Boston and were confined to the newly arrived immigrant population. The same attempts to add the poor to the dissection pools in Connecticut and New Hampshire occurred, but these laws were soon repealed. Outside of New England, it was only New York State, with its "Bone Bill" passed in 1854, that included vagrants and the poor.

Following the Civil War, Maine (1869), New Hampshire (1869), Connecticut (1871), and finally Vermont (1884) added anatomy laws that now included the poor.[34] Not content with access to the poor, the anatomists continued to complain that the laws were discretionary and that many officials refused to comply and deliver bodies to the medical schools. Of course, this was not just in New England but also occurred in most of the new anatomical laws in other states. Although against the wishes of the poor they had been able to expand the pool of potential cadavers in the anatomical laws, the physicians still found themselves battling with officials who, for either religious reasons, as something considered morally corrupt, or for mercenary reasons, refused to turn over the dead to physicians who believed they were legally entitled to acquire them.

As I noted previously, following the Civil War conditions had changed, and the ready acceptance among the elites that the poor owed society a benefit for the charity shown toward them became more acceptable as a justification for including them in the dissection pool. Also, the uproar in the latter part of the nineteenth century over body snatching from cemeteries and the stealing of corpses of respectable and prominent persons as well as wholesale stealing of corpses from cemeteries required a solution.

Oddly enough, it was not until after the carnage of the Civil War and the transformation of antebellum American society in the Gilded Age that physicians, their elite supporters, and by the end of the century even the lower classes, including the Black population and the respectable poor, were willing to sacrifice the desperately poor and the unclaimed, for the good of society, in death to the ignominy of dissection. Not only should the poor repay society for its charity by serving as raw material for medical research, but as we can see from these new anatomy laws, a second goal was that they helped resolve the problem of the wholesale robbing of graveyards!

On the Nation's Capital

Initially there was a Philadelphia-like scandal in Washington, D.C., where it was admitted body snatching was an ongoing enterprise involving the medical schools, the District of Columbia government, and the federal medical services. In response, the medical schools asked Congress to enact an anatomy law for Washington, D.C., to obtain legal cadavers and allow them to get out of the loathsome business of dealing with "resurrection" men and the rampant trafficking in illegal corpses going on in D.C. There were two attempts that failed. By the time of the third attempt in 1892, the medical schools had discovered that what would work in a state might not be feasible in the small land area comprising the District of Columbia, with three medical schools.

The medical schools in the District of Columbia may have had second thoughts and realized that the demand for cadavers would exceed the supply with such a proposed restrictive anatomy act. To meet their "subject" needs, they would still depend on the "resurrectionists" possibly obtaining bodies from both the private and public cemeteries in D.C. Putting the latter out of business by strict imprisonment laws would threaten both the availability of cadavers and their affordability. Likely this may have caused the medical schools to lose interest in pushing the anatomy law proposed in 1892.[35]

Because there was no anatomy law in the District of Columbia during the last two decades of the nineteenth century, the city government of Washington, D.C., and federal authorities actively supported the body-snatching activities of the D.C. medical schools.

The medical schools had free rein over "Potter's Field," even calling it the "Scientific Ground" while using a procedure to ensure deniability and anonymity to protect themselves if bodies were obtained from other cemeteries.

The states that passed recent anatomy laws expanded their reach of subjects, and by this time it had become acceptable to acquire the bodies of paupers who had lived off the charity of the states and purpose their bodies for dissection in the medical schools. Whereas the states with anatomy laws obtained their indigent subjects from institutions prior to burial, the District of Columbia medical schools obtained most of their indigent subjects from the graves in the D.C. Potter's Field. The snatching of bodies from Potter's Field was tolerated. In keeping with the new value put on the funeral industry and the investment in the proper burial of family and friends, body snatching from respectable cemeteries was not acceptable. Those cemeteries did have security, and as we saw, although body snatchers in those cemeteries were actively discouraged by force if necessary, the superintendents of the cemeteries admitted that body snatching did occur in their cemeteries.

In the early 1890s, officials admitted that of the ten thousand graves in the Potter's Field, there were fewer than four hundred in 1892, while at Harmony Cemetery if the graves were opened, they estimated that it would "reveal hundreds of empty coffins" and that the number of "graves robbed in the Congressional Cemetery can never be told unless an examination is made of each grave." There is also evidence that bodies were shipped out of the District of Columbia to Virginia and likely up north. Even in those states where anatomy laws were in place, there were always shortages due to restrictions in the law or the manner of distribution. The traffic in illegal bodies was certainly reduced but not altogether eliminated even in those states. There is no doubt that the District of Columbia was an avid supplier.[36]

The medical schools in Washington finally supported the passage of an anatomy act for Washington, D.C., in 1902. The new law reduced the punishment for anyone transgressing the law, ensuring that the schools could continue to work with their suppliers if ever there was a shortage of corpses.

Because of the circumstances of the requirements in Washington, D.C., for subjects due to its three medical schools, its lack of an anatomy law, and the collaboration of the D.C. government during the last two decades of the nineteenth century in supporting body-snatching activity in D.C., it was not only the political capital of the nation but also the body snatching capital of the nation.

In conclusion, the century-long struggle between the medical profession and the elites and popular opinion was settled in favor of the former. Yet, the arguments and the implications in opposition to the anatomy laws continued to focus on the poor as an exploited underclass of raw material for the medical profession. For example, in the debate in the House of Representatives on the proposed anatomy house bill of the Fiftieth Congress, although it was for the District of Columbia, it "had similar provisions" to laws enacted in sixteen states. Therefore, the criticism went beyond the District bill. The main complaint from those opposed to the bill was like many of the state anatomy laws "the unclaimed bodies shall be those which are buried at the public expense" and were to be sent to the dissection table.[37]

For "persons dying in the almshouses or asylums," it was argued that "unless of their own accord they request the privileges of Christian burial, [they] shall be handed over to the savage, soulless science of the medical schools. Imagine for a moment a poor, homeless, friendless, suffering man in the very throes of dissolution, his faculties deserting him, eternity with its awful possibilities before him, the earth and its ties receding, and just as he is about to penetrate the veil of the tremendous future, he is obliged ... asking that his body may not be handed over to the surgeons to be mutilated after his death.... Every poor waif of humanity who wants the benefit of this act (or state anatomy statutes) must spend his last moments arguing law to the hospital or conventionally cold-hearted almshouse attendants."[38]

As one Congressional representative concluded, "Science, in this utilitarian age, selects its victims by reason of their poverty." As far as the role of these hospitals, doctors and officials are concerned, we can infer those opposed to this bill probably believed their own state anatomy laws were likewise simply measures "to send the Jerry Crunchers from the grave yards into the hospitals." The "ghoul of the grave-yard is by this act dignified into the legalized 'body snatcher' of the hospital."[39]

As for the supporters of these anatomy bills, even in the debate in the House of Representative over the 1888/89 failed anatomy bill, Representative Hemphill of South Carolina, a member of the District Committee, answered the argument coldly about the disposition of the poor and as to whether there should be some regulation of "resurrectionists." He stated, "There is not so much difference in being cut up after death and buried afterwards, and being buried and cut up afterwards." Most importantly for the public, another member noted in the state of Michigan, because of the anatomy law, "people now lay the bodies of their relatives and friends in the grave with the most absolute assurance they will repose where they are laid."[40]

As one historian noted, anatomy legislation expanded the number of bodies available to the medical profession and lessened the anguish over the fate of loved ones but continued to be a "humiliation" inflicted on "social outcasts," the impoverished and wards of the state.[41] Of course, it was more than this; by the end of the nineteenth century it had become acceptable to consign what was formerly a protected group of "in care" and prisoners to post-mortem dissection, creating a permanent "underclass" of victims by legislative statute.

By the beginning of the twentieth century, body snatching was not eliminated. However, the "procurement, dissection, and disposal of cadavers became for most citizens an invisible process and a distant issue."[42] Newspapers continued to report instances of body snatching throughout the nation; in retrospect, these were rare but made good copy for the papers. The medical profession and state laws had made it economically impractical to continue the business on the same scale as it had been practiced in the past.[43]

In 1935, Alan F. Guttman (ironically a future president of Planned Parenthood) confidently wrote, "Body snatching is now a memory which will be kept alive by literary allusions, as in Jerry Cruncher's discourse—in which he explains to his son that a 'resurrectionist is an honest tradesman' whose wares are a 'branch of scientific goods.'"[44]

However, trade and interest in the human body and body parts as a commodity to be exploited and trafficked has taken on a whole new meaning in the twenty-first century beyond anything Charles Dickens' nineteenth-century character Cruncher the body snatcher could have imagined.

Chapter Notes

Introduction

1. Michael E. Bell, *Food for the Dead, On the Trail of New England's Vampires* (New York: Carroll and Graf, 2001).

2. For example, Edgar Allan Poe's short story "The Premature Burial." See Jan Bondeson, *Buried Alive: The Terrifying History of Our Most Primal Fear* (New York: Norton, 2002), 177 and 208.

3. William Tebb and Edward P. Vollum, *Premature Burial and How It May Be Prevented ...* (London: Sonenshein & Co., 1897), 157.

4. David Walsh, MD, *Premature Burial: Fact or Fiction* (London: Bailliere, Tindall & Cox, 1897), 5, 17–19.

5. Suzanne Shultz, *Body Snatching: The Robbing of Graves for the Education of Physicians in Early Nineteenth Century America* (Jefferson, NC: McFarland, 1992); and Michael Sappol, *A Traffic of Dead Bodies* (Princeton: Princeton University Press, 2002).

6. "Medical Schools in Boston," *Boston Medical and Surgical Journal* 50, no. 14 (1854): 260.

7. Frederick C. Waite, "Grave Robbing in New England," *Bulletin of the Medical Library Association* 33 (1945): 276–77.

8. *Morning Advertiser*, January 16, 1893, 1–2.

9. See Seán Columb, *Trading Life: Organ Trafficking, Illicit Networks, and Exploitation* (Stanford: Stanford University Press, 2020).

10. See especially Shultz, *Body Snatching*; and Sappol, *A Traffic of Dead Bodies*.

11. See, for example, Craig Steven Wilder, *Ebony and Ivy: Race, Slavery, and the Troubled History of American Universities* (New York: Bloomsbury, 2013).

12. LeRoy Bowman, *The American Funeral: A Study in Guilt* (Washington, D.C.: Public Affairs, 1959), 114.

13. John Knott, "Popular Attitudes to Death and Dissection in Early Nineteenth Century Britain: The Anatomy Act and the Poor," *Labour History: A Journal of Labour and Social History*, no. 49 (1985): 6.

14. Frederick C. Waite, "The Development of Anatomical Laws in the States of New England," *New England Journal of Medicine* 233 (1945): 722. Even when the Johns Hopkins Medical School opened in 1893, the law in Maryland did not compel officials to provide corpses. To obtain bodies it was "necessary to have the goodwill of the Health Commissioner and a strong Anatomical Board." Franklin P. Mall, "Anatomical Material: Its Collection and Its Preservation at the Johns Hopkins Anatomical Laboratory," *Bulletin of the Johns Hopkins Hospital* 16, no. 167 (February 1905): 38.

15. Peter Linebaugh, "The Tyburn Riot against Surgeons," in *Albion's Fatal Tree: Crime and Society in Eighteenth-Century England*, ed. Douglas Hay et al. (New York: Pantheon Books, 1975), 117. For a standard interpretation on the meaning of death and burial customs for the living, see Bronisław Malinowski, *Magic, Science and Religion, and Other Essays* (Boston: Beacon, 1948), 29–32.

16. Knott, "Popular Attitudes to Death and Dissection in Early Nineteenth Century Britain," 7.

Chapter 1

1. "The Resurrectionists of Old," *Hospital: A Journal of Medical Sciences and Hospital Administration* 21 (1896): 193; and E.C. Brewer, *Dictionary of Phrase and Fable* (London: Cassel & Co., 1896), 1052.

2. Frederick C. Waite, "Grave Robbing in New England," *Bulletin of the Medical Library Association* 33 (1945): 279–81. For an example of clothes being identified as belonging to a victim of Burke and Hare, who usually "destroyed the clothes of their victims," see Lisa Rosner, *The Anatomy Murders* (Philadelphia: University of Pennsylvania Press, 2010), 189.

3. "Resurrectionists," *Literary Cadet and Saturday Evening Bulletin* 2 (Providence, RI, 1828): 2.

4. Waite, "Grave Robbing in New England," 281.

5. William Blackstone, *Commentaries on the Laws of England*, 4 vols. ed. Edward Christianson (Philadelphia, 1825), 4:241. Cited in Waite, "Grave Robbing in New England," 272–273.

6. David L. Freedman, "Practicing on the Newly Dead: Is a Corpse Considered Property?," *ED Legal Letter*, February 1, 2000, https://www.reliasmedia.com/articles/44628-practicing-on-the-newly-dead-is-a-corpse-considered-property#:~:text=Courts%20generally%20have%20held%20that%20either%3A%201%29%20There,body%20for%20purposes

%20of%20burial%20%28a%20%22quasi-property%22%20right%29.

7. Blackstone, *Commentaries on the Laws of England*, 2:457.

8. Richard S. Ross, *Before Salem: Witch Hunting in the Connecticut River Valley, 1647–1663* (Jefferson, NC: McFarland, 2017), 118.

9. A.D.J. Macfarlane, *Witchcraft in Tudor and Stuart England* (New York: Harper Torchbooks, 1970), 15.

10. Edward Coke, *Institutes of the Laws of England*, Vol. 3 (London: Fletcher, W. Lee, and Pakeman, 1644), 45.

11. Great Britain. *The Law Reports: The Public General Statutes ... Passed in the Fifty Ninth Year and Sixtieth Year of Her Majesty Queen Victoria*, Vol. 33 (London: William Clowes and Sons Ltd., 1896), 23.

12. Waite, "Grave Robbing in New England," 274; and "An Act to Protect the Sepulchers of the Dead, March 2, 1815," in *The Public General Laws of the Commonwealth of Massachusetts*, Vol. 4 (Boston: Wells and Lilly, 1816), 477.

13. D. Hamilton Hurd, *History of Essex County, Massachusetts*, 2 vols. (Philadelphia: J.W. Lewis & Co., 1888), 2:1188.

14. Joseph B. Felt, *History of Ipswich, Essex and Hamilton* (Cambridge, MA: Charles Folsom, 1834), 270.

15. Frederick C. Waite, "An Episode in Massachusetts in 1818 Related to Teaching of Anatomy." *New England Journal of Medicine* 220 (1939): 224.

16. Christopher Benedetto, "A Most Daring and Sacrilegious Robbery: The Extraordinary Story of Body Snatching at Chebacco Parish in Ipswich, Massachusetts." *New England Ancestors: Newsmagazine of the New England Historical Society* 6 (Spring 2005): 32; and Waite, "An Episode in Massachusetts," 224.

17. Robert Crowell, *Interment of the Dead, a Dictate of Natural Affection, Sanctioned by the Word of God, and the Examples of the Good in Every Age: A Sermon Delivered in Ipswich, Second Parish, July 23, 1818, on the Occasion of Reinterring the Coffins Which Had Been Robbed of Their Contents* (Andover, 1818), iii.

18. Benedetto, "A Most Daring and Sacrilegious Robbery," 32.

19. Crowell, *Interment of the Dead*, iii.

20. Benedetto, "A Most Daring and Sacrilegious Robbery," 32; and Robert Crowell, *History of the Town of Essex from 1634–1868* (Springfield, MA: Samuel Bowles & Co., 1868), 470. On Mary Millet, see Crowell, *Interment of the Dead*, iii. However, Robert Crowell, *History of the Town of Essex*, 470, lists her as Mrs. Polly Millet. She may have gone by Polly, as it was a diminutive for Mary. On Allen, see Crowell, *Interment of the Dead*, iii.

21. Crowell, *Interment of the Dead*, iv.

22. *Salem Gazette*, April 21, 1818, 3.

23. Salem, April 21, reprinted from the *Salem Gazette*. Generally, the missing body in Gloucester is not mentioned in the Chebacco story in most histories of this incident. It is interesting that the newspaper in which the story was reported indicated that it had the names of some of the corpses taken from the burial ground and that as early as April 24 the townspeople already had their suspicions about who was responsible for the grave robbing. *New-England Palladium*, April 24, 1818, 1.

24. *Records of the Second Parish Church of Ipswich, Massachusetts Beginning in 1752*, cited in Waite, "An Episode in Massachusetts," 224.

25. Harry M. Brooks, *The Olden Times Series: Quaint and Curious Advertisements* (Boston: Ticknor and Co., 1886), 140. See also *Salem Gazette*, April 28, 1818, 3.

26. Waite, "An Episode in Massachusetts," 224; and Benedetto, "A Most Daring and Sacrilegious Robbery," 32.

27. Christopher Benedetto, "A Most Daring and Sacrilegious Robbery: The Extraordinary Story of Body Snatching at Chebacco Parish in Ipswich, Massachusetts." *New England Ancestors: Newsmagazine of the New England Historical Society* 6 (Spring 2005): 32.

28. See below the discussion of Crowell's sermon *Interment of the Dead*; and Edward Warren, *Life of John Collins Warren, M.D.*, 2 vols. (Boston: Ticknor and Fields, 1860), 1:420.

29. *Essex Register*, May 9, 1818, 2.

30. *Essex Register*, May 9, 1818, 2.

31. William Bentley, *The Diary of William Bentley, Pastor of the East Church of Salem, Massachusetts, 1811–1819*, Vol. 4 (Salem, MA: Essex Institute, 1914) 4:516.

32. Bentley, *Diary of William Bentley*, 4:559.

33. Warren, *Life of John Collins Warren, M.D.*, 1:406.

34. Warren, 1:406.

35. Bentley, *Diary of William Bentley*, 4:629.

36. Crowell, *Interment of the Dead*, 35.

37. Michael Sappol, *A Traffic of Dead Bodies* (Princeton: Princeton University Press, 2002), 87.

38. Hurd, *History of Essex County, Massachusetts*, 2:1188.

39. Waite, "An Episode in Massachusetts," 224.

40. Hurd, *History of Essex County, Massachusetts*, 2:1188.

41. Murderers' bodies, if ordered by a judge by Massachusetts law, could be dissected following their execution. In 1805, when a duelist was convicted of "murder committed in a duel" a judge could order the body to be "dissected and anatomized." But because judges were "not compelled to assign the bodies of criminals for dissection," the number of bodies was sometimes only two per year. Waite, "An Episode in Massachusetts," 222.

42. Bentley, *Diary of William Bentley*, 4:558–59, 629, 631. Later one minister would write of Crowell that he was "loyal to the doctrines of that Word[,] ... not led by any speculations a step beyond[;] ... the need of any departure from the faith which was then taught does not command itself to serious regard." See First Congregational Church (Essex, Mass.), "Two Centuries of the Two Hundredth ... " (Salem, MA: Choate & Co., 1884), 157.

43. Crowell, *Interment of the Dead*, 8.
44. Crowell, 15–16.
45. Crowell, 11.
46. Crowell, 9.
47. Crowell, 12.
48. Crowell, 24.
49. Crowell, 24–26.
50. Crowell, 27–28.
51. Crowell, 28.
52. Crowell, 29.
53. Crowell, 31–33. And there were those who argued, according to Crowell, that "we have no right to examine our sepulchers, to see if our dead are there, or not. It is enough for us that we have decently buried them. And if we officiously examine, and find them gone, then we are the guilty authors of our own distress, and of all the difficulty that ensues; since, if we had not examined, all would have been peace and quietness." Crowell, *Interment of the Dead*, 33.
54. Crowell, 34–35.
55. Crowell, 35.
56. Crowell, 35–36.
57. Sappol, *A Traffic of Dead Bodies*, 322.
58. S. LeBlond, "Les Anatomists et les Résurrectionistes aux Etat-Unis," *Canadian Medical Association Journal* 101 (August 23, 1969): 221.
59. William E. Horner, *Necrological Notice of Dr. Philip Syng Physick, Delivered before the American Philosophical Society, May 4, 1838*, Vol. (Philadelphia: Haswell, 1838), 369.
60. Sappol, *A Traffic of Dead Bodies*, 382. Unfortunately, there is no source given here.
61. Warren, *Life of John Collins Warren, M.D.*, 2:359.
62. See Chapter 11, note 8, on Judge Israel Keith's reference to St. Paul and John Locke on the resurrection of the body. Keith attended Dr. John Warren's (John C. Warren's father) anatomy demonstrations and was a partisan supporter of dissection.
63. Crowell, *Interment of the Dead*, 19–21.
64. Crowell, 38–39.
65. Crowell, 40. Ironically, Robert Crowell would bury his wife Hannah (Frost) Crowell, who died five months later on December 11, 1818, in the same burying ground where the eight bodies were previously stolen. *Vital Records of Ipswich Massachusetts: Marriages and Deaths to the End of 1849*, 3 vols. (Salem, MA: Essex Institute, 1910), 3 vols. (Salem, MA: Essex Institute, 1910), 2:534.
66. First Congregational Church, "Two Centuries of the Two Hundredth," 158.
67. Henry Raymond, "Editor's Table, The Sacredness of the Human Body," *Harper's New Monthly Magazine* 8 (April 1854): 690.
68. Raymond, "Editor's Table," 691–92.
69. Raymond, "Editor's Table," 692.

Chapter 2

1. Christopher Benedetto, "A Most Daring and Sacrilegious Robbery: The Extraordinary Story of Body Snatching at Chebacco Parish in Ipswich, Massachusetts." *New England Ancestors: Newsmagazine of the New England Historical Society* 6 (Spring 2005): 31.
2. *Vital Records of Ipswich Massachusetts: Marriages and Deaths to the End of 1849*, 3 vols. (Salem, MA: Essex Institute, 1910), 2:315.
3. Henry Bowditch, *Memoir of Amos Twitchell M.D.* (Boston: John Wilson, and Son, 1851), 35; on his procurement of bodies for Dr. Nathan Smith, see 37 and 38. Dr. Mussey was also with Dr. Nathan Smith at Dartmouth. John B. Hamilton, "Life and Times of Doctor Reuben D. Mussey," *Journal of the American Medical Association* 26 (April 1896): 650.
4. D. Hamilton Hurd, *History of Essex County, Massachusetts*, 2 vols. (Philadelphia: J.W. Lewis & Co., 1888), 2:1190.
5. Frederick C. Waite, "An Episode in Massachusetts in 1818 Related to Teaching of Anatomy," *New England Journal of Medicine* 220 (1939): 225.
6. Hurd, *History of Essex County, Massachusetts*, 2:1190; and Edward Warren, *Life of John Collins Warren, M.D.*, 2 vols. (Boston: Ticknor and Fields, 1860), 1:123.
7. Waite, "An Episode in Massachusetts," 225.
8. Edward M. Hartwell, "The Progress of Anatomical Study in Massachusetts with Remarks upon its Legal Status," *Annals of Anatomy and Surgery* 3 (1881): 267.
9. Warren, *Life of John Collins Warren, M.D.*, 1:404.
10. Warren, 1:405.
11. Warren, 1:406.
12. Warren, 1:407–408.
13. Warren, 1:409.
14. See also Benedetto, "A Most Daring and Sacrilegious Robbery," 32. Clearly, Sewall was an accomplished grave robber and learned his craft as a student. As noted earlier by Bowditch, "It was the fixed fate of every medical student to do this," Bowditch, 35-36.
15. Bentley, William Bentley, *The Diary of William Bentley, Pastor of the East Church of Salem, Massachusetts, 1811–1819*, Vol. 4 (Salem, MA: Essex Institute, 1914), 4:629.
16. Tyler Parsons, *Truth Espoused, Relative to the Difficulties That Existed in the Town of Manchester, Massachusetts* (Dedham, MA: M & W M Mann, 1823), 69.
17. Samuel G. Brown, *Life of Rufus Choate* (Boston: Little, Brown, 1879), 10; and Benedetto, "A Most Daring and Sacrilegious Robbery," 34.
18. *Chebacco Parish Tax Records*, cited in Benedetto, "A Most Daring and Sacrilegious Robbery," 32.
19. Robert Crowell, *History of the Town of Essex from 1634–1868* (Springfield, MA: Samuel Bowles & Co., 1868), 279.
20. Benedetto, "A Most Daring and Sacrilegious Robbery," 32.
21. Benedetto, 32.
22. According to Frederick Waite, Dr. Sewall also had "a group of students at the time under his

instruction in operative surgery." Waite does not cite where he obtained this information. Frederick C. Waite, "Grave Robbing in New England," *Bulletin of the Medical Library Association* 33 (1945): 286. However, Crowell does mention that Dr. Sewall did have a student, Asa Story, the son of Captain John Story, who had to leave Dartmouth at the end of his sophomore year due to an eye disease. Asa soon "began the study of medicine in his native place with Dr. Thomas Sewall." Yet, there is no mention of other students in any of the proceedings. Asa returned to Hanover, New Hampshire, and attended medical lectures there in 1816 and 1817. For most of 1818 and 1819 he was in Frederick City, Maryland. Crowell, *History of the Town of Essex*, 276–77.

23. Waite, "Grave Robbing in New England," 278.

24. Warren, *Life of John Collins Warren, M.D.*, 1:420.

25. Thomas Francis Harrington, *The Harvard Medical School*, 3 vols. (New York: Lewis Publishing, 1905), 2:654.

26. Harrington, *The Harvard Medical School*, 2:654.

27. *The Public General Laws of the Commonwealth of Massachusetts*, Vol. 4 (Boston: Wells and Lilly, 1816), 477.

28. Harrington, *The Harvard Medical School*, 2:655.

29. Bowditch, *Memoir of Amos Twitchell M.D.*, 34.

30. Harrington, *The Harvard Medical School*, 2:656–57.

31. Joseph B. Felt, *History of Ipswich, Essex and Hamilton* (Cambridge, MA: Charles Folsom, 1834), 198; and Waite, "An Episode in Massachusetts," 224.

32. *Records of the Supreme Judicial Court, Commonwealth vs. Sewall*, Manuscript 1817–1818, vol. 1, docket 541–42, Massachusetts Supreme Judicial Court Archives.

33. Cited in Benedetto, "A Most Daring and Sacrilegious Robbery," 32.

34. Bentley, *Diary of William Bentley*, 4:516.

35. Daniel Webster, *Private Correspondence of Daniel Webster*, 2 vols. (Cambridge, MA: John Wilson and Son, 1826), 1:292.

36. Benedetto, "A Most Daring and Sacrilegious Robbery," 33.

37. *Records of the Supreme Judicial Court*, vol. 1, docket 541.

38. *Records of the Supreme Judicial Court*, vol. 1, docket 542.

39. *Records of the Supreme Judicial Court*, vol. 1, docket 542.

40. Bentley, *Diary of William Bentley*, 4:558.

41. Bentley, 4:559.

42. Bentley, 4:559–60.

43. Bentley, 4:561.

44. *Records of the Supreme Judicial Court*, vol. 1, docket 542.

45. Bentley, *Diary of William Bentley*, 4: 629.

46. Bentley, 4:631.

47. Waite, "An Episode in Massachusetts," 225.

48. *Records of the Supreme Judicial Court*, vol. 1, docket 542.

49. Benedetto, "A Most Daring and Sacrilegious Robbery," 34.

50. "Medical School in Boston," *Boston Medical and Surgical Journal* 35, no. 31 (December 26, 1846): 417.

51. Prior to the trial on May 25, 1819, Rufus Choate wrote to his brother David Choate that "I am rejoiced that brother S. [Sewall] settles in about to leave his people. Do write particularly about [it] and give me all the politics of the place in detail." H.D. Foster, "Some Unpublished Letters of Rufus Choate," *Dartmouth Alumni Magazine* 17, no. 4 (February 1925): 309.

52. *Resolves of the General Court of the Commonwealth of Massachusetts* (Boston: Russell and Gardner, 1820), 126–27.

53. *Essex County, Court of Common Pleas*, March 1820, March 1822, and June 1822 terms. Cited in Benedetto, "A Most Daring and Sacrilegious Robbery," 34.

54. Bentley, *Diary of William Bentley*, 4:629.

55. Brown, *Life of Rufus Choate*, 28.

56. *Celebration of the Two Hundredth Anniversary of the Organization of the Congregational Church and Parish in Essex, Massachusetts, August 19–20, 1883* (Salem, MA: J.H. Choate, and Co., 1884), 101.

57. For a good discussion of the events leading up to the disestablishment of the Congregational church in Massachusetts in 1833, see Jacob C. Meyer, *Church and State in Massachusetts from 1740–1833* (New York: Russell, and Russell, 1930), 133–59.

58. *Celebration of the Two Hundredth Anniversary of the Organization of the Congregational Church and Parish in Essex*, 15.

59. Francis Wright D'Arusmont, *Views of Society and Manners in America: In a Series of Letters from That Country* (London: Longman, Hurst, Rees, and Brown, 1821), 513–14.

Chapter 3

1. It is most unusual to find clergy involved in or advocating body snatching for dissection. Llewellin Eliot, who wrote on body snatching in Washington, D.C., mentions the following. "There was a negro preacher: he taught salvation and repentance to the limit on Sundays, buried the dead of his congregation; but the strain on his nervous system was so great that he was compelled to let off steam by stealing the bodies he so faithfully buried." Dr. Llewellin Eliot, "Comment on Frank Baker's 'A History of Bodysnatching,'" *Washington Medical Annals* 15 (1916): 247–53. Of course, the conversations between the Jesuits at Georgetown and the medical department at the college regarding the stealing of cadavers for

the dissecting tables in the last half of the nineteenth century would be of great interest also. On the Catholic Church and dissection, see James J. Walsh, *World's Debt to the Catholic Church* (Boston: Stratford Co., 1924), 309. It is unlikely that there was any disagreement over dissection itself, but there must have been some soul searching over the school's involvement in the sordid business of trafficking in stolen corpses.

2. D. Hamilton Hurd, *History of Essex County, Massachusetts*, 2 vols. (Philadelphia: J.W. Lewis & Co., 1888), 2:1255.

3. Hurd, *History of Essex County, Massachusetts*, 2:1255.

4. Darius Francis Lamson, *History of the Town of Manchester, Essex County, Massachusetts, 1645–1895* (Published by the Town, 1895), 265.

5. Lamson, *History of the Town of Manchester*, 230.

6. See Richard S. Ross, *Before Salem: Witch Hunting in the Connecticut River Valley, 1647-1663* (Jefferson, NC: McFarland, 2017), 194–96.

7. Lamson, *History of the Town of Manchester*, 230–31.

8. Joseph Buckminster, *A Sermon Preached at the Installation of the Reverend James Thurston, to the Pastoral Charge of the Church of Manchester* (Portsmouth, NH: Oracle, 1809), 22–23, 25, 27.

9. Lamson, *History of the Town of Manchester*, 232–33.

10. Tyler Parsons, *Truth Espoused, Relative to the Difficulties That Existed in the Town of Manchester, Massachusetts* (Dedham, MA: M & W M Mann, 1823), 5–6.

11. Parsons, *Truth Espoused*, 16.

12. Parsons, 16.

13. Letter, Mussey to Sewall, Hanover, October 26, 1818, in Parsons, *Truth Espoused*, 16.

14. Letter, Parsons to Mussey, Manchester, November 24, 1818, in Parsons, *Truth Espoused*, 17.

15. Parsons, *Truth Espoused*, 4.

16. Letter, Mussey to Parsons, Hanover, November 26, 1818, in Parsons, *Truth Espoused*, 17.

17. Parsons, *Truth Espoused*, 7.

18. Testimony of Major Burley Smith before the Manchester Town Committee, February 15, 1819, Parsons, *Truth Espoused*, 25.

19. Parsons, 25.

20. Parsons, 25.

21. Parsons, 26. Also, Dr. Dewey could not settle makes sense even though the difficulty of setting up a rural practice was realized. On this, see Michael Sappol, "The Odd Case of Charles Knowlton: Anatomical Performance, Medical Narrative, and Narrative Identity in Antebellum America," *Bulletin of the History of Medicine* 83 (2009): 488–89. For general challenges and the social status of New England physicians, see Barnes Riznik, "The Professional Lives of Early Nineteenth Century New England Doctors," *Journal of the History of Medicine and Allied Sciences* 19 (1964): 3–9.

22. Mr. John Dewey studied under Nathan Smith at Dartmouth and earned his medical degree there. For more on Nathan Smith and his emphasis on dissection in teaching, see Chapter 4 in this volume. See also E.C. Benton, *A History of Guildhall, VT* (Waverly, MA: E.C. Benton, 1886), 221.

23. Letter, Mussey to Sewall, Hanover, October 26, 1818, in Parsons, *Truth Espoused*, 16.

24. Testimony of Major Burley Smith before the Manchester Town Committee, February 15, 1819, in Parsons, *Truth Espoused*, 26–27.

25. William Bentley, *The Diary of William Bentley, Pastor of the East Church of Salem, Massachusetts, 1811–1819*, Vol. 4 (Salem, MA: Essex Institute, 1914), 4:558.

26. Affidavit of Captain John Girdler, March 9, 1823, in Parsons, *Truth Espoused*, 59–60.

27. Affidavit of Dr. Reuben Mussey, March 7, 1820, in Parsons, *Truth Espoused*, 69.

28. Affidavit of Captain John Girdler, March 9, 1823, in Parsons, *Truth Espoused*, 60–61.

29. Parsons, *Truth Espoused*, 61.

30. Parsons, 59–60.

31. Parsons, 59.

32. Parsons, 59.

33. Parsons, 62–63.

34. Parsons, 31.

35. Bentley, *The Diary of William Bentley*, 4:561.

36. Letter, James Thurston to Dr. John Dewey, Manchester, January 19, 1819, in Parsons, *Truth Espoused*, 20.

37. Deposition of Daniel Annable, Manchester, March 3, 1823, in Parsons, *Truth Espoused*, 68.

38. Parsons, *Truth Espoused*, 31.

39. Parsons, 32.

40. Parsons, 33; and Burgess, in Parsons, 67.

41. Deposition of Dr. John Dewey, Lancaster, New Hampshire, March 13, 1820, in Parsons, *Truth Espoused*, 70–71.

42. Deposition of Dr. John Dewey, Lancaster, New Hampshire, April 20, 1820, in Parsons, *Truth Espoused*, 72–73.

43. Frederick C. Waite, "Grave Robbing in New England," *Bulletin of the Medical Library Association* 33 (1945): 274; Arthur M. Lassek, *Human Dissection: Its Drama and Struggle* (Springfield, IL: Charles C. Thomas, 1958), 186–87; and Edward M. Hartwell, "The Progress of Anatomical Study in Massachusetts with Remarks upon Its Legal Status," *Annals of Anatomy and Surgery* 3 (1881): 276.

44. Sappol, "Odd Case of Charles Knowlton," 476.

45. Robert E. Riegel, "American Father of Birth Control," *New England Quarterly* 6 (1937): 478. And for Knowlton's early student experiences with grave robbing and his jail time, see Stephen J.W. Tabor, "The Late Dr. Knowlton's Autobiography," *Boston Medical and Surgical Journal* 45 (1851): 115–17, 151–52.

46. Besides calling for the ecclesiastical council for advice, some church members were hoping that Thurston would be willing to quit the his pastorate in their church before the council met. Parsons, *Truth Espoused*, 35.

47. Parsons, 35.

48. Parsons, 36.

49. James Thurston, "To the brethren…, April 3, 1819," Parsons, *Truth Espoused*, 36.
50. Parsons, *Truth Espoused*, 38.
51. James Thurston, "To the brethren…, April 5, 1819," Parsons, *Truth Espoused*, 39.
52. Parsons, *Truth Espoused*, 39.
53. Tyler Parsons and Richard Allen, "To the Gentlemen of the Committee of the First Baptist Church in Beverly…, Manchester, 19 April 1919" in Parsons, *Truth Espoused*, 40.
54. Parsons, *Truth Espoused*, 40..
55. For a copy of the minutes of the meeting held by the Manchester church on May 6, 1819, presented to the town by Reverend Thurston, see James Thurston, "Proceedings of the Church, and Their Pastor, Laid before the Town at Their Meeting Held 15, May 1819," see Parsons, *Truth Espoused*, 40.
56. Parsons, *Truth Espoused*, 42–43.
57. Council members consisted of pastors and brother delegates from churches in the Massachusetts towns of Hamilton, Newbury, Marblehead, Danvers, Essex, Salem, and Gloucester. Council Paper No. 1, in Parsons, *Truth Espoused*, 50.
58. Parsons, *Truth Espoused*, 50–51.
59. Parsons, 49.
60. Affidavit of Captain John Girdler, in Parsons, *Truth Espoused*, 64.
61. Council Paper No. 1, in Parsons, *Truth Espoused*, 50–51.
62. Samuel Dana, scribe of the council, "To the Ecclesiastical council now in session in Manchester, June 17, 1819," in Parsons, *Truth Espoused*, 51–52.
63. Parsons, *Truth Espoused*, 53.
64. Parsons, 56.
65. Bentley, *The Diary of William Bentley*, 4:559.
66. Henry Raymond, "Editor's Table: The Sacredness of the Human Body," *Harper's New Monthly Magazine* 8 (April 1854): 691.
67. Ironically, Crowell's wife had died on December 11, 1818, and was buried in the same cemetery as Sewall's victims. Crowell married Hannah Choate on September 2, 1822, the sister of Rufus Choate, becoming the brother-in-law of Dr. Thomas Sewall. *Vital Records of Ipswich Massachusetts: Marriages and Deaths to the End of 1849*, 3 vols. (Salem, MA: Essex Institute, 1910), 2:98, 176, 534. On the status of New England clergy, see R.W. Dale, "Impressions of America," *Nineteenth Century* 4 (July–December 1878): 724. On New England physicians, see Riznik, "Professional Lives of Early Nineteenth Century New England Doctors," 2–3.
68. Affidavit of Captain John Girdler, in Parsons, *Truth Espoused*, 64.
69. "Agreeably to the Advice of the Ecclesiastical Council Here Convened, at the Request of the Pastor and Church of Manchester, 17 June 1819," in Parsons, *Truth Espoused*, 54.
70. Selectmen of Manchester to Rev. James Thurston, December 24, 1819, in Parsons, *Truth Espoused*, 95.
71. Parsons, *Truth Espoused*, 74.
72. Parsons, 75.
73. On the trial, see Parsons, *Truth Espoused*, 74–92.
74. *Essex Register*, November 1, 1820, 2.
75. Parsons, *Truth Espoused*, 85.
76. Parsons, 80 (emphasis added).
77. Cyrus M. Tracey, *Standard History of Essex County, Massachusetts* (Boston: Jewett & Co., 1878), 291; and Charles Henry Bell, *History of the Town of Exeter, New Hampshire* (Exeter, 1888), chap. 9 and 10.

Chapter 4

1. William H. Welch, "From the Address of William H. Welch," in Emily Anna Smith, *The Life and Letters of Nathan Smith* (New Haven: Yale University Press, 1914), 153.
2. Oliver S. Hayward and Constance E. Putnam, *Improve, Perfect, & Perpetuate: Nathan Smith and Early American Medical Education* (Hanover, NH: University Press of New England, 1998), 81.
3. Letter, Nathan Smith (Hanover, NH) to New Hampshire governor John Langdon, June 19, 1806 (facsimile), in John Waite, "The Doctor, the Murderer, and the Governor," *The New Antiquarian, the Blog of the Antiquarian Booksellers of America*, February 9, 2015, https://www.abaa.org/blog/post/the-doctor-the-murderer-and-the-governor.
4. The hanging was termed a glorious occasion, with nearly ten thousand persons attending. For a description of the event, see Rev. John Quincy Bittinger, *A History of Haverhill, New Hampshire* (Haverhill, NH: Cohos Steam Press, 1888), 396. The hanging was also reported on by numerous New England newspapers of the day.
5. *Weekly Wanderer*, August 18, 1806, 3.
6. Josiah Burnham was in the Haverhill, New Hampshire, jail with Russell Freeman and Captain Starkweather for debt. There was an argument, and Burnham, who had a knife, stabbed Freeman in the bowels and cut Starkweather's throat. Both men subsequently died. The sheriff of the jail, David Webster, prepared to move the bodies. A lawyer who represented the "parties at whose suit the two men dead had been imprisoned cautioned the sheriff as to the steps about to be taken." He advised the sheriff "to be careful about moving the bodies until they were "discharged by due process of the law." The lawyer told the sheriff he could be charged with an escape if the bodies were moved. Otherwise, he would have to "settle with their creditors." His only choice was to leave the bodies. "Am I to leave these two bodies to rot and stink in the jail … ?" The lawyer replied, "Barrel up and salt those two bodies." The sheriff, unpleased, rode all night to consult with a judge who "relieved him of his fears." It appears that in the northern part of England up to the end of the eighteenth century, "the body of the imprisoned debtor, whether dead or alive, belonged to the creditor." No doubt the lawyer, perhaps through legal legerdemain, hoped to convince the families of the slain men to

sell their bodies to pay off their creditors. William F. Whitcher, ed., *Josiah Burnham: His Trial and Execution for Murder with a Sermon Preached at Haverhill New Hampshire at the Time and Place of His Execution, August 12, 1806* (Woodsville, NH: New Books and Job Print, 1909), 5–6, 11–12. For a discussion on why corpses in the United States "have been more frequently arrested for debts due from the deceased" and on why even in Massachusetts "as late as 1811, a statute was enacted to prevent, imposing a fine upon the sheriff or other officers who did so," see R. S. Guernsey, "Ownership of a Corpse," *Central Law Journal* 10 (January–June 1880): 326–7. Later by law a dead body was not owned by creditors but instead was part of the deceased's estate and under the direction of probate courts (326).

7. Whitcher, *Josiah Burnham*, 15; and Bittinger, *A History of Haverhill*, 395.

8. Hayward and Putnam, *Improve, Perfect, & Perpetuate*, 86.

9. For example, there is a letter dated September 25, 1830, from Nathan Smith's son, Nathan R. Smith, to Parker Cleaveland, a former colleague of Nathan Smith at Bowdoin College, who wrote, "I shall immediately invoke Frank, our body snatcher (a better man never lifted a spade), ...We get them here without any difficulty at the present." He adds, he would not want anyone to know some bodies have been shipped out of state. As for the shipping terms, he puts the bodies in "barrels [of] whiskey" then enumerates the cost of the whiskey, barrels, and three cadavers for a sum of $50.00 each. Parker Cleaveland Papers, Special Collections, Bowdoin College Library, cited in Hayward and Putnam, 86. The text of this letter is posted in Davidge Hall, University of Maryland, Baltimore, next to a barrel like those filled with whiskey and then used for shipping the purloined bodies.

10. Hayward and Putnam, 86.

11. Henry I. Bowditch, *Memoir of Amos Twitchell* (Boston: John Wilson and Son, 1851), 37. For a description of Twitchell and Smith's close relationship and influence on his pupil, see 30–31.

12. Letter, Nathan Smith to Governor John Langdon, June 19, 1806, in John Waite, "The Doctor, the Murderer, and the Governor," *The New Antiquarian, the Blog of the Antiquarian Booksellers of America*, February 9, 2015, https://www.abaa.org/blog/post/the-doctor-the-murderer-and-the-governor.

13. Letter, Nathan Smith to George C. Shattuck, May 14, 1810, in Smith, *The Life and Letters of Nathan Smith*, 51–52.

14. Dr. James Alfred Spalding, *Dr. Lyman Spalding: The Originator of the United States Pharmacopoeia* (Boston: W.M. Leonard, 1916), 153.

15. Hayward and Putnam, *Improve, Perfect, & Perpetuate*, 95.

16. Letter, Ezekiel D. Cushing to Nathaniel Cushing, December, 2, 1809, EDC Papers (Folder 4), Manuscripts and Archives, Yale University Library.

17. Letter, Ezekiel D. Cushing to Nathaniel Cushing, December, 2, 1809, EDC Papers (Folder 4), Manuscripts and Archives, Yale University Library.

18. Letter, Ezekiel D. Cushing to Mehetabel Cushing (mother), December 5, 1809, EDC Papers (Folder 4), Manuscripts and Archives, Yale University Library.

19. Medical instruction at Dartmouth was given in the fall. The grave-robbing incident likely occurred in late November. On the medical instruction calendar, see Frederick C. Waite, "Grave Robbing in New England," *Bulletin of the Medical Library Association* 33 (1945): 278. Oddly enough, in his extensive article the Dartmouth "grave robbing" incident of 1809 is not mentioned.

20. Letter, Nathan Smith to Lyman Spalding, February 13, 1810, in Spalding, *Dr. Lyman Spalding*, 186.

21. Letter, Ezekiel D. Cushing to Mehetabel Cushing (sister), February 11, 1810, Francis A. Countway Library of Medicine, Harvard University, https://nrs.lib.harvard.edu/urn-3:hms.count:26856034?n=4.

22. For example, both Ezekiel D. Cushing and Ruggles Sylvester received their bachelor of medicine degrees from Dartmouth in 1811. Amos Twitchell also received his doctor of medicine degree. See *Washingtonian*, September 9, 1811, 3.

23. Hayward and Putnam, *Improve, Perfect, & Perpetuate*, 97.

24. Letter, Ebenezer Adams to George C. Shattuck, December 6, 1809, Shattuck Papers, Massachusetts Historical Society, in Hayward and Putnam, *Improve, Perfect, & Perpetuate*, 97.

25. Letter, Ezekiel D. Cushing to Mehetabel Cushing (mother), December 15, 1809, Ezekiel D. Cushing Papers (Folder 4), Yale University Manuscripts and Archives, Yale University Library, in Hayward and Putnam, *Improve, Perfect, & Perpetuate*, 97.

26. Mills Olcott, Account Books, Hanover, 41, MO Accounts of His Law Practice, 1800–1840, Vol. 2, 1807–1825, 9, Rauner Library, Dartmouth College Archives, Baker Library.

27. Edward M. Hartwell, "American Anatomy Acts," *Boston Medical Surgical Journal* 103 (1880): 361.

28. Carleton B. Chapman, *Dartmouth Medical School: The First 175 Years* (Hanover, NH: University Press of New England, 1973), 37.

29. President John Wheelock to the Hon. Benjamin J. Gilbert, December 6, 1809 (#809668), Resolutions Made at the Meeting of the President and Other Officers of Dartmouth College, December 18, 1809 (#809668.1), [Student Committee] to the Honorable President and Professors of Dartmouth College, ca. 1810 (#810900.6), in Craig Steven Wilder, *Ebony and Ivy: Race, Slavery, and the Troubled History of American Universities* (New York: Bloomsbury, 2013), 205.

30. Wilder, *Ebony and Ivy*, 205.
31. Wilder, 205.
32. Hayward and Putnam, *Improve, Perfect, & Perpetuate*, 101.
33. Letter, Dr. Nathan Smith to Dr. George C. Shattuck, January 7, 1821, in Smith, *The Life and Letters of Nathan Smith*, 109–10.
34. Chapman, *Dartmouth Medical School*, 18.
35. *Concord Gazette*, February 13, 1810, 3.
36. Letter, Ezekiel D. Cushing to Nathaniel Cushing, December 27, 1809, Francis A. Countway Library, Harvard University, https://nrs.lib.harvard.edu/urn-3:hms.count:26856044?n=11.
37. Letter, Ezekiel D. Cushing to Nathaniel Cushing, May 23, 1810, Francis A. Countway Library, Harvard University, https://nrs.lib.harvard.edu/urn-3:hms.count:26856044?n=11.
38. Letter, Ezekiel D. Cushing to Nathaniel Cushing, October 7, 1810, Francis A. Countway Library, Harvard University, https://nrs.lib.harvard.edu/urn-3:hms.count:26856044?n=11.
39. Deposition, Ezekiel D. Cushing, November 18, 1810, Shattuck Papers, Massachusetts Historical Society, in Hayward and Putnam, *Improve, Perfect, & Perpetuate*, 98–99.
40. Hayward and Putnam, 99.
41. Hayward and Putnam, 98.
42. Letter, Ezekiel D. Cushing to Nathaniel Cushing, November 28, 1810, Francis A. Countway Library, Harvard University, https://nrs.lib.harvard.edu/urn-3:hms.count:26856044?n=11.
43. Letter, George Shattuck to Ezekiel Dodge Cushing, December 10, 1810, Ezekiel D. Cushing Papers (Folder 4), Yale University Manuscripts and Archives, Yale University Library.
44. Letter, Ezekiel Dodge Cushing to Nathaniel Cushing, January 22, 1811 (Folder 4), Yale University Manuscripts and Archives, Yale University Library.
45. Hayward and Putnam, *Improve, Perfect, & Perpetuate*, 98–99.
46. Chapman, 39 and *Catalogus... Harvardiani*, 1830, 45.
47. Hayward and Putnam, 89.
48. Letter, Nathan Smith to Dr. George C. Shattuck, May 14, 1810, in Smith, *The Life and Letters of Nathan Smith*, 51–52.
49. Letter, Nathan Smith to George C. Shattuck, December 20, 1811, in Smith, *The Life and Letters of Nathan Smith*, 71–72.
50. Hayward and Putnam, 101.
51. *Washingtonian*, September 9, 1811, 3.
52. *Mt. Lebanon Fiftieth Anniversary, 1912–1962* (Mt. Lebanon, PA: Mt. Lebanon News, 1912), 24.
53. Stephen West Williams, *American Medical Biography: Or Memoirs of Eminent Physicians; Embracing* ... (Greenfield, MA: L. Merriam, and Co., 1845), 117–18.
54. Letter, Timothy J. Gridley to Jonathan Knight, November 20, 1810, in Hayward and Putnam, 195, 199; *Memorial of the Centennial of the Yale Medical School*, 1915, 24.
55. Michael O. Dumas, MD, "The Evolution of Medicine and Surgery," *Journal of the National Medical Association* 18 (1926): 6.
56. Hayward and Putnam, 100.

Chapter 5

1. Hannibal Hamlin, "The Dissection Riot of 1824 and the Connecticut Anatomical Law," *Yale Journal of Biology and Medicine* 7, no. 4 (1934–1935): 275–89; and "Interment of the Dead," *Connecticut Herald*, June 19, 1824, 3.
2. Hamlin, "The Dissection Riot of 1824," 282–83.
3. Charles E. Cunningham, *Timothy Dwight: A Biography, 1752–1817* (New York: Macmillan, 1941), 220–222.
4. Letter, Dr. Nathan Smith to Dr. George C. Shattuck, May 14, 1810, in Emily Anna Smith, *The Life and Letters of Nathan Smith* (New Haven: Yale University Press, 1914), 51.
5. Smith, *The Life and Letters of Nathan Smith*, 98.
6. John Morison Duncan, *Travels through Part of the United States and Canada in 1818 and* ... 2 vols. (Glasgow: Hurst, Robinson & Co., 1823), 1:102. Perhaps Duncan had learned of this provision from Benjamin Silliman, professor of chemistry at Yale and one of the most "earnest advocates for establishing a medical school at Yale" and to whom Duncan dedicated his book. Nevertheless, there were persistent rumors that "the medical school had been put near the Grove Street cemetery so that bodies could be snatched, and that there was an underground tunnel between the building and the grave yard." See Loomis Untermeyer, "Out of Yale's Past: A Story of Undergraduate Traditions" (New Haven, CT: n.p., 1960), 18. The provision may have been part of the negotiations when Nathan Smith, who had rented a building near the burying ground, called on the state legislature to help him purchase the building. The "Medical School was opened in the fall of 1813, in the building at the head of College Street, familiar to us as Sheffield Hall ... [and was] ... at first leased, but its purchase was soon made possible by a grant from the State Legislature." I suspect that Smith may have found this requirement insulting to him and other medical school faculty members. General Joseph L. Chamberlain, *Yale University: Its History, Influence, Equipment and Characteristics* ... (Boston: R. Herndon Company, 1900), 136.
7. Dr. James Lyman Spalding, *The Originator of the United States Pharmacopoeia* (Boston: W.M. Leonard, 1916), 293.
8. Letter, Ezekiel D. Cushing to Nathaniel Cushing, December 2, 1809, in Oliver S. Hayward and Constance E. Putnam, *Improve, Perfect, & Perpetuate: Nathan Smith and Early American Medical Education* (Hanover, NH: University Press of New England, 1998), 96.
9. James A. Spalding, MD "The Friendship of Dr. Nathan Smith and Dr. Lyman Spalding," *Bulletin of the American Academy of Medicine* 7, no. 10 (1906), 727–28.

10. Jonathan Knight attended the school of medicine at the University of Pennsylvania, and he—along with Dr. Nathan Smith—would be founding members of the medical school at Yale. Knight was appointed professor of anatomy and physiology in 1813. Yale Medical School, *Memorial of the Centennial of the Yale Medical School* (New Haven: Yale University School of Medicine, 1915), 16.

11. Letter, Timothy J. Gridley to Jonathan Knight, November 20, 1810, in Hayward and Putnam, *Improve, Perfect, & Perpetuate*, 199 (emphasis added).

12. Hayward and Putnam, *Improve, Perfect, & Perpetuate*, 199. Gridley also implies in the letter that not only would Smith help establish the reputation of the new medical school but also could bring in tow "the 60 students at Hanover ... [who] ... would largely follow him to New Haven." Yale Medical School, *Memorial of the Centennial of the Yale Medical School* (New Haven: Yale University, School of Medicine, 1915), 24.

13. *Connecticut Courant*, February 16, 1819, 3–4.

14. *Connecticut Herald*, February 23, 1819, 3.

15. Thomas Day, *Reports of the Cases Argued and Determined in the Supreme Court of Errors of the State Connecticut*, Vol. 4 (New York: Banks, Gould, and Co., 1848), 71–70; Yale University, *Catalogue of Officers and Graduates of Yale University* (New Haven: Tuttle, Morehouse, and Taylor, 1910), 253; and *Connecticut Herald*, September 13, 1819, 3.

16. Hayward and Putnam, 100; and Letter, Nathan Smith to Mills Olcott, May 1819, Mss. 819340.2, Dartmouth College Archives, Baker Library.

17. *Hartford Courant*, May 25, 1819, 2.

18. On Dr. Jonathan Knight's inexperience and rationale for hiring him, see Cunningham, *Timothy Dwight*, 220.

19. The threat of a mob may have brought back memories of Knight's early days, previously discussed. Cunningham, *Timothy Dwight*, 222.

20. *New London Gazette*, June 1, 1819, 3.

21. *Hartford Courant*, May 25, 1819, 2.

22. *American Mercury*, June 1, 1819, 2

23. *Hartford Courant*, June 8, 1819, 2.

24. Thomas Southwood Smith, *Use of the Dead to the Living* (London: Craddock and Paternoster Row, 1828), 43–44.

25. Craig Steven Wilder, *Ebony and Ivy: Race, Slavery, and the Troubled History of American Universities* (New York: Bloomsbury, 2013), 204.

26. T.F. Harrington, *The Harvard Medical School*, 3 vols. (New York: Lewis Publishing, 1905), 2:662.

27. *Middlesex Gazette*, June 2, 1824, 2.

28. *New England Palladium*, February 26, 1819, 1.

29. The Charles R. Hale Collection, Hale Collection of Connecticut Cemetery Inscriptions, Hartford, Connecticut State Library; Hartford, Connecticut, Connecticut Newspaper Notices, Vol. 17, 272, accessed at Ancestry.com; Connecticut, U.S., Hale Collection of Cemetery Inscriptions and Newspaper Notices, 1629–1934 [database online], Provo, UT; and *Middlesex Gazette*, January 14, 1824, 3.

30. For Peck's sources, see Henry Peck, *The New Haven State House with Some Accounts of the Green* (New Haven, CT: Henry Peck and George H. Coe, 1889), 118–121.

31. Peck, *New Haven State House*, 118–19.

32. Hamlin, "The Dissection Riot of 1824," 280. For a more terse obituary, see "In Orange, Miss Bathsheba Smith, 19, Daughter of Laban S.," *Connecticut Herald*, January 18, 1824, 3. The town of Orange was incorporated in 1822 and included the parishes of West Haven and North Milford.

33. Peck, *New Haven State House*, 119.

34. Perhaps in a similar manner, in Manchester, England, in 1832 it was reported that a brick was used to replace the stolen head of the corpse of a young boy, probably to avoid a telltale depression at the grave site. The gruesome act was discovered by the father and set off a riot. John Knott, "Popular Attitudes to Death and Dissection in Early Nineteenth Century Britain: The Anatomy Act and the Poor," *Labour History* (1985): 8.

35. Obviously, I cannot identify whose chaise was used, but for the record Dr. Nathan Smith did own a chaise. "I left a chaise at Middletown in Connecticut with orders to send it on to Boston," Dr. Nathan Smith to Samuel Shattuck, Brunswick, April 17, 1823, in Smith, *The Life and Letters of Nathan Smith*, 121. And "if you are willing ... the captain of the vessel who may bring my chaise," Dr. Nathan Smith to Samuel Shattuck, Brunswick, May 5, 1823, in Smith, *The Life and Letters of Nathan Smith*, 123.

36. Ironically, it was in Southbury, Connecticut, in 1819 where there had been a storm of protest and outrage over the body-snatching episode of Mr. Major Tiff. The justice of the peace in the Joseph T. Waldo case was named Shadrach Osborn Esq., who does not seem to be related to Erastus Osborn. See William Cothren, *History of Ancient Woodbury, Connecticut: From the First ...*, 2 vols. (Waterbury, CT, Bronson Brothers, 1854), 1:390–91.

37. Erastus Osborn to Shadrach Osborn, January 12, 1824, Yale University Library, https://imageserver.library.yale.edu/digcoll:4342544/guest2708120bc940472caf3fab55a4dc8923@yaleguest.edu/YEcXdYQ10qTHqcrUf3cle83ApOU/1500.jpe?authroot=findit.library.yale.edu&parentfolder=digcoll:4342544&ip=32.214.70.86; and Hamlin, "The Dissection Riot of 1824," 278.

38. Peck, *New Haven State House*, 118.

39. Erastus Osborn to Shadrach Osborn, January 12, 1824, Yale University Library.

40. Peck, *New Haven State House*, 118–19.

41. Second Company Governor's Foot Guard, *A Souvenir of New Haven Connecticut: Connecticut Governor's Foot Guard Second Company*, 2nd ed. (New Haven, CT: Governor's Foot Guard, 1908), 97. The times given for the appearance of the militia is "ten o'clock" on the evening of January 12, 1824. Other sources indicate that the militia was called out during the morning of the search. See, for example, Erastus Osborn to Shadrach Osborn, 12 January 1824, https://imageserver.library.yale.

edu/digcoll:4342544/guest2708120bc940472caf3fab55a4dc8923@yaleguest.edu/YEcXdYQ10qTHqcrUf3cle83ApOU/1500.jpe?authroot=findit.library.yale.edu&parentfolder=digcoll:4342544&ip=32.214.70.86. The local military group called the New Haven Grays was also put on alert and were "put under arms [and] provided with ammunition at summons of the authorities to keep the people within boundaries." See Jerome Bonaparte Luckè, *History of the New Haven Grays from Sept. 13, 1816, to Sept. 13, 1876* (New Haven, CT: Tuttle, Morehouse, and Taylor, 1876), 38.

42. Peck, *New Haven State House*, 118–19.

43. Henry Blake Taylor, *Chronicles of the New Haven Green from 1638 to 1862* (New Haven, CT: Tuttle, Morehouse, and Taylor, 1898), 238.

44. Erastus Osborn to Shadrach Osborn, January 12, 1824, Yale University Library.

45. Taylor, *Chronicles of the New Haven Green*, 238.

46. Erastus Osborn to Shadrach Osborn, January 12, 1824, Yale University Library.

47. *Norwich Courier*, January 21, 1824, 3.

48. Peck, *New Haven State House*, 121.

49. "A Card," West Haven, January 15, 1824, *Connecticut Herald*, January 20, 1824, 3.

50. Peck, *New Haven State House*, 121.

51. Erastus Osborn to Shadrach Osborn, January 12, 1824, Yale University Library.

52. For example, according to Peck, "There were found, however, four or five bodies concealed under some charcoal" during the first search. See Peck, *New Haven State House*, 119. Could this have been what Osborn was referring to when he wrote "found just as I suppose usually to be found at such institutions"? The bodies under charcoal would make sense to help conceal the odor of the decaying corpses, those bodies having been legally obtained. Letter, Erastus Osborn to Shadrach Osborn, January 12, 1824, Yale University Library.

53. *New Haven Register*, January 17, 1824, 3.

54. Erastus Osborn to Shadrach Osborn, January 12, 1824, Yale University Library.

55. Peck, *New Haven State House*, 120.

56. Erastus Osborn to Shadrach Osborn, January 19, 1824, Yale University Library.

57. I have specifically used this term because in a letter to his lawyer and friend Mills Olcott in Hanover, New Hampshire, Dr. Smith wrote that "her body had been placed by the person who got it & our sweeper." Nathan Smith to M. Olcott, January 30, 1824, MS-436, Box 4 (Folder 62), Dartmouth College Archives, Baker Library. According to the "Laws of the Government of the Medical Institution" at Yale in 1815, "A sweeper shall be appointed, whose duty it shall be to cause the public and private rooms, passages, and appurtenances to be kept clean and in decent order." In the medical school the duty likely included taking care of the "equipment" (appurtenances) such as bodies for the dissection room. Yale University, School of Medicine, *Memorial of the Centennial of the Yale Medical School* (New Haven: Yale University Press, 1915), 35, 39.

58. Erastus Osborn to Shadrach Osborn, January 19, 1824, Yale University Library.

59. Michael Sappol, *A Traffic of Dead Bodies* (Princeton: Princeton University Press, 2002), 322.

60. Elizabeth Klaver, *Sites of Autopsy in Contemporary Culture* (Albany: State University of New York Press, 2005), 19.

61. Sappol, *A Traffic of Dead Bodies*, 323.

62. Sappol, 87–88.

63. Crowell, Robert Crowell, *Interment of the Dead, a Dictate of Natural Affection, Sanctioned by the Word of God, and the Examples of the Good in Every Age: A Sermon Delivered in Ipswich, Second Parish, July 23, 1818, on the Occasion of Reinterring the Coffins Which Had Been Robbed of Their Contents* (Andover, 1818), 37. For a discussion on one of the last anatomy riots also involving the "honor" of a young woman in Cleveland in 1852, see Sappol, *A Traffic of Dead Bodies*, 137.

64. Peck, *New Haven State House*, 117–18; and *Connecticut Herald*, January 20, 1824, 3.

65. "Letter to the Editor," *Middlesex Gazette*, January 21, 1824, 3.

66. *Middlesex Gazette*, January 14, 1824, 3; and *Boston Commercial Gazette*, January 19, 1824, 2.

67. *Middlesex Gazette*, January 14, 1824, 3.

68. Hamlin, "The Dissection Riot of 1824," 281–82; and *Boston Commercial Gazette*, January 19, 1824, 2.

69. Peck, *New Haven State House*, 120–21.

70. *Middlesex Gazette*, January 21, 1824, 3.

71. On medical students, see Sappol, *A Traffic of Dead Bodies*, 80–88.

72. Dr. Nathan Smith to Dr. George C. Shattuck, January 7, 1821, in Smith, *The Life and Letters of Nathan Smith*, 109–10.

73. James Knight, *An Eulogium on Nathan Smith Late Professor of the Theory and Practice of Physic and Surgery...* (New Haven, CT: Hezekiah Howe, 1829), 21–22.

74. Wilder, *Ebony and Ivy*, 199. These exploits were doubtless no exaggeration. As noted earlier, similar medical student hijinks helped precipitate the New York Doctors Riot in 1788. Similar activities took place in London in 1810. A medical student took an amputated leg and threw it down a nearby chimney. It fell into a "cooking pot in which the wife of a chimney sweep was boiling up some stew." The woman went into hysterics, and a riot broke out. See Hubert Cole, *Things for the Surgeon: A History of the Resurrection Men* (London: Heinemann, 1964), 22.

75. "Dr. Isaac Wood and Dissection Material in the Early Days," *Medical News* 82 (May 7, 1903): 851.

76. Hayward and Putnam, 81–82.

77. Edward Warren, *Life of John Collins Warren, M.D.*, 2 vols. (Boston: Ticknor and Fields, 1860), 1:404; and Samuel Ward Francis, *Biographical Sketches of Distinguished Living New York Physicians* (New York: Putnam, 1867), 99.

78. Letter, Nathan Smith to Mills Olcott,

January 30, 1824, MS-436, Box 4 (Folder 62), Dartmouth College Archives, Baker Library.

79. Letter, Nathan Smith to Mills Olcott, January 30, 1824.

80. Hamlin, "The Dissection Riot of 1824," 282–83, *Connecticut Herald*, February 10, 1824, 3, and February 20, 1824, 3. Fortunately, there was no smallpox outbreak in New Haven at the time. There were two people sickened with a disease, but as one newspaper reported the disease did not exhibit the "distinctive characteristics" of smallpox, but "care should be taken to prevent contagion," as inoculation did not prevent it. *Connecticut Herald*, January 20, 1824, 3.

81. *Portsmouth Journal*, , January 24, 1824, 3.

82. Letter, Nathan Smith to Mills Olcott, February 28, 1824, MS-436, Box 4 (Folder 62), Dartmouth College Archives, Baker Library.

83. Peck, *New Haven State House*, 121.

84. On the position and duties of the waiters, see Yale University School of Medicine, *Memorial of the Centennial of the Yale Medical School*, 43.

85. Erastus Osborn to Shadrach Osborn, January 19, 1824, Yale University Library.

86. Hamlin, "The Dissection Riot of 1824," 285.

87. Hamlin, 285.

88. *Connecticut Courant*, November 9, 1824, 3.

89. *Connecticut Herald*, January 18, 1824, 3, and April 20, 1824, 3.

90. *Sentinel and Witness*, February 11, 1824, 2. Seth P. Staples also founded Yale's law school. See Luckè, *History of the New Haven Grays*, 18.

91. *Connecticut Courant*, May 18, 1824, 2; and *Connecticut Herald*, April 27, 1824, 1.

92. *Connecticut Herald*, February 10, 1824, 3. The *Salem Gazette*, familiar with the earlier Seward body-snatching episode and trial, introduced this report with the headline "Medical Students Look at This." This headline and story were repeated in many newspapers throughout the United States. See the *Salem Gazette*, February 17, 1824, 3.

93. Hamlin, "The Dissection Riot of 1824," 285.

94. Edward M. Hartwell, *The Study of Anatomy, Historically, and Legally Considered* (Boston: Tolman & White, 1881), 31.

95. I have paraphrased the sentiments found in a letter published in the *Middlesex Gazette*, January 21, 1824, 3.

Chapter 6

1. Edward M. Hartwell, *The Study of Anatomy, Historically, and Legally Considered* (Boston: Tolman & White, 1881), 30–31.

2. *Hartford Courant*, May 25, 1819, 2.

3. Oliver Wolcott, *Message of His Excellency Oliver Wolcott: To the Senate and House of Representatives of the State of Connecticut, at the Commencement of the Session of the General Assembly, in New-Haven, May, A.D. 1824* (Hartford, CT: Joseph Barber, 1924), 13; and *Connecticut Courant*, May 11, 1824, 2–3.

4. Michael Sappol, *A Traffic of Dead Bodies* (Princeton: Princeton University Press, 2002), 57–58.

5. *Connecticut Courant*, May 11, 1824, 3.

6. *American Mercury*, May 11, 1824, 3.

7. *American Mercury*, May 25, 1824, 3.

8. *Norwich Courier*, June 2, 1824, 2.

9. *Connecticut Herald*, June 15, 1824, 3.

10. *Connecticut Herald*, June 22, 1824, 3.

11. "Remarks by the Editor of the Nat Democrat," *Connecticut Herald*, July 27, 1824, 2, reprinting an article from the *Connecticut Register*, n.d.

12. Franklin Bowditch Dexter, *Biographical Sketches of the Graduates of Yale College with Annals of the College History*, Vol. 6 (New Haven: Yale University Press, 1912), 714–15.

13. Dexter, *Biographical Sketches of the Graduates of Yale College*, 715.

14. *New London Gazette*, September 3, 1823, 3.

15. *Baltimore Patriot*, October 20, 1823, 2.

16. *Middlesex Gazette*, May 12, 1824, 2.

17. *Connecticut Mirror*, May 17, 1824, 2.

18. *Baltimore Patriot*, September 3, 1823, 2.

19. For the term "democrat republican," see *Connecticut Mirror*, October 20, 1823, 2. In addition, the same paper noted that it had to accept Wolcott's temporary choice "until the Legislature should ratify the appointment or make another." *Connecticut Mirror*, October 20, 1823, 2; and Jarvis Means Morse, *A Neglected Period of Connecticut's History, 1818–1850* (New York: Octagon Books, 1979), 69–70.

20. "Remarks by the Editor of the Nat Democrat," 2.

21. "Remarks by the Editor of the Nat Democrat," 2.

22. Ironically, in 1831 the term unclaimed was substituted for the word "paupers" or "poor" and was included in the 1831 Massachusetts anatomy act. The law required "civil officials to surrender any body that was to be buried at public expense (with some exceptions), for dissection." Frederick C. Waite, "The Development of Anatomical Laws in the States of New England," *New England Journal of Medicine* 233 (1945): 721. This provision would appear later in the Connecticut anatomy law of 1833, which was admittedly at the time based on the Massachusetts Act, setting off a storm of controversy in Connecticut (see below).

23. See Rosemary Stevens, *American Medicine and the Public Interest* (Berkeley: University of California Press, 1998), 26–28. This is an excellent discussion on the changing nature of anti-elitism and general distrust of the medical profession and its impact on medical legislation in Jacksonian America.

24. *Connecticut Herald*, August 3, 1824, 3.

25. On Colburn, see Hannibal Hamlin, "The Dissection Riot of 1824 and the Connecticut Anatomical Law," *Yale Journal of Biology and Medicine* 7 (1934–1935): 286.

26. *Public Statutes of the State of Connecticut*

(Hartford, CA: C. Babcock, 1824), 51; and *Connecticut Herald*, June 22, 1824, 1.

27. Edward Augustus Kendall, *Travels through the Northern Parts of the United States, in the Years 1807 and 1808*, 2 vols. (New York: I. Riley, 1809), 1:211.

28. Kendall, *Travels through the Northern Parts of the United States*,. 210–11.

29. Kendall, 211.

30. In 1821 a law was passed stating that "any woman convicted of a crime punishable with imprisonment in New-Gate Prison, must be confined with the female prisoners in the common workhouse of the county where such offense is tried, or she might be confined in the county jail.... The indescribable condition of this underground prison is sufficient justification for such a law." However, because there were no county workhouses, "such women were to be sent to jail, unless they might perhaps have been confined in a town workhouse at the county seat. There they would have been with beggars and stubborn children." See Edward W. Capen, *The Historical Development of the Poor Law of Connecticut* (New York: Columbia University Press, 1905), 152.

31. Kendall, *Travels through the Northern Parts of the United States*, 212–13.

32. Kendall, 213.

33. *Public Statutes of the State of Connecticut* (Hartford, CA: C. Babcock, 1824), 51–52; and *Connecticut Herald*, June 22, 1824, 1.

34. The old Newgate prison was abandoned in 1827, and a new state prison replaced it in Wethersfield, Connecticut. The new prison resulted from the prison reform movement and came to be considered a "model penitentiary." See Richard H. Phelps, *Newgate, a History of the Prison: Its Insurrections, Massacres ...* (Albany, NY: J. Mussel, 1860), 117, 125–27.

35. *Public Statutes of the State of Connecticut*, 52; and *Connecticut Herald*, June 22, 1824, 1.

36. Hamlin, "The Dissection Riot of 1824," 286. Waite makes the point that it was the first law to provide for the "anatomical study of bodies other than those of murderers and duelists," though, as argued here, hardly providing enough to meet the demand. Waite, "The Development of Anatomical Laws," 720.

37. William Mackenzie, "An Appeal to the Public and to the Legislatures on the Necessity of Affording Dead Bodies to the Schools of Anatomy, by Legislative Enactment," *Westminster Review* 2 (July–August): 89.

38. Elisha North, MD, *Outlines of the Science of Life: Which Treats Physiologically of Both Body and Mind; Designed Only for Philosophers, and Other Candid Persons, to Which Are Added Essays on Other Subjects* (New York: Collins and Co., 1829), 140.

39. North, *Outlines of the Science of Life*, 133.

40. North, 134.

41. North, 137.

42. North 158.

43. North, 156.

44. North, 153.

45. North, 153–54.

46. North, 153–54.

47. North, 160–61.

48. North, 162.

49. *Columbian Register*, April 27, 1833, 3.

50. The article has no title but is signed "A Physician." See *Connecticut Courant*, April 30, 1833, 2, from *the Columbian Register*.

51. "An Act Regarding Anatomical and Medical Science," *Connecticut Courant*, July 8, 1833, 1.

52. *New London Gazette*, May 21, 1834, 2.

53. *Columbian Register*, July 20, 1833, 3.

54. *Norwich Courier*, July 24, 1833, 3.

55. *New London Gazette*, October 9, 1833, 3.

56. *New London Gazette*, April 30, 1834, 3.

57. *Connecticut Courant*, May 5, 1834, 2.

58. *Connecticut Courant*, May 19, 1834, 3.

59. *New London Gazette*, May 21, 1834, 2.

60. *New London Gazette*, July 2, 1834, 1.

61. Edward M. Hartwell, *The Study of Anatomy, Historically, and Legally Considered* (Boston: Tolman & White, 1881), 29; and Sappol, *A Traffic of Dead Bodies*, 122–23.

62. Waite has attributed the success of the Massachusetts anatomy law to two factors: "the education of the public concerning the desirability of the anatomical law in Massachusetts made by the Massachusetts Medical Society" leading up to its passage and that the Massachusetts legislature was composed of many Harvard graduates who were unlikely to repeal a law "that much concerned the medical school of that university." Waite, "The Development of Anatomical Laws," 721. I believe it more likely that it was the way the law was written. It was limited to Boston, and the "subjects" were the poor and newly arrived Irish immigrants who were not missed, a fact recognized by the legislators in Connecticut during debates over the repeal of the Connecticut anatomical law. See my discussion below as to the factors that led to the repeal of the Connecticut law of 1833.

63. Michele Goodwin, *The Global Body Market Altruism's Limits* (Cambridge: Cambridge University Press, 2013), 134; and Sappol, *A Traffic of Dead Bodies*, 123.

64. William Jeremy Bromwell, *History of Immigration to the United States, Exhibiting the Number, Sex, Age ...* (New York: Redfield, 1856), 61, 105, 145.

65. Morse, *A Neglected Period of Connecticut's History*, 181. After 1820 the "state thus divested itself of as much responsibility for the care of the poor as it could. Connecticut's system became so decentralized that it assumed the nearest approach to a purely town system that could be found anywhere in America" (182).

66. The immigrant population in Connecticut until the middle of the century was minimal. Any immigrants tended to avoid settling in Connecticut because "local sentiment was hostile to them," the laws made it difficult for them to own real estate, and local officials were reluctant to make them eligible to vote. During this time

Connecticut was witnessing an outflow of its population and retained its agricultural base. Newcomers were simply not welcome. In addition, because the young men were leaving for the West and larger cities, by 1818 "many towns were already declining toward the feeble and half-deserted parishes of today." See Morse, *A Neglected Period of Connecticut's History,* 22–23. One can see the devastating impact of the 1833 anatomical law on the morale of a rural population caught up in a demographic and economic decline, confirming their worst fears if they were to slide into poverty and become dependent on the town.

67. Edward Warren Capen, *Historical Development of the Poor Law in Connecticut* (New York: Columbia University Press, 1905), 171.

68. Morse, *A Neglected Period of Connecticut's History,* 293–94.

Chapter 7

1. Frederick C. Waite, *The First Medical College in Vermont: Castleton. 1818–1862* (Montpelier: Vermont Historical Society, 1949), 52.

2. Castleton Academy was the first of what became known as "propriety medical schools," the term that was traced back to Castleton's founding document with the use of the term "proprietor." These were private schools not attached to a college, as was the traditional pattern in America. Generally founded by private doctors, the schools did not require prerequisites and depended on student fees. "Standards ranged from inadequate to excellent." The physicians were trained "on a parochial basis for the county practitioner." State legislatures "saw no difficulty in chartering such colleges," since they chartered schools teaching homeopathy. In the case of Castleton, the school did affiliate with Middlebury College to confer a degree, as it had inadvertently omitted this action in its founding document. This was remedied in October 1819. However, it has been suggested since all schools up to then had been affiliated with a college. The trustees of Castleton continued the partnership until December 27, 1827, when it was finally dissolved. See Rosemary Stevens, *American Medicine and the Public Interest* (Berkeley: University of California Press, 1998), 25; Waite, *The First Medical College in Vermont,* 55, 57–58, 78; and Joshua Bates, *Address Delivered in Castleton December 2, 1823, at the Commencement of the Vermont Academy of Medicine, with an Appendix Containing an Historical Sketch of the Medical School in Castleton, by One Fully Acquainted with Its Origin and Progress* (Poultney, VT, 1824), 11.

3. "Medical Science," *Rutland Daily Herald,* July 25, 1820, 2, in Waite, *The First Medical College in Vermont,* 53.

4. Waite, *The First Medical College in Vermont,* 55.

5. Waite, *The First Medical College in Vermont,* 60.

6. Bates, *Address Delivered in Castleton December 2, 1823,* 11; and Waite, *The First Medical College in Vermont,* 62.

7. Waite, *The First Medical College in Vermont,* 69.

8. Bates, *Address Delivered in Castleton December 2, 1823,* 12–14. In Waite, *The First Medical College in Vermont,* 64–65.

9. Waite, *The First Medical College in Vermont,* 66.

10. Interestingly, the legislatures in both New Hampshire and Vermont reference thirty-nine lashes. The punishment is biblical in nature, forty lashes less one, or thirty-nine lashes. Both the Old Testament and Roman law determined that forty lashes was enough to kill a man; therefore, thirty-nine lashes were the most you could give a man without it being considered a death sentence.

11. *Th Laws of the State of Vermont* (Randolph, VT: Serena Wright, 1808), 368.

12. Waite, "Grave Robbing in New England," 274 and Lassek, 185–186.

13. Bingham H. Stone, "One Hundred Years of Medicine in Vermont," *Vermont Medical Monthly* 19, no. 10 (October 15, 1913): 241.

14. Waite, *The First Medical College in Vermont,* 72.

15. Waite, *The First Medical College in Vermont,* 77.

16. Stone, "The First Medical College in Vermont," 241; and Henry S. Dana, *History of Woodstock, Vermont* (Boston: Houghton Mifflin, 1889), 233–34.

17. Waite, *The First Medical College in Vermont,* 123.

18. Waite, *The First Medical College in Vermont,* 123–24.

19. MS Records of the Corporation of the Vermont Academy of Medicine, I, 74, January 20, 1824, in Frederick C. Waite, "Grave Robbing in New England," *Bulletin of the Medical Library Association* 33 (1945): 283.

20. Waite, *The First Medical College in Vermont,* 124.

21. *Middlesex Gazette,* December 8, 1824, 2.

22. Dana, *History of Woodstock, Vermont,* 233.

23. Stone, "One Hundred Years of Medicine in Vermont," 242; and *Woodstock Observer,* July 21, 1829, 3, in Dana, *History of Woodstock, Vermont,* 234; and Waite, *The First Medical College in Vermont,* 123.

24. Stone, "One Hundred Years of Medicine in Vermont," 242.

25. James Sanford, "Recollections of Castleton Medical College," *Rutland Daily Herald and Globe,* July 21, 1879, 3, in Waite, *The First Medical College in Vermont,* 124.

26. Waite, "Grave Robbing in New England," 283.

27. Frederick C. Waite, *The Story of a Country Medical College: A History of the Clinical School of Medicine and the Vermont Medical College, Woodstock, Vermont* (Brattleboro: Vermont Printing Company, 1945), in Arthur M. Lassek, *Human Dissection Its: Drama and Struggle* (Springfield, IL: Charles C. Thomas, 1958), 213–14.

28. Gardner H. Churchill, *The Churchill Family in America* (Boston: Gardner Family, 1904), 453. *New York Spectator*, December 10, 1830, 1.

29. Abby M. Hemenway, *The Vermont Historical Gazetteer: A Magazine, Embracing a History of Each Town, Civil, Ecclesiastical, Biographical, and Military*, 5 vols. (Claremont, NH: Claremont Publishing Co., 1877), 3:770.

30. John M. Currier, MD, *Song of Hubbardton Raid: Delivered on the 50 (-I)th anniversary of the citizens of Hubbardton, Vermont, on Castleton Medical College, Held at the Residence of J. Sanford, M.D. Castleton, Vt. November 29, 1879* (Castleton, VT: Tuttle and Co., 1880), 19.

31. Hemenway, *The Vermont Historical Gazetteer*, 770–71.

32. Waite, *The First Medical College in Vermont*, 124.

33. Waite, *The First Medical college in Vermont*, 124–25.

34. *Vermont Statesman*, New York Spectator, December. 10, 1830, 1.

35. Hemenway, *The Vermont Historical Gazetteer*, 770–71.

36. At the annual meeting of the Rutland County Medical and Surgical Society, held at the Otter Creek House in Pittsford on July 9, 1879, Dr. James Sanford of Castleton delivered "an address, entitled, *Reminiscences of Castleton Medical College.*" He spoke on "the raid of the citizens of Hubbardton on Castleton Medical College to recover the body of Mrs. Penfield Churchill, which had been stolen from the graveyard in Hubbardton." The address was printed in the *Rutland Herald & Globe*. Students and others questioned some of the facts in this article. The next meeting of the Rutland County Medical and Surgical Society, held in Castleton, was on October 9, 1879, to celebrate the raid. "Song of the Hubbardton Raid" was read at this meeting. There were many persons present who had a knowledge of this event and would likely have had firsthand experience or spoken to those that did. See Currier, *Song of Hubbardton Raid*, 4–6.

37. This description is not exaggerated. According to the English doctor William Dale, who described dissecting rooms in the 1830s in England in the same way, there was a "total want of order … even of ordinary decency in conducting dissections at many medical schools…. There was "drinking, smoking, and brawling[;] … it was no uncommon thing to see a regular battle among the students, parts of the human body forming their weapons," and the more orderly "might expect to have the bowels or other viscera flying about their ears." See William Dale, *The Present State of the Medical Profession in Great Britain and Ireland* (London: A.W. Bennett, 1860), 42.

38. Currier, *Song of Hubbardton Raid*, 29.

39. Currier, 30.

40. Currier, 31–32.

41. Currier, 33.

42. Currier, 34.

43. Donald R. Sondergeld, *History of Hubbardton, Vermont* (Collierville, N: Instant Publisher, 2005), 2.

44. *New Hampshire Sentinel*, January 21, 1831, 2.

45. *Brattleboro Messenger*, January 29, 1831, 2.

46. *National Gazette*, February 1, 1831, 3.

47. *Catalogue of the Officers and Students of the Vermont Academy of Medicine* (Castleton, VT: H.H. Houghton, 1830), 8; and Waite, *The First Medical College in Vermont*, 274, 261.

48. "Dr. Almon Lull," Hartland Historical Society (Hartland, VT), https://hartlandhistory.org/?p=1063.

49. *Wisconsin Enquirer* (Madison, WI), March 2, 1838, 4.

50. Wisconsin Department of Health and Family Services, Wisconsin Vital Records Index Pre-1907, Vol. 1, 1, 4, https://www.wisconsinhistory.org/Records/Article/CS15307.

51. *Wisconsin Democrat*, March 30, 1850, 3.

52. *Wisconsin State Journal*, June 7, 1881, 8.

53. Hilah Violet Eddy, *The Lull Book* (Detroit, 1926), 16.

54. "Dr. Almon Lull," Hartland Historical Society (Hartland, VT), https://hartlandhistory.org/?p=1063.

55. *San Francisco Bulletin*, August 28, 1861, 3.

56. "Dr. Almon Lull"; "Death of Doctor Almon Lull, Obituary," *Vermont Journal*, April 7, 1894, 8; and "An Improvident Son" [Will of Almond Lull], *San Francisco Call*, March 25, 1894, 9.

57. State of Vermont, Vermont Vital Records through 1870, https://www.ancestry.com/discoveryui-content/view/487590:4661?tid=&pid=&queryId=a9ab6384d8a4a2d9a0f3c68dbb7cf74b&_phsrc=oMP5711&_phstart=successSource. Other sources have his birth erroneously as occurring in Windsor, Connecticut.

58. Lewis Darling, MD, *Papers and Proceeding of the Tioga County Historical Society*, Vol. 1 (Wellsboro: Pennsylvania, Agitator, 1906), 158. For more information on Dr. Lewis Darling, Sr., see 156–57.

59. John Daggett, *A Sketch of the History of Attleborough: From Its Settlement to the Division …* (Boston: Samuel Fisher, 1894), 642.

60. D.H. Hurd, *History of Bristol County…* (Philadelphia: J.W. Lewis, 1883), 36.

61. Daggett, *Sketch of the History of Attleborough*, 642.

62. Currier, *Song of Hubbardton Raid*, 1–8.

63. Waite, *The First Medical College in Vermont*, 228, 223, 177. In 1841 the Castleton Medical Academy was renamed Castleton Medical College.

64. G.D. Spencer, *A Poem on the Hubbardton Raid* (Rutland, VT: Tuttle and Co., 1880), 3–4.

65. It was not until the opening of Johns Hopkins Hospital (1889) and Johns Hopkins Medical School (1893) marking a new era in medical education that "Hopkins took all that was best in English and French medical education, which was based on clinical experience in hospitals, and combined it with all that was best in German medical education, which was based on research-oriented universities" and that medical education began to

achieve a new respect among the general population. See U.S. House of Representatives, *Subcommittee on Health, Panel Discussions on National Health Insurance* (Washington, D.C.: U.S. Government Printing Office, 1975), 27. For the original quote on the worth of doctors, see Daniel Drake, *Practical Essays on Medical Education, and the Medical Profession in the United States* (Cincinnati: Rolfe & Young, 1832), 6–7.

66. Spencer, *Poem on the Hubbardton Raid*, 6–7.

67. Spencer, 7. The snake is associated with Asclepius, the ancient Greek God of medicine.

68. Spencer, 8.

69. Spencer, 8–9.

70. Spencer, 10.

71. During most of the nineteenth century there was little progress in medicine. The diagnosis of diseases was "unsystematic and superficial." There were few "useful drugs"; some, such as the poison strychnine (used in tonics) and mercury for syphilis, were freely dispensed. Operations were rarely performed because they generally led to death from infection. William G. Rothstein, *American Medical Schools and the Practice of Medicine: A History* (New York: Oxford University Press, 1987), 41; and Samuel D. Gross, *Autobiography of Samuel D. Gross, with a Sketch of His ...* , 2 vols. (Philadelphia: George Barrie Publishers, 1887), 1:56.

72. Spencer, *Poem on the Hubbardton Raid*, 11.

73. Spencer, 12.

74. Spencer, 13.

75. Spencer, 13.

76. The complaint by the religiously inclined was not that the body does not undergo dissolution but rather its treatment in the dissecting room and the aftermath, as cremation hurries the process along. There is the further belief that in the entombed body "there is a mysterious preservation of surviving identity." Henry Raymond, "Editor's Table: The Sacredness of the Human Body," *Harper's New Monthly Magazine* 8 (April 1854): 691.

77. Spencer, *Poem on the Hubbardton Raid*, 14–15.

78. Spencer, 16.

79. Spencer, 18–19. Her body might be described as once the "temple" of her spirit, now in the dissecting room "lying mangled, debased, deformed," the raw material for "some cold materializing lecturer and ruder hands of a ... licentious student." Raymond, "Editor's Table," 691. For more on this, see Chapter 12 in this volume.

80. Spencer, 19–20.

81. Spencer, 21–22.

82. Spencer, 23.

83. Spencer, 26.

84. Spencer, 27.

85. Spencer, 28.

86. Spencer, 29.

87. For example, from an advertisement in the *Charleston Mercury*, October 12, 1838, "Wanted fifty negroes. Any person having sick negroes considered incurable ... and willing to dispose of them. Dr. S. will pay cash." Presumably, Dr. S. and others would be experimenting on them as living slaves and dissecting their bodies as owned goods upon their death. In Theodore E. Weld, *American Slavery as It Is: Testimony of a Thousand Witnesses* (New York: American Slavery Society, 1839), 171.

88. Spencer, *Poem on the Hubbardton Raid*, 30.

89. Spencer, 31.

90. Spencer, 32–33.

91. The doctor mentioned here was William Crary Fox, born on July 4, 1811. He studied under his father, John Fox, a doctor at Castleton Medical Academy. See William A. Ellis and Granville M. Dodge, *Norwich University, 1819–1911...* , 3 vols. (Montpelier, VT: Capital City Press, 1911) 2:113; and Horace Houghton, *Catalogue of the Officers and Students of the Vermont Academy of Medicine* (Castleton, VT: H.H. Houghton, 1830), 4. William C. Fox, MD, spent nearly fifty years in Wallingford, Vermont. He was noted for a "life of great usefulness" and served in the Vermont legislature from 1852 and 1853 and took a great interest in military affairs, serving as an officer in the state militia. See Walter Thorpe, *History of Wallingford Vermont* (Rutland, VT: Tuttle Co., 1911), 52; and Ellis and Dodge, *Norwich University, 1819–1911*, 113. Interestingly, at the same session in 1830, Amos Twitchell served as an instructor at Castleton. He was notorious for procuring subjects for himself and Dr. Nathan Smith. See Henry Bowditch, *Memoir of Amos Twitchell M.D.* (Boston: John Wilson and Son, 1851), 36–37. However, the only mention of William C. Fox being connected with the Hubbardton Raid appears at the end of the "Poem of the Hubbardton Raid."

92. Spencer, *Poem on the Hubbardton Raid*, 34.

93. Hemenway, *The Vermont Historical Gazetteer*, 770.

94. According to an article in the *Burlington Gazette*, J.F. Daggett had "just commenced the study of medicine" at the college when he was arrested. After he was freed, he "returned to the Woodstock School of Medicine and graduated in June 1837. This is, apparently, the only case on record in the New England states where a student was sentenced to a state prison." From the *Burlington Gazette*, reported in the *Alexandria Gazette*, September 16, 1834, 3; and Waite, *Grave Robbing in New England*, 276.

95. Waite, in Arthur M. Lassek, *Human Dissection: Its Drama and Struggle* (Springfield, IL: Charles C. Thomas, 1958), 214–15.

96. Waite, in Lassek, *Human Dissection*, 214.

97. From the *Burlington Gazette*, reported in the *Alexandria Gazette*, September 16, 1834, 3; and Waite, *Grave Robbing in New England*, 276.

98. Stone, "One Hundred Years of Medicine in Vermont," 242.

99. Clarence Pitkin et al., *The Revised Laws of Vermont, 1880, with the Public Acts of the ...* (Rutland, VT: Tuttle Co., 1881), 807.

100. Waite, *Grave Robbing in New England*, 276.

101. Waite, *The First Medical College in Vermont*, 124.

102. The canal from Albany to Whitehall was reported finished in September 1829. *Daily*

Richmond Whig, September 24, 1829, 3; and James Sanford, "Recollections of Castleton Medical College," *Rutland Daily Herald and Globe*, July 21, 1879, 3, in Waite, *The First Medical College in Vermont*, 124.

103. *The Vermont Statutes, 1894: Including the Public Acts of 1894* ... (Rutland, VT: Tuttle Co., 1895), 833–34; and Frederick C. Waite, "The Development of Anatomical Laws in New England," *New England Journal of Medicine* 233 (1945): 723.

Chapter 8

1. Elmer L. Kayser, *A Medical Center: The Institutional Development of the Medical Education in George Washington University* (Washington, D.C.: George Washington University Press, 1973), 7, 10.

2. Kayser, *A Medical Center*, 14 and fourth unnumbered page between pages 14 and 15.

3. Frederick C. Waite, "An Episode in Massachusetts in 1818 Related to Teaching of Anatomy," *New England Journal of Medicine* 220 (1939): 223.

4. Kayser, *A Medical Center*, 17–19; and Thomas Sewall MD, "A Lecture Delivered at the Opening of the Medical Department of the Columbian College in the District of Columbia, March 30, 1825," 2nd ed. (Washington City, 1826), passim.

5. Sewall, "Lecture Delivered at the Opening of the Medical Department of the Columbian College," 5.

6. Sewall, 15.

7. Kayser, *A Medical Center*, 21–22.

8. Kayser, 29–30.

9. Frederick C. Waite, "Grave Robbing in New England," *Bulletin of the Medical Library Association* 33 (1945): 281–82; Thomas Francis Harrington, *The Harvard Medical School*, 3 vols. (New York: Lewis Publishing, 1905), 2:664; and "Medical School in Boston," 261.

10. Waite, "An Episode in Massachusetts," 223.

11. Waite, "Grave Robbing in New England," 281–82.

12. Harrington, *The Harvard Medical School*, 2:654.

13. Waite, "Grave Robbing in New England," 282.

14. *Memorial of Sundry Citizens of the District of Columbia Praying That a Charter May Be Granted by Congress to Enable Them to Institute a Medical College, February 13, 1826* (Washington: Gab and Seaton, 1826), 19th Congress, 1st Session, Memorial No. 35, Vol. 2, 1–4.

15. *Memorial of the Professors of the Medical Department of the Columbian College in the District of Columbia, February 13, 1826* (Washington, D.C.: Gab and Seaton, 1826), 19th Congress, 1st Session, Memorial No. 36, Vol. 2, 1–5.

16. *Memorial of the Professors of the Medical Department of the Columbian College*, 2:4.

17. *Memorial of the Professors of the Medical Department of the Columbian College*, 2:4.

18. *The Times*, December 19, 1807, 6; and E.M. Hartwell, "The Hindrances to Anatomical Study in the United States, Including a Special Record of the Struggles of Our Early Anatomical Teachers," *Annals of Anatomy and Surgery* 3 (1881): 224.

19. *The Times*, December 19, 1807, 6.

20. *Georgetown Metropolitan*, March 25, 1826, 2 and Kayser, 37. It should be noted that for most people and many older physicians, dissection and the source of supply of bodies was thoroughly distasteful. Following the riot, the doctors organized and, with the help of the Maryland legislature, founded a medical school. Davidge became dean of anatomy at the school. The fear that the people would attack the school was so great that the new building in which the dissection room was placed ensured that the activity was done "in stealth." There were "concealed dissecting areas behind the sloping seats in the anatomy theater ... [that were] used, when necessary, [and] the construction ... [included] ... hidden exits, stairways, and cubby holes in anticipation of surprise attacks by irate citizens." Lassek, *Human Dissection*, 226–227.

21. *The Times*, December 19, 1807, 6.

22. Corpses for research and dissection were provided by the city's charity hospitals. Michael Sappol, *A Traffic of Dead Bodies* (Princeton: Princeton University Press, 2002), 111.

23. Sappol, *A Traffic of Dead Bodies*, 59.

24. Sappol, 116.

25. In Philadelphia, anatomists were entitled to "all subjects buried in the two public grounds." This constituted a yearly rate of about 450 bodies. Sappol, *A Traffic of Dead Bodies*, 111.

26. James Webster, *Facts Concerning Anatomical Instruction in Philadelphia* (Philadelphia, 1833), 11.

27. Webster, *Facts Concerning Anatomical Instruction in Philadelphia*, 1–94.

28. Sappol, *A Traffic of Dead Bodies*, 112–15.

29. Edward Dixon, "Scenes in a Medical Student's Life," *Scalpel: An Entirely Original Quarterly Expositor of the Laws of Health* 7 (1855): esp. 93.

30. *Counter Memorial of Sundry Citizens of the District of Columbia Praying That a Charter May Be Granted by Congress to Enable Them to Institute a Medical College, February 20, 1826* (Washington, D.C.: Gab and Seaton, 1826), 19th Congress, 1st Session, Memorial No. 44, 1–8.

31. *Memorial of Sundry Citizens of the District of Columbia Praying That Another Medical School May Not Be Incorporated in the City of Washington, February 22, 1826* (Washington, D.C.: Gab and Seaton, 1826), 19th Congress, 1st Session, Senate Documents, No. 48, v. 2, 1–4.

32. Joseph M. Toner, "Anniversary Oration Delivered before the Medical Society of the District of Columbia, September 26, 1866," in *Medical Society of the District of Columbia: Societies* (Washington, D.C.: Cunningham & McIntosh, 1869), 50–51.

33. James Joseph Walsh, *The History of Medicine in New York*, 5 vols. (New York: National

Americana Society, J.J. Little, and Ives, 1919), 2:390.

34. For an excellent overview of the murders and the trial, see Lisa Rosner, *The Anatomy Murders Being the True and Spectacular History of Edinburgh's Burke and Hare and the Man of Science Who Abetted Them in the Commissions of Their Most Heinous Crimes* (Philadelphia: University of Pennsylvania Press, 2010).

35. Alan F. Guttmacher, "Bootlegging Bodies: A History of Body Snatching," *Bulletin of the Society of Medical History of Chicago* 4 (1935): 397–98.

36. Frederick C. Waite, "The Development of Anatomical Laws in New England," *New England Journal of Medicine* 233 (1945): 720–21.

37. Walsh, *The History of Medicine in New York*, 2:391; and Waite, "The Development of Anatomical Laws," 721.

38. E.M. Hartwell, "The Present Legal Status of Human Anatomy in the United States, *Annals of Anatomy and Surgery 4* (1881): 14. Massachusetts, General Court, House of Representatives, J.B. Davis et al., "Report 4 of the Select Committee of the House of Representatives on So Much of the Governors Speech, at the June Session, 1830 as It Relates to Legalizing the Study of Anatomy," in *Massachusetts House of Representatives, January 1831* (Boston: Dutton and Wentworth, 1831), 106.

39. J.B. Davis et al., "Report 4 of the Select Committee of the House of Representatives On so Much of the Governors Speech, at the June Session, 1830 as it relates to Legalizing the Study of Anatomy," Massachusetts House of Representatives, January 1831 (Dutton and Wentworth, 1831), 106.

40. Davis et al., "Report 4 of the Select Committee of the House of Representatives," 94–95.

41. Davis et al., 101.

42. Davis et al., 103.

43. "Medical School in Boston," *Boston Medical and Surgical Journal* 35, no. 31 (December 26, 1846): 417.

44. William Bensing Webb, *Centennial History of the City of Washington, D.C.* (Dayton, OH: W.J. Shuey, 1892.) 593.

45. Webb, *Centennial History of the City of Washington, D.C.*, 593.

46. Toner, "Anniversary Oration Delivered before the Medical Society of the District of Columbia, September 26, 1866," 56–57.

47. For a fuller explanation, see Richard S. Ross, *Contagion in Prussia, 1831: The Cholera Epidemic and the Threat of the Polish Revolt* (Jefferson, NC: McFarland, 2015), 9–12.

48. Ross, *Contagion in Prussia, 1831*, 593.

49. "D.C. Board of Health, 14 August 1832," *D.C. Board of Health Minutes 1822–1878, District of Columbia Archives* (D.C. Office of Public Records and Archives), Vol. 1, in Max Lee, "Long before Prohibition, D.C. Had a Brief Ban on Liquor," *Boundary Stones*, October 11, 2016, https://boundarystones.weta.org/2016/10/11/long-prohibition-dc-had-brief-ban-liquor#footnote-2.

50. Thomas Sewall, *An Address Delivered before the Washington City Temperance Society, November15, 1830* (Washington, D.C.: Washington City Temperance Society, 1830), 4.

51. Thomas Sewall, *The Pathology of Drunkenness, or the Effects of Alcoholic Drinks, with Drawings of the Drunkard's Stomach* (Albany, NY: C. Van Benthuysen, 1841), 15.

52. "D.C. Board of Health, 26 July 1832," in Lee, "Long before Prohibition."

53. "D.C. Board of Health, 14 August 1832," in Lee, "Long before Prohibition."

54. "D.C. Board of Health, 16 August 1832," in Lee, "Long before Prohibition."

55. Webb, *Centennial History of the City of Washington, D.C.*, 594.

56. Webb, 595.

57. Webb, 596.

58. Webb, 596.

59. Charles Hurd, *Washington Cavalcade* (New York: E.P. Dutton and Co., 1948), 79.

60. Webb, *Centennial History of the City of Washington, D.C.*, 597.

61. Toner, "Anniversary Oration Delivered before the Medical Society of the District of Columbia, September 26, 1866," 78.

62. Samuel Kline Cohen, Jr., *Epidemics: Hate and Compassion from the Plague of Athens to AIDS* (Oxford: Oxford University Press, 2018), 189.

63. *Cobbett's Political Register* 16 (7 April 1832): 15.

64. R.J. Morris, *Cholera 1832: The Social Response to an Epidemic* (New York: Holmes and Meier, 1976), 109. Body snatching and the cholera epidemic in Britain are discussed in Knott, "Popular Attitudes to Death and Dissection in Early Nineteenth Century Britain," 8; Sean Burrell and Geoffrey Gill, "The Liverpool Cholera Epidemic of 1832 and Anatomical Dissection—Medical Mistrust and Civil Unrest," *Journal of the History of Medicine and Allied Sciences* 60 (October 2005): 478–98; and Michael Durey, *The Return of the Plague, British Society and the Cholera, 1831–2* (Dublin: Gill and MacMillan, 1979), 178–80.

65. *Newburyport Herald*, August 17, 1832, 1.

66. D. Hayes Agnew et al., *History and Reminiscences of the Philadelphia Almshouse and Philadelphia Hospital*, Vol. 1 (Philadelphia: Detre and Blackburn, 1890), 48–49.

67. Paul Starr, *The Social Transformation of American Medicine: The Rise of A Sovereign Profession and the Making of a Vast Industry* (New York: Basic Books, 1982), 152.

68. J.C. Ladenheim, "The Doctors Mob of 1788," *Journal of the History of Medicine and Allied Sciences* 5 (1950): 23–43.

69. Toner, "Anniversary Oration Delivered before the Medical Society of the District of Columbia, September 26, 1866," 47.

70. A.W. Woodruff and S. Bell, *Synopsis of Infectious Tropical Diseases* (Baltimore: Williams and Wilkins, 1968), 103–4; and Ross, *Contagion in Prussia, 1831*, 9.

71. "François-Joseph-Victor Broussais,"

Encyclopedia Britannica, December 13, 2020, https://www.britannica.com/biography/Francois-Joseph-Victor-Broussais (accessed July 6, 2021).

72. François-Joseph-Victor Broussais, *Cours de Phrénologie* (Paris: J.B. Bailliere, 1836), ix.

73. Thomas Sewall, *An Examination of Phrenology: In Two Lectures, Delivered to the Students of Columbian College, District of Columbia, February 1837* (Washington City: B. Homans Printer, 1837), 15–16.

74. Sewall, *An Examination of Phrenology*, 38. On phrenology and its interest in skull snatching to evaluate "genius," see Bess Lovejoy, *Rest in Pieces: The Curious Fates of Famous Corpses* (London: Duckworth, 2021).

75. Sewall, *An Examination of Phrenology*, 62.

76. Sewall, 66.

77. Sewall, 66–67.

78. "John Frederick May," obituary: *Critic and Record*, May 2, 1891; R.E. Mansel, David J.T. Webster, and H.M. Sweetland, *Hughes, Mansel & Webster's Benign Disorders and Diseases of the Breast*, 3rd ed. (New York: Elsevier, 2009), 9; and "Francois Magendie," *World Biographical Encyclopedia*, https://prabook.com/web/francois.magendie/2446583.

79. "Dr. Hun's and Dr. May's Introductory Lectures," in Robley Dunglison, *American Medical Intelligencer, April 1, 1839–April 1, 1840*, Vol. 3 (Philadelphia: A. Waldie, 1840): 314–17.

80. Thomas Hun, *Introductory Lecture before the Albany Medical College, Delivered November 12, 1839*, in Dunglison, *American Medical Intelligencer*, 314–15.

81. John F. May, *An Introductory Lecture, Delivered at the Opening of the Medical Department of Columbian College, November 4, 1839*, in Dunglison, *American Medical Intelligencer*, 316–17. As for Dr. May, he did become a distinguished physician in Washington. "Dr. May was one of President Lincoln's attending physicians at the time of the assassination by John Wilkes Booth, and, by a singular coincidence, was called upon, some days later, to perform an autopsy on the corpse of the assassin." "John Frederick May," obituary, *Critic and Record*, May 2, 1891, 2.

82. Toner, "Anniversary Oration Delivered before the Medical Society of the District of Columbia, September 26, 1866," 55.

83. District of Columbia Board of Commissioners, *Annual Report of the Commissioners of the District of Columbia: Year Ended June 30, 1913*, Vol. 1 (Washington, D.C.: Board of Commissioners, 1914), 260.

84. District of Columbia Board of Commissioners, *Annual Report of the Commissioners of the District of Columbia*, 1913, 55.

85. District of Columbia Board of Commissioners, 1913, 56.

86. District of Columbia Board of Commissioners, 1913, 261.

87. One newspaper in January 1893 published an exposé on body snatching in Washington, D.C., noting that "there is no other city in the Union where, in proportion to its size, grave robbing is so extensively carried on as it is in the Capital of the Nation. The crime is fostered by men of science and winked at by the authorities." Efforts had been made in the past to "suppress it" but with little success. *Morning Advertiser*, January 16, 1893, 1.

88. Dr. Llewellin Eliot, "Comment on Frank Baker's 'A History of Bodysnatching,'" *Washington Medical Annals* 15 (1916): 247–48.

89. Eliot, "Comment on Frank Baker's 'A History of Bodysnatching,'" 248.

90. "Dr. Thomas Sewall," obituary, *Niles' National Register*, May 17, 1845, 164. See also the abbreviated obituary in Robert Crowell, *History of the Town of Essex from 1634–1868* (Springfield, MA: Samuel Bowles & Co., 1868), 322–23.

91. "Dr. Thomas Sewall," obituary, *Niles' National Register*, May 17, 1845, 164.

92. Waite, "Grave Robbing in New England," 286.

93. "Dr. Thomas Sewall," obituary, *Niles' National Register*, May 17, 1845, 164.

94. The Methodist Episcopal Burying Ground was part of what is now known as the Mt. Zion Cemetery in Georgetown, Washington, D.C. Originally, white and Black burials occurred in the cemetery. After 1849, only Black persons were buried there. Mary Choate Sewall, Thomas Sewall's wife, died in 1855. Since he is buried with her in Oak Hill Cemetery in Georgetown, today it seems that at some point his body was exhumed and he was buried with Mary. This explains the discrepancy between the obituary and his final resting place at Oak Hill.

95. Anne O. Brockett, *Gone but Not Forgotten: Cemeteries in the Nation's Capital* (Washington, D.C.: U.S. Department of the Interior, National Park Service, 2012), 23, and see throughout on the conditions of various cemeteries in nineteenth century Washington, D.C.

96. *Morning Advertiser*, January 16, 1893, 1.

97. George Alfred Townsend, *Washington Outside and Inside: A Picture and a Narrative* (Hartford, CT: James Betts & Co., 1876), 256–57.

98. Eliot, "Comment on Frank Baker's 'A History of Bodysnatching,'" 248–49.

99. "The Innocent Man" written concurrently with Sewall's body snatching affair. Hurd, *History of Essex County, Massachusetts*, 2:1188.

100. Hurd, 1188, 1190.

101. Polleys refers to a poem "given me some years ago by an old lady whose parents were present when the graves were opened, and who knew the person who wrote the 'lines' about the time of the event in 1818." Maidee P. Polleys, "Robbed the Graveyard," RootsWeb, http://sites.rootsweb.com/~macessex/cemetery/ref3.html (accessed August 29, 2021).

Chapter 9

1. Frederick C. Waite, "The Development of Anatomical Laws in New England," *New England Journal*

of Medicine 233 (1945): 722; and Rosemary Stevens, *American Medicine and the Public Interest* (Berkeley: University of California Press, 1998), 30–31.

2. Shauna Devine, *Learning from the Wounded: The Civil War and the Rise of American Medical Science* (Chapel Hill: University of North Carolina Press, 2014), 54. For the handling of the overwhelming number of the dead, see Drew Gilpin Faust, *This Republic of Suffering: Death and the American Civil War* (New York: Vintage Books, 2008).

3. Waite, "The Development of Anatomical Laws in New England," 722.

4. David C. Humphrey, "Dissection and Discrimination: The Social Origins of Cadavers in America, 1760–1915," *Bulletin of the New York Academy of Medicine* 49 (1973): 823; and Frederick C. Waite, "Grave Robbing in New England," *Bulletin of the Medical Library Association* 33 (1945): 283–84.

5. As for the Black population, the addition of Howard University's medical school only added to their paranoia about the "night doctors" and body snatchers. They feared the Howard medical students too. Perhaps some of the fear could be attributed to the makeup of the student population. According to Montague Cobb, "Howard has always had some white students and in the early years a large percentage of a class was sometimes white." W. Montague Cobb, "Surgery and the Negro Physician: Some Parallels in Background," *Journal of the National Medical Association* 43 (1951): 150–51.

6. Thomas Dwight, "Anatomy Laws versus Bodysnatching," *The Forum* 21 (1896): 499.

7. Dwight, "Anatomy Laws versus Bodysnatching," 499.

8. Dr. Llewellin Eliot, "Comment on Frank Baker's 'A History of Bodysnatching,'" *Washington Medical Annals* 15 (1916): 249.

9. *Evening Star* (Washington, DC), December 15, 1873, 7. Maryland did not pass an anatomy law until 1882. See Arthur M. Lassek, *Human Dissection: Its Drama and Struggle* (Springfield, IL: Charles C. Thomas, 1958), 226.

10. *Evening Star*, January 15, 1872, 4. Interestingly, in an article published in 1885 the author asserts that it was more than just Black people who feared the night doctors. It was also the "superstitious dread of 'night doctors' which is universal among the common people." Francis King Carey, "The Disposition of the Body after Death, *American Law Review* 19 (1855): 267. On the continued exploitation of body snatching today, see Catherine Saldago, "Uncovered HHS Docs Reveal Federal Funding to Harvest Human Fetal Organs," *National Pulse*, August 5, 2021. https://thenationalpulse.com/breaking/uncovered-hhs-docs-reveal-federal-funding-to-harvest-human-fetal-organs/.

11. "Burking in Baltimore," *Cecil Whig*, December 18, 1886, 2.

12. Alan F. Guttmacher, "Bootlegging Bodies: A History of Body Snatching," *Bulletin of the Society of Medical History of Chicago* 4 (1935): 401.

13. Suzanne Shultz, *Body Snatching: The Robbing of Graves for the Education of Physicians in Early Nineteenth Century America* (Jefferson, NC: McFarland, 1992), 73.

14. *Evening Star*, December 16, 1886, 5.

15. Shultz, *Body Snatching*, 73–74.

16. *Evening Star*, December 16, 1886, 5,

17. *Evening Star*, December 15, 1873, 8.

18. Eliot, "Comment on Frank Baker's 'A History of Bodysnatching,'" 250; and Shultz, *Body Snatching*, 61.

19. *Evening Star*, December 17, 1873, 4.

20. On the text of Christian's diary and an explication of its contents, see especially Shultz, *Body Snatching*, 62–68.

21. Newly located from the previous site in 1870, it was described as "a smart brick building, four stories high, with green trimmings.... The Potter's Field preceded the Poor-house.... [T]he main part is the almshouse ... and the number of inmates is less than two hundred, the females preponderating in the proportion of three to one. Under the same roof are the Almshouse; and the Work- house." George A. Townsend, *Historic Sketches at Washington* (Hartford, CT: Jas. Betts & Co., 1877), 253–54.

22. Townsend, *Historic Sketches at Washington*, 256–57.

23. Benjamin P. Poore, *Congressional Directory* (Washington D.C.: U.S. Government Printing Office, 1875), 126; *General Register of Georgetown University* (Washington, D.C.: Georgetown University, 1916), 340; and *A Catalogue of the Officers and Students of Georgetown University, 1872–1873* (Baltimore: John Murray, 1873), 39. I have confirmed Schleimer's identity. See Shultz, *Body Snatching*, 61.

24. *General Register of Georgetown University*, 472. See also Shultz, *Body Snatching*, 66.

25. United States Department of the Treasury, *Annual Report of the Secretary of the Treasury on the State of the Finances* (Washington, D.C.: U.S. Government Printing Office, 1875), 111; and *General Register of Georgetown University*, 472.

26. For this description of Wright's execution see "President Grant Stays an Execution of African-American Who Murdered a Jewish Peddler," Shapell, May 29, 1873, https://www.shapell.org/manuscript/ulysses-grant-capital-punishment-minorities/.

27. The *Evening Star* gave a long and detailed account of the trial and execution of Thomas Wright. *Evening Star*, June 6, 1873, 4.

28. Allen C. Clark, *Beau Hickman (Robert S. Hickman)*, Records of the Columbia Historical Society, Washington, DC, 1940, Vol. 5, 40/41, 1940, 79–96.

29. "Washington Biography of Beau Hickman," *Evening Star*, September 2, 1873, 4. See also Clark, *Beau Hickman*, 93.

30. *Alexandria Gazette*, September 4, 1873, 2.

31. Clark, *Beau Hickman*, 94.

32. Shultz, *Body Snatching*, 66.

33. Shultz, 66.

34. Board of Health District of Columbia, *Third Annual Report of the Board of Health of the District*

of Columbia, 1874 (Washington, D.C.: Chronicle Publishing Co., 1874), 161, 165.

35. Anne O. Brockett, *Gone but Not Forgotten: Cemeteries in the Nation's Capital* (Washington, D.C.: U.S. Department of the Interior, National Park Service, 2012), 6.

36. Shultz, *Body Snatching*, 66; and Brockett, *Gone but Not Forgotten*, 6.

37. *Morning Advertiser*, January 16, 1893, 2.

38. *Morning Advertiser*, January 16, 1893, 2; and Shultz, *Body Snatching*, 66.

39. United States Army, *Annual Report of the Quartermaster-General to the Secretary of War* (Washington, D.C.: U.S. Government Printing Office, 1872), 152.

40. Brockett, *Gone but Not Forgotten*, 19.

41. Shultz, *Body Snatching*, 67.

42. Shultz, 67.

43. "Rock Creek Cemetery," Find a Grave, https://www.findagrave.com/cemetery/104448/Rock-Creek-Cemetery.

44. District of Columbia Board of Health, *Third Annual Report of the Board of Health of the District of Columbia, 1874* (Washington, D.C.: Chronicle Publishing Co., 1874), 166.

45. Medical Society of the District of Columbia, *History of the Medical Society of the District of Columbia, 1817–1909* (Washington, D.C.: Medical Society of the District of Columbia, 1909), 297; and Shultz, *Body Snatching*, 67.

46. For the close relationship of the demonstrators at the National Medical College, see Chapter 10: A.C. Adams, with the convicted body snatcher Vigo Jansen Ross, and William P. Carr, with another body snatcher, Dr. W.W. Beall.

47. Shultz, *Body Snatching*, 67.

48. District of Columbia Board of Commissioners, *Fourth Annual Report of the Commissioners of the District of Columbia, November 30, 1876, to November 1, 1877* (Washington, D.C.: U.S. Government Printing Office, 1877), 226.

49. District of Columbia Board of Commissioners, *Fourth Annual Report of the Commissioners of the District of Columbia*, 209.

50. District of Columbia Board of Commissioners, *Fourth Annual Report of the Commissioners of the District or Columbia*, 226.

51. On August 3, 1874, the *Evening Star* reported that the offices of physicians to the poor had been abolished. The commissioners wanted more documentation, contrary to in the past. Now the police force was responsible for determining the necessity of each "respective case, when found meritorious[,] [to] send them to the secretary of the commission, who will give them tickets of admission to the asylum or an order for medicine. *Evening Star*, August 3, 1874, 4.

52. *Evening Star*, August 3, 1874, 4.

53. Townsend, *Historic Sketches at Washington*, 225.

54. On Frothingham and Quimby, see Shultz, *Body Snatching*, 67.

55. For a full description of the arrest, trial, and execution of Henry Young, see *Evening Star*, November 28, 1873, 4.

56. Lassek, *Human Dissection*, 231, 234–35, 244.

57. Michael Sappol, *A Traffic of Dead Bodies* (Princeton: Princeton University Press, 2002), 317.

58. Young Men's Cemetery, also known as Free Young Men's Burial Ground, was a Black cemetery. See Shultz, *Body Snatching*, 67. It was established by the Free Young Men's Benevolent Association, in Washington, D.C., in 1849 and operated until 1870. See "The Benevolent Association, 1838–1923," Walter Pierce Park Cemeteries, https://walterpierceparkcemeteries.org/the-free-young-mens-colored-union-benevolent-association/.

59. Edith Abbott, "The Wages of Unskilled Labor in the United States, 1850–1890," *Journal of Political Economy* (June 5, 1905): 363.

60. Shultz, *Body Snatching*, 67–68.

61. Brockett, *Gone but Not Forgotten*, 19.

62. Daina Ramey Berry, *The Price for Their Pound of Flesh* (Boston: Beacon, 2017), 174–78.

63. *Evening Star*, February 9, 1874, 4.

64. *The Papers of Ulysses S. Grant*, Vol. 25, *1874*, Digital edition (Charlottesville: Rotunda, 2018), https://rotunda.upress.virginia.edu/founders/GRNT-01-25-03-0001-0256 (accessed July 24, 2021), which covers the interment of a private individual. The pardon did not absolve him of all his criminal activities. On December 9, 1874, Christian was charged with "removing dead bodies" and charged $700 for an earlier crime. *Evening Star*, December 9, 1874, 1.

65. David H. Beckwith, "History of the Cleveland Homeopathic College," *Cleveland Homeopathic Reporter* (1900): 10–12.

66. *Cincinnati Daily Gazette*, June 16, 1852, cited in Linden F. Edwards, "Resurrection Riots during the Heroic Age of Anatomy in America," *Bulletin of the History of Medicine* 25, no. 2 (March–April 1951): 181.

67. Beckwith, "History of the Cleveland Homeopathic College," 12.

68. Sappol, *A Traffic of Dead Bodies*, 317.

69. Lassek, *Human Dissection*, 239; and Harry J. Sievers, *The Harrison Horror* (Fort Wayne, IN: Public Library of Fort Wayne and Allen County, 1956).

70. Lassek, *Human Dissection*, 240–41.

71. On Cincinnati as a distribution center, see Shultz, *Body Snatching*, 37.

Chapter 10

1. Arthur M. Lassek, *Human Dissection: Its Drama and Struggle* (Springfield, IL: Charles C. Thomas, 1958), 247; The *Evening Star* stated that "Vigo Jansen, called the King of Resurrectionists, will lecture at the Comique Sunday evening on the lives, eccentricities, [and] incidents of the lives of the most noted resurrectionists." *Evening Star*, May 17, 1884, 2.

2. For a second review, see "How to Rob a Grave, the Business Publicly Illustrated by Jansen, 'the Resurrectionist,'" *National Republican*, May 19, 1884, 6.

3. "The Ghoul at Work," *Evening Critic*, May 19, 1884, 2.

4. "The Ghoul at Work," 2.

5. Besides the topic itself, Jansen spoke in broken English, was nervous onstage, and appeared to be drunk, causing laughter and howls from the audience. See especially "How to Rob a Grave, the Business Publicly Illustrated by Jansen, 'the Resurrectionist,'" *National Republican*, May 19, 1884, 6.

6. Edward Sylvester, *District of Columbia: A Retrospective of the Police Organization of the Cities of Washington, Georgetown, and the District of Columbia* (Washington, D.C.: Gibson Bros., 1894), 243.

7. "Graves of Two Females Robbed of Their Contents," *Evening Critic*, October 11, 1884, 1.

8. Sylvester, *District of Columbia*, 243.

9. "Graves of Two Females Robbed of Their Contents," 1.

10. Dwight, "Anatomy Laws versus Bodysnatching," 499.

11. *Alexandria Gazette*, November 4, 1887, 3.

12. There was no grave-robbing law in Washington, D.C. As late as 1893 the applicable statute in the *Crimes and Offenses of the Revised Statutes of the District of Columbia* only forbade the "desecration of cemeteries, specifying the grounds, tombs, and fencing." As we saw with Jansen, in order to charge a grave robber, the authorities had to fall back on English common law. "Ghouls at Work," Morning *Advertiser*, January 16, 1893, 2.

13. *Morning Advertiser*, January 16, 1893, 1–2.

14. *Evening Star*, December 23, 1889, 5.

15. *Evening Star*, June 6, 1890, 5.

16. *Evening Star*, December 23, 1889, 5.

17. *Evening Star*, December 23, 5 and June, 6, 5.

18. *Baltimore Sun*, January 9, 1890, 4.

19. *Evening Star*, January 6, 1890, 7.

20. *Evening Star*, January 6, 1890, 7.

21. *Baltimore Sun*, January 9, 1890, 8; and *Evening Star*, January 9, 1890, 8.

22. *Evening Star*, June 10, 1890, 5; *Daily Critic*, June 12, 1890, 5; and *Evening Star*, June 12, 1890, 7.

23. *Evening Star*, June 12, 1890, 8.

24. *Morning Advertiser*, January 16, 1893, 2.

25. John Rauch, *Report on Medical Education, Medical Colleges… 1765–1889* (Springfield, IL: H.W. Roker, 1889), 38. Also, Columbian College became Columbian University in 1873.

26. The article involved undercover work by the newspaper, sending in its man with letters of introduction from a medical college in Richmond, Virginia; the man interviewed cemetery superintendents and health officials. The findings and information agreed with earlier material I previously discussed. Why a New York newspaper undertook this can only be speculated on; perhaps some people felt that too many Washington officials were involved and would have shut down any hometown investigation. Based on the earlier Beall case, for the Washington public much of this had been covered in the Washington newspapers during the Beall trial and was old news. *Morning Advertiser*, January 16, 1893, 1–2.

27. *Evening Star*, November 13, 1893, 8.

28. Evidence for the cozy relationship between the medical colleges and the police is illustrated in the following report. About six years prior to 1892, the resurrectionists were so bold that they brought their cadavers through the front door of the National Medical College. A young policeman witnessing this "interfered, and the subject was removed to the morgue." The demonstrator at the time "talked to the Superintendent of Police and complained against the young officer." The "subject was restored to the college. Since that time the reception of subjects at the National Medical College has not been interfered with." *Morning Advertiser*, January 16, 1893, 2. See also Dr. King's March 1888 letter, United States Congress, Senate, "Argument in Support of the Bill (No. 1566) for the Promotion of Anatomical Science, and to Prevent the Desecration of Graves in the District of Colombia, March 7, 1890," *Reports of Committees for the First Session of the Senate of the United States of the Fifty-First Congress 1889–90*, Vol. 2, Rep. 411 (Washington, D.C.: U.S. Government Printing Office, 1890), 1.

29. Morning *Advertiser*, January 16, 1893, 1–2.

30. *Evening Star*, December 6, 1882, 1.

31. *Alexandria Gazette*, March 19, 1883, 1.

32. United States Congress, Senate, "Argument in Support of the Bill (No. 1566) for the Promotion of Anatomical Science," 3. For a transcript of Cleveland's veto see Grover Cleveland, "Veto Message," April 26, 1886, American Presidency Project, https://www.presidency.ucsb.edu/documents/veto-message-379.

33. United States Congress, Senate, "Argument in Support of the Bill (No. 1566) for the Promotion of Anatomical Science,"Vol. 2, Rep. 411, 1.

34. "The Ghoul at Work," 2.

35. United States Congress, Senate, "Argument in Support of the Bill (No. 1566) for the Promotion of Anatomical Science," Vol. 2, Rep. 411, 2. It appears the Naval Medical Corps was concerned with the use of illegally obtained bodies for dissection, because on May 10, 1876, a "draft of a bill regulating dissecting material in this District, was presented to the [District of Columbia Medical] Society" by "the Naval Medical Corps." It was referred to a Society committee, however, no report was ever made, and "it does not appear the subject ever again came before the Society." Medical Society of the District of Columbia, *History of the Medical Society of the District of Columbia 1817–1909* (Washington, D.C.: The Society, 1909), 116.

36. United States Congress, Senate, Vol. 2, Rep. 411, 3.

37. United States Fifty First Congress, Senate, Vol. 2, Rep. 411, 2–3.

38. United States Congress, *Congressional Record Containing the Proceedings and Debates of the Fiftieth Congress, First Session*, Vol. 19 (Washington, D.C.: U.S. Government Printing Office, 1888), 2419–2420.

39. Many of the arguments in support of the

1888 bill that was defeated are found in United States Congress. *Congressional Record Containing the Proceedings and Debates of the Fiftieth Congress, First Session*, Vol. 19. Washington, D.C.: U.S. Government Printing Office, 1888) 2412–2423. They would be included in the 1902 bill.

40. A similar argument was made in the Pennsylvania legislature in 1883 regarding the potential loss of prestige to cities such as Boston and New York because their states had more progressive anatomy laws (see Chapter 11).

41. United States Congress, Senate, "Argument in Support of the Bill (No. 1566) for the Promotion of Anatomical Science," Vol. 2, Rep. 411, 7.

42. The letter was signed by A.F.A. King, Dean of the Medical Department of Columbian University; the surgeon general of the Marine Hospital, John B. Hamilton; the surgeon general of the U.S. Navy; F.M. Gunnell, professor of surgery, Georgetown University; D.D. Lamb, professor of anatomy, Howard University Medical College; George William West, professor of anatomy in the Medical Department of National University; and Jacob L. Wortman, Department of Anatomy, Georgetown University, Anatomist, U.S. Army Medical Museum and professor of anatomy, Medical Department, Columbian University. It is of interest that George Christian had worked for the Office of the Surgeon General, according to Suzanne Shultz, *Body Snatching: The Robbing of Graves for the Education of Physicians in Early Nineteenth Century America* (Jefferson, NC: McFarland, 1992), 61. Note that one of the signers of the letter was the anatomist at the U.S. Army Medical Museum. "Christian would inject and pack the bodies in whiskey barrels at the college, roll these barrels up in front of the Army Medical Museum, where the express company would call for them; Christian was always on hand to pay charges and direct the shipments; in this way the company did not suspect the fraud." One cannot help but suspect that someone was in on his scheme at the museum in the early 1870s. Dr. Llewellin Eliot, "Comment on Frank Baker's 'A History of Bodysnatching,'" *Washington Medical Annals* 15 (1916): 249.

43. United States Congress, "An Act for the Promotion of Anatomical Sciences, and to Prevent the Desecration of Graves in the District of Columbia, February 1, 1892," *Congressional Record Containing the Proceedings and Debates of the Fifty Second Congress, First Session*, Vol. 22 (Washington, D.C.: U.S. Government Printing Office, 1892), 730.

44. Interestingly, in the same article this New York newspaper reported on a body-snatching scandal in Washington, D.C. It did not seem to gain any traction and was not reported on in the local press. *Morning Advertiser*, January 16, 1893, 2.

45. Lassek, *Human Dissection*, 231.

46. United States Congress, "An Act for the Promotion of Anatomical Sciences, and to Prevent the Desecration of Graves in the District of Columbia, April 29, 1901," *Public Laws of the United States of America Passed at the First Session of the Fifty-Seventh Congress, 1901–1902* (Washington, D.C.: U.S. Government Printing Office, 1902), 173–75.

47. United States Congress, Senate, "Argument in Support of the Bill (No. 1566) for the Promotion of Anatomical Science," Vol. 2, Rep. 411, 1.

48. For example, the Washington newspaper the *Morning Times* on February 22, 1896, reported on Dr. Fallon's body-snatching ring and noted that even when caught and convicted "the punishment was light." *Morning Times*, February 22, 1896, 1, 3.

49. *Morning Advertiser*, January 16, 1893, 1.

50. Eliot, "Comment on Frank Baker's 'A History of Bodysnatching,'" 253. Also of interest is that Dr. Llewellin Eliot was so familiar with body snatching and especially his knowledge of George Christian. As I noted earlier, many of the doctors involved in Christian's activities were graduates of the Georgetown medical school in 1873–1874. Eliot was a classmate of Daily and also graduated from the Georgetown University medical school in 1874. See Will J. Maxwell, *General Register of Georgetown University* (Washington, D.C.: Georgetown University, 1916), 472.

Chapter 11

1. Steven Robert Wilf, "Anatomy and Punishment in Late Eighteenth Century New York," *Journal of Social History* 2, no. 3 (1989): 511–12.

2. See chapters 9 and 10.

3. *New York Daily Advertiser*, April 23, 1788, cited in Wilf, "Anatomy and Punishment in Late Eighteenth Century New York," 511.

4. "Keith was admitted to practice before the Superior Court in March, 1780.... In the same year he took Dr. John Warren's ... course of lectures and subscribed for a copy of the Revere; diploma." On Israel Keith's life, see Clifford K. Shipton and John L. Sibley, *Sibley's Harvard Graduates: Biographical Sketches of Those Who Attended Harvard College ...*, Vol. 17 (Boston: Massachusetts Historical Society, 1873–19__), 1768–71, 552. For a general biography, see 549–52. The second diploma was for Levi Bartlett dated June 8, 1785. For current information on both men and the diplomas, see "Anatomical Lecture, 1780," American Antiquarian Society, https://www.americanantiquarian.org/Inventories/Revere/anatomical.PDF.

5. Benjamin Curtis is the only physician by this name listed in Boston at this time. See Philip Cash, "The Professionalization of Boston Medicine," *Medicine in Colonial Massachusetts, 1620–1680*, Vol. 57 (Boston: The Society, 1980), 95.

6. "Case of Doctor Curtis and Anthony Frederick, 1782," Israel Keith papers II, MS. N-1521, Massachusetts Historical Society. See also Joanne Pope Melish, *Disowning Slavery: Gradual Emancipation and "Race" in New England, 1780–1860* (Ithaca: Cornell University Press, 2016), 186.

7. "Boston was noted for the homogeneity of its permanent inhabitants, and its medical

community was no exception. Of the forty-seven physicians who practiced in Boston between 1760 and 1798 … all but four were New England born of English stock. Many Boston doctors of this era could trace their ancestry back to the Puritan migration of 1630–1680." Cash, "The Professionalization of Boston Medicine," 71–72.

8. Locke's paraphrase of St. Paul on why the earthly body cannot be resurrected: "Because … flesh and blood cannot inherit the kingdom of God; [at] … Christ's coming… those, that are in their graves, shall be changed likewise at the instant of their being raised; … shall be put into a state of incorruptibility, ver. 51, in a new sort of bodies." John Locke, *A Paraphrase and Notes on the Epistles of St. Paul to the Galatians, First and Second Corinthians, Romans, and Ephesians: To Which Is Prefixed an Essay for the Understanding of St. Paul's Epistles, by Consulting St. Paul Himself* (Cambridge, UK: Brown, Shattuck, and Company, 1832), 174.

9. "Case of Doctor Curtis and Anthony Frederick, 1782."

10. Edward M. Mussey, "The Early American Anatomists and the Legal Status of Anatomy in Massachusetts before 1800," *New England Journal of Medicine* 103 (July–December 1880): 540. See also Samuel A. Forman, *Dr. Joseph Warren: The Boston Tea Party, Bunker Hill, and the Birth of American Liberty* (Gretna, LA: Pelican, 2012), 10, 43.

11. Forman, *Dr. Joseph Warren*, 363.

12. Warren's body "was identified on the 4th of April, covered with about three feet of ground, much disfigured; yet it was sufficiently known by two artificial teeth; which were set for him a short time before his glorious exit." Richard Frothingham, *Life and Times of Joseph Warren* (Boston: Little, Brown, 1865), 522. On Paul Revere's role, see Mike F. Nola, "Paul Revere and Forensic Dentistry," *Military Medicine* 181, no. 7 (July 2016): 714–15.

13. "Case of Doctor Curtis and Anthony Frederick, 1782."

14. Melish, *Disowning Slavery*, 187.

15. No doubt Frederick's lawyer may have originally convinced him that he had a case even though "common law" and statutory law of England did not provide "any penalty for the exhumation of a human body." According to Blackstone "stealing the corpse itself, which has no owner [though a matter of great indecency], is no felony, unless some of the grave clothes be stolen with it." However, "any person who has a freehold of the soil may bring an action of trespass against such as dig or disturb it." Keith's interest in common law was such that the first book he recommended when asked what law students should read was Mathew Hale's *Advice for the Study of Common Law*. See Charles Warren, *A History of the American Bar* (Boston: Little, Brown, 1911), 182.

16. "Case of Doctor Curtis and Anthony Frederick, 1782."

17. "Certificate of Attendance at Dr. John Warren's Course of Anatomical Lectures," Massachusetts Historical Society, March 28, 1782, https://www.masshist.org/database/248.

18. Transcription, "Certificate of Attendance at Dr. John Warren's Course of Anatomical Lectures," https://www.masshist.org/database/viewer.php?item_id=248&img_step=1&mode=transcript#.

19. For a corrective on Keith's partisan views at the time, see Mussey, "The Early American Anatomists and the Legal Status of Anatomy in Massachusetts before 1800."

20. John Warren and Aaron Dexter, "Memorial and Petition for the Removal of the Med. Lec. to Boston," February 20, 1810, J.C. Warren Papers, MHS, cited in Harriet Washington, *Medical Apartheid: The Dark History of Medical Experimentation on Blacks* (New York: Harlem, Moon, 2006), 133.

21. Suzanne Shultz, *Body Snatching: The Robbing of Graves for the Education of Physicians in Early Nineteenth Century America* (Jefferson, NC: McFarland, 1992), 29.

22. J.C. Ladenheim, "The Doctor's Mob of 1788," 22.

23. Craig Steven Wilder, *Ebony and Ivy: Race, Slavery, and the Troubled History of American Universities* (New York: Bloomsbury, 2013), 199.

24. Letter, Ezekiel D. Cushing to Mehetabel Cushing (sister), February 11, 1810, Francis A. Countway Library of Medicine, Harvard University, https://nrs.lib.harvard.edu/urn-3:hms.count:26856034?n=4.

25. Wilder, *Ebony and Ivy*, 199.

26. Frederick C. Waite, "Grave Robbing in New England," *Bulletin of the Medical Library Association* 33 (1945): 283–84.

27. Michael Sappol, *A Traffic of Dead Bodies* (Princeton: Princeton University Press, 2002), 107.

28. Sappol, *A Traffic of Dead Bodies*, 346n27.

29. "Petitions 1700–1795, Records of the City Clerk, New York," in Isaac Newton Phelps, *The Iconography of Manhattan Island, 1498–1909: Compiled from Original Sources and Illustrated by Photo-Intaglio Reproductions of Important Maps, Plans, Views, and Documents in Public and Private Collections*, Vol. 6 (New York: Robert H. Dodd, 1915), 46; and Wilf, "Anatomy and Punishment in Late Eighteenth Century New York," 511.

30. Sappol, *A Traffic of Dead Bodies*, 107; Phelps, 46.

31. Phelps, *The Iconography of Manhattan Island, 1498–1909*, 46.

32. *New York Daily Advertiser*, February 2, 1788, cited in Sappol, *A Traffic of Dead Bodies*, 107.

33. Sappol, *A Traffic of Dead Bodies*, 107.

34. Mary Roach, *Stiff: The Curious Lives of Human Cadavers* (New York: Norton, 2004), 40.

35. Ruth Richardson, *Death Dissection and the Destitute*, 2nd ed. (Chicago: University of Chicago Press, 2000), 174, Humphrey, 822 and Halperin, 494.

36. Steven Robert Wilf, *Law's Imagined Republic: Popular Politics and Criminal Justice in Revolutionary America* (New York: Cambridge University Press, 2010), 174; Humphrey, 822; and Halperin, 494.

37. Wilf, "Anatomy and Punishment in Late Eighteenth Century New York," 511–12.

38. Additionally, at the time of Turner's execution there was a high demand for corpses at the medical department of the University of Virginia. On Turner, see Kenneth Greenberg, "Name, Face, Body," in Kenneth Greenberg, ed., *Nat Turner: A Slave Rebellion in History and Memory*, ed. Kenneth Greenberg (New York: Oxford University Press, 2003), 18–19. For an interesting account of the distribution of Nat Turner's body parts, see Greenberg, 18–23.

39. Thomas Dwight, "*Anatomy Laws versus Bodysnatching*," 499.

40. *Evening Star*, December 15, 1873. Maryland did not pass an anatomy law until 1882. See Arthur M. Lassek, *Human Dissection: Its Drama and Struggle* (Springfield, IL: Charles C. Thomas, 1958), 226.

41. Gladys-Marie Fry, *Night Riders in Black Folk History* (Chapel Hill: University of North Carolina Press, 1975), 210; and Edward C. Halperin, "The Poor, the Black, and the Marginalized as the Source of Cadavers in United States Anatomical Education," *Clinical Anatomy* 20 (2007): 490.

42. Francis King Carey, "The Disposition of the Body After Death," *American Law Review* 19 (1855): 267. See also Dr. Samuel C. Busey in his book published in 1898 regarding the way people in Washington had traditionally buried their dead "to protect the bodies from resurrection by 'Night Doctors.'" Samuel Claggett Busey, *Pictures of the City of Washington in the Past*, (Washington, D.C.: Wm. Ballard & Sons, 1898), 94.

43. Fry, *Night Riders in Black Folk History*, 178. On the "Night Doctor" tradition in Washington, D.C., in the late nineteenth century and the twentieth century, see 182–87.

44. Halperin, "The Poor, the Black, and the Marginalized," 493; and Sanford B. Hunt, "The Negro as a Soldier," *Anthropological Review* 7, no. 24 (1869): 51.

45. William J. McKnight, *Jefferson County Pennsylvania: Her Pioneers and People, 1800*–1915, 2 vols. (Chicago: J.H. Beers & Co. 1917), 1:261.

46. Horace Montgomery, "A Body Snatcher Sponsors Pennsylvania's Anatomy Act," *Journal of the History of Medicine and Allied Sciences* 21, no. 4 (October 1966): 383.

47. *Philadelphia Inquirer*, December 6, 1882, 8.

48. *Philadelphia Public Ledger*, December 6, 1882, cited in Montgomery, "A Body Snatcher Sponsors Pennsylvania's Anatomy Act," 383; and *Philadelphia Inquirer*, December 6, 1882, 8.

49. *Philadelphia Inquirer*, December 6, 1882, 8.

50. *Philadelphia Inquirer*, December 6, 1882, 8.

51. *Philadelphia Inquirer*, December 6, 1882, 8.

52. *Cincinnati Daily Gazette*, December 6, 1882, 1.

53. *Philadelphia Inquirer*, December 6, 1882, 8

54. *Philadelphia Inquirer*, December 6, 1882, 8.

55. *Philadelphia Inquirer*, December 8, 1882, 2.

56. *Philadelphia Inquirer*, December 8, 1882, 2.

57. *Philadelphia Public Ledger*, December 8, 1882, cited in Montgomery, "A Body Snatcher Sponsors Pennsylvania's Anatomy Act," 386–87.

58. *Philadelphia Inquirer*, December 16, 1882, 2.

59. *Reading Daily Eagle*, December 7, 1882, cited in Montgomery, "A Body Snatcher Sponsors Pennsylvania's Anatomy Act," 386.

60. *Philadelphia Inquirer*, December 16, 1882, 2; and Shultz, *Body Snatching*, 81.

61. *Philadelphia Inquirer*, December 16, 1882, 2; and Shultz, *Body Snatching*, 81.

62. *Philadelphia Inquirer*, December 20, 1882, 3.

63. See George Edward Vickers, *The Fall of Bossism: A History of the Committee of One Hundred and the Reform Movement in Philadelphia*, Vol. 1 (Philadelphia: A.C. Bryson, 1883), 1. See also *Philadelphia Inquirer*, December 21, 1882, 2.

64. *Philadelphia Inquirer*, March 30, 1883, 2.

65. *Evening Star*, December 6, 1882, 2.

66. *Philadelphia Inquirer*, December 6, 1882, 8.

67. *Philadelphia Inquirer*, December 8, 1882, 2.

68. *Philadelphia Inquirer*, December 20, 1882, 3.

69. Montgomery, "A Body Snatcher Sponsors Pennsylvania's Anatomy Act," 387.

70. McKnight, *Jefferson County Pennsylvania*, 1:259.

71. McKnight, 1:261.

72. Montgomery, "A Body Snatcher Sponsors Pennsylvania's Anatomy Act," 389.

73. *Philadelphia Inquirer*, March 19, 1883, 4.

74. *Philadelphia Inquirer*, March 17, 1883, 2.

75. Dr. Forbes received a victors' celebration back at the college, with students, faculty, and administrators in full support of their demonstrator of anatomy. For a full description, see the *Philadelphia Inquirer*, March 19, 1883, 2. For a more critical description of Forbes as "callous, whose popular image was that of an evil genius in a glistening silk topper," see *Reading Daily Eagle*, December 17, 1882, cited in Montgomery, "A Body Snatcher Sponsors Pennsylvania's Anatomy Act," 387.

76. *Philadelphia Inquirer*, March 19, 1883, 4.

77. Cited in Erin McLeary, "The Curious Case of Body Snatching at Lebanon Cemetery," *Hidden City*, April, 13, 2015, https://hiddencityphila.org/2015/04/the-curious-case-of-body-snatching-at-lebanon-cemetery/.

78. McKnight, *Jefferson County Pennsylvania*, 1:261–62.

79. *Legislative Record: Proceedings of the General Assembly of Pennsylvania*, 1883, 658–59, 669–71, in Montgomery, "A Body Snatcher Sponsors Pennsylvania's Anatomy Act," 391.

80. Charles Lyell, *Principles of Geology* (1830–1833); Charles Darwin, *Origin of the Species* (1854); Jeremy Bentham, his various writings on "utilitarianism"; and Herbert Spencer, *Principles of Biology* (1864), who coined the term "survival of the fittest."

81. For a full discussion, see Sappol, *A Traffic of Dead Bodies*, 322–23.

82. Sappol, 314.

83. *Legislative Record: Proceedings of the General Assembly of Pennsylvania*, 1883, 658, 659, 671, in Montgomery, "A Body Snatcher Sponsors Pennsylvania's Anatomy Act," 391.

84. *Legislative Record: Proceedings of the General Assembly of Pennsylvania*, 670, 672–74, in Montgomery, "A Body Snatcher Sponsors Pennsylvania's Anatomy Act," 391.

85. *Legislative Record: Proceedings of the General Assembly of Pennsylvania*, 674–75, in Montgomery, "A Body Snatcher Sponsors Pennsylvania's Anatomy Act," 392. For more on his arguments, see McKnight, *Jefferson County Pennsylvania*, 1:264–66.

86. Montgomery, "A Body Snatcher Sponsors Pennsylvania's Anatomy Act," 392–93. For more detail, see Venetia M. Guerrasio, "Dissecting the Pennsylvania Anatomy Act: Laws, Bodies, and Science, 1880–1960," 38–40, PhD dissertation, University of New Hampshire, Durham Scholars Repository, https://scholars.unh.edu/cgi/viewcontent.cgi?article=1375&context=dissertation.

87. William S. Forbes, "History of the First Anatomy Act of Pennsylvania," *Philadelphia Medical Journal* 2 (July–December 1898): 1135.

88. *Wheeling Register*, March 29, 1883, 1

89. *Philadelphia Inquirer*, March 15, 1883, 2.

90. *Wheeling Register*, March 29, 1883, 1.

91. Montgomery, "A Body Snatcher Sponsors Pennsylvania's Anatomy Act," 393; and McKnight, *Jefferson County Pennsylvania*, 1:263.

92. McKnight, 1:263–64.

93. Guerrasio, "Dissecting the Pennsylvania Anatomy Act," 17.

94. Mears J. Ewing, J.D. Bryant, and Thomas Dwight, "Report of the Committee on the Collection and Preservation of Anatomical Material," Report of the Eighth Annual Meeting of the Association of American Anatomists, *Science* 3 (January 17, 1896): 84.

95. William Keen, *Addresses and Other Papers* (Philadelphia: W.B. Saunders, 1905), 14.

96. David C. Humphrey, "Dissection and Discrimination: The Social Origins of Cadavers in America, 1760–1915," *Bulletin of the New York Academy of Medicine* 49 (1973): 821. See Edward D. Bangs, "Executions Which Have Taken Place in Massachusetts January 1, 1800, to December 31, 1830 … from the Records in the Secretary of State's Office," Massachusetts General Court, "Report of the Select Committee of the House of Representatives, on So Much of the Governor's Speech at the June Session 1830, to Legalizing the Study of Anatomy," House Document No. 4, Session 2, 1830–1931, Boston, 1831, 91–93.

97. Humphrey, "Dissection and Discrimination," 819–20. See also "Report of the Select Committee … to Legalizing the Study of Anatomy," Massachusetts House Document no. 4, session 2, 1830/31, 67, 91–92.

98. *Columbian Register*, April 27, 1833, 3.

99. Humphrey, "Dissection and Discrimination," 821.

100. John B. Blake, "The Development of American Anatomy Acts," *Journal of Medical Education* 30, no. 8 (1955): 436.

101. Edward Warren, *Life of John Collins Warren, M.D.*, 2 vols. (Boston: Ticknor and Fields, 1860), 1:411; E.M. Hartwell, *The Study of Anatomy, Historically and Legally Considered*" (Boston: Tolman and White, 1881), 29. On the Irish in Boston, see Oscar Handlin, *Boston's Immigrants: A Study in Acculturation* (Cambridge: Harvard University Press, 1991), 114–16.

102. Hartwell, *The Study of Anatomy*, 30. It appears that when the Massachusetts Anatomy Act of 1831 was passed, one physician from Stow, Massachusetts, about twenty-one miles west of Boston, wrote to the *Boston Medical and Surgical Journal* in October 1831 that the change in public opinion of the law was dramatic: "four years ago had people known that a person here, was dissecting a human body, I think his personal safety could not have been insured from the mob." He then went on to describe how a proper burial was held for a pauper in Stow: "the grave left unfilled, the body removed, dissected, and returned to the grave"; a second ceremony was held, and then he was buried. However, the new law did not pertain to the towns and cities outside of Boston, so it is curious that his enthusiasm for the public support of the new law and its implications had gotten ahead of the actual basis of the law. See Isaac W. Mulliken, "Letter to the Editor: Popular Feeling Respecting the Anatomy Law," *Boston Medical and Surgical Journal* 5 (October 31, 1831): 190–191.

103. Linden F. Edwards, "Dr. Frederick C. Waite's Correspondence with Reference to Grave Robbery," *Ohio State Medical Journal* 54 (1958): 602.

104. L.B. Arey, *Northwestern University Medical School, 1859–1959: A Pioneer in Educational Reform* (Evanston: Northwestern University Medical School, 1959), 128.

105. Humphrey, "Dissection and Discrimination," 822.

106. T.S. Sozinsky, "Grave-Robbing and Dissection," *Penn. Monthly* 10 (1879): 216.

107. *Bureau of the Census: Paupers in Almshouses* (Washington, D.C.: U.S. Government Printing Office, 1904), 6.

108. George B. Jenkins, "The Legal Status of Dissecting," *Anatomical Record* 7 (1913): 395.

109. Humphrey, "Dissection and Discrimination," 824; and Bureau of the Census, *Tuberculosis in the United States* (Washington, D.C.: U.S. Government Printing Office, 1908), 18.

110. Humphrey, "Dissection and Discrimination," 824.

111. Humphrey, 824.

112. Willard Bean, *A.B.C. History of Palmyra, and the Beginning of "Mormonism"* (Palmyra, NY: Palmyra Courier Co., 1938), 34.

113. Sappol, *A Traffic of Dead Bodies*, 113.

114. Frederick L. Hoffmann, *Pauper Burials and the Interment of the Dead in Large Cities* (Newark, NJ: Prudential Press, 1919), 57. The fear of a pauper burial has even been cited as the reason for the growth of the life insurance industry, beginning in the 1875 with the formation of the Prudential

Friendly Society that became the Prudential Insurance Company of America. "The abhorrence of a pauper burial is so universal that it may be said to form the foundation of life insurance as represented in the more humble sphere of burial clubs and friendly societies" (11–12).

115. Humphrey, "Dissection and Discrimination," 824. On the humiliation imposed on the pauper dead, see Appendix G, "Potter's Field Graves Opened in Indianapolis, 1918), in Hoffman, *Pauper Burials and the Interment of the Dead in Large Cities*, 113–23.

116. Humphrey, "Dissection and Discrimination," 824.

Conclusion

1. William G. Rothstein, *American Medical Schools and the Practice of Medicine: A History* (New York: Oxford University Press, 1987), 39–41.

2. Samuel D. Gross, *Autobiography of Samuel D. Gross, with a Sketch of His...*, 2 vols. (Philadelphia: George Barrie Publishers, 1887), 1:56.

3. Rothstein, *American Medical Schools*, 40.

4. Frederick C. Waite, "The Development of Anatomical Laws in New England," *New England Journal of Medicine* 233 (1945): 722.

5. William C. Wigglesworth, "Surgery in Massachusetts, 1620–1800," in *Medicine in Colonial Massachusetts, 1620–1820* (Boston: The Society, 1980), 220.

6. John Jones, *Plain Concise Practical Remarks on the Treatment of Wounds and Fractures...* (Philadelphia: Robert Bell, 1776), 10.

7. Waite, "The Development of Anatomical Laws in New England," 719.

8. "The Development of Anatomical Laws in New England," 720–21.

9. "Medical Schools in Boston," *Boston Medical and Surgical Journal* 50, no. 14 (1854): 260.

10. Waite, "The Development of Anatomical Laws in New England," 722.

11. Mark S. Schantz, *Awaiting the Heavenly Country: The Civil War and America's Culture of Death* (Ithaca: Cornell University Press, 2011), 39–40, 53. For a full discussion on bodily resurrection in antebellum America, see 38–69.

12. Henry Raymond, "Editor's Table," *Harper's New Monthly Magazine* 8 (April 1854): 690.

13. Raymond, "Editor's Table," 691–92.

14. Sarah Gould, *The Guardian Angels: Or, Friends in Heaven* (Boston: Higgins and Bradley, 1857), 214.

15. Drew Gilpin Faust, *This Republic of Suffering: Death and the American Civil War* (New York: Vintage Books, 2008), xi–xii.

16. Faust, *This Republic of Suffering*. Faust's book is replete with examples of confronting the dead during the war and the consequences of its aftermath (xvi–xvii).

17. Faust, 173–210.

18. Gary Laderman, "The Sacred Remains: American Attitudes toward Death, 1799–1883" (New Haven: Yale University Press, 1996), 169.

19. Laderman, "The Sacred Remains," 169.

20. Laderman, 166, 169.

21. Laderman, 173.

22. Laderman, 165.

23. Laderman, 175.

24. James J. Farrell, *Inventing the American Way of Death, 1830–1920* (Philadelphia: Temple University Press, 1980), 136.

25. Farrell, *Inventing the American Way of Death, 1830–1920*, 136.

26. Farrell, 136–137.

27. Farrell, 149.

28. *Philadelphia Inquirer*, 1 March 1883, 3 and 6 March 1883, 3.

29. Laderman, 164.

30. Waite, "The Development of Anatomical Laws in New England," 722–23.

31. *Morning Advertiser*, January 16, 1893, 1–2.

32. Franklin P. Mall, "Anatomical Material: Its Collection and Its Preservation at the Johns Hopkins Anatomical Laboratory," *Bulletin of the Johns Hopkins Hospital* 16, no. 167 (February 1905), 38.

33. Mears J. Ewing, J.D. Bryant, and Thomas Dwight, "Report of the Committee on the Collection and Preservation of Anatomical Material," Report of the Eighth Annual Meeting of the Association of American Anatomists, *Science* 3 (January 17, 1896): 84.

34. Waite, "The Development of Anatomical Laws in New England," 722.

35. *Morning Advertiser*, January 16, 1893, 1–2.

36. *Morning Advertiser*, January 16, 1893, 1–2.

37. United States Government, *Congressional Record Containing the Proceedings and Debates of the Fiftieth Congress, First Session* (Washington, D.C.: Government Printing Office, 1888), v. 19, 2416.

38. United States Government, *Congressional Record*, Fiftieth Congress, First Session, v. 19, 2418.

39. United States Government, *Congressional Record*, Fiftieth Congress, First Session, v. 19, 2418.

40. United States Government, *Congressional Record*, Fiftieth Congress, First Session, v. 19, 2416 and 2421. Of course, there was push-back on the decline of body snatching once these laws were passed. See *Congressional Record*, Fiftieth Congress, First Session, v. 19, 2414.

41. Humphrey, "Dissection and Discrimination," Fiftieth Congress, First Session, v. 19, 824.

42. Humphrey, 824.

43. Mall, "Anatomical Material," 39. See on the measures taken to virtually eliminate "the trafficking in dead bodies" in Baltimore by 1900.

44. Guttmacher, "Bootlegging Bodies," 402.

Bibliography

Manuscripts

Erastus Osborn to Shadrach Osborn, January 12, 1824, Yale University Library. https://imageserver.library.yale.edu/digcoll:4342544/guest2708120bc940472caf3fab55a4dc8923@yaleguest.edu/YEcXdYQ10qTHqcrUf3cle83ApOU/1500.jpe?authroot=findit.library.yale.edu&parentfolder=digcoll:4342544&ip=32.214.70.86.

Erastus Osborn to Shadrach Osborn, January 19, 1824, Yale University Library. https://imageserver.library.yale.edu/digcoll:4342544/guest2708120bc940472caf3fab55a4dc8923@yaleguest.edu/YEcXdYQ10qTHqcrUf3cle83ApOU/1500.jpe?authroot=findit.library.yale.edu&parentfolder=digcoll:4342544&ip=32.214.70.86.

Ezekiel D. Cushing to Mehetabel Cushing [mother], December 5, 1809. EDC Papers, folder 4, Manuscripts and Archives, Yale University Library.

Ezekiel D. Cushing to Mehetabel Cushing [sister], February 11, 1810. Francis A. Countway Library of Medicine, Harvard University. https://nrs.lib.harvard.edu/urn-3:hms.count:26856034?n=4.

Ezekiel D. Cushing to Nathaniel Cushing, December 2, 1809. EDC Papers, folder 4, Manuscripts and Archives, Yale University Library.

Ezekiel D. Cushing to Nathaniel Cushing, December 27, 1809. Francis A. Countway Library, Harvard University. https://nrs.lib.harvard.edu/urn-3:hms.count:26856044?n=11.

Ezekiel D. Cushing to Nathaniel Cushing, May 23, 1810. Francis A. Countway Library, Harvard University. https://nrs.lib.harvard.edu/urn-3:hms.count:26856044?n=11.

Ezekiel D. Cushing to Nathaniel Cushing, October 7, 1810. Francis A. Countway Library, Harvard University. https://nrs.lib.harvard.edu/urn-3:hms.count:26856044?n=11.

Ezekiel D. Cushing to Nathaniel Cushing, November 28, 1810. Francis A. Countway Library, Harvard University. https://nrs.lib.harvard.edu/urn-3:hms.count:26856044?n=11.

Ezekiel D. Cushing to Nathaniel Cushing, January 22, 1811. Ezekiel D. Cushing Papers, folder 4, Yale University Manuscripts and Archives, Yale University Library,

George Shattuck to Ezekiel Dodge Cushing, December 10, 1810. Ezekiel D. Cushing Papers (folder 4), Yale University Manuscripts and Archives, Yale University Library.

Israel Keith, Case of Doctor Curtis, and Anthony Frederick, 1782. Israel Keith papers II, MS. N-1521. Massachusetts Historical Society.

Mills Olcott, Account Books, Hanover, 41. MO Accounts of His Law Practice, 1800–1840, v. 2, 1807–1825, 9. Rauner Special Collections Library, Dartmouth College, Hanover, New Hampshire.

Nathan Smith to Mills Olcott, May 1819. Mss. 819340.2, Rauner Special Collections Library, Dartmouth College, Hanover, New Hampshire.

Nathan Smith to Mills Olcott, January 30, 1824. MS-436, box 4 (folder 62), Rauner Special Collections Library, Dartmouth College, Hanover, New Hampshire.

Nathan Smith to Mills Olcott, February 28, 1824. MS-436, box 4 (folder 62), Rauner Special Collections Library, Dartmouth College, Hanover, New Hampshire.

Records of the Supreme Judicial Court. Commonwealth vs. Sewall, Manuscript 1817–1818, Vol. 1, docket 541–542. Massachusetts Supreme Judicial Court Archives.

Primary Sources

"An Act to Protect the Sepulchers of the Dead, March 2, 1815." *The Public General Laws of the Commonwealth of Massachusetts*, Vol. 4. Boston: Wells and Lilly, 1816.

Agnew, D. Hayes, et al. *History and Reminiscences of the Philadelphia Almshouse and Philadelphia Hospital*. Philadelphia: Detre and Blackburn, 1890.

"Agreeably to the advice of the Ecclesiastical Council here convened, at the request of the pastor and Church of Christ in Manchester, ... 17 June 1819." In Tyler Parsons, *Truth Espoused, Relative to the Difficulties That Existed in the Town of Manchester, Massachusetts*, 54. Dedham, MA: M & W M Mann, 1823.

Alexandria Gazette (Alexandria, VA). 1834, 1873,1877, and 1883.

American Association for the Advancement of Science. "Anatomical Law of the State of Pennsylvania Enacted June 13, 1883." *Science*, New Series, 3, no. 55 (January 17, 1896): 84–86.

American Mercury (Hartford, CT), 1819, 1824.
Annable, Daniel. "Deposition." March 3, 1823. In Tyler Parsons, *Truth Espoused, Relative to the Difficulties That Existed in the Town of Manchester, Massachusetts*, 67–68. Dedham, MA: M & W M Mann, 1823.
Baltimore Patriot. 1823.
Bangs, Edward D. "Executions which have taken place in Massachusetts. January 1, 1800, to December 31, 1830 ... from the Records in the Secretary of State's Office." In Massachusetts General Court, *Report of the Select Committee of the House of Representatives, on so much of the Governor's Speech at the June Session 1830, to Legalizing the Study of Anatomy*. House Document no. 4, session 2, 1830/1831. Boston: Dutton and Wentworth, 1831.
Barber, Orion M., Lavant M. Read, and John Young. *The Vermont Statutes, 1894: Including the Public Acts of 1894....* Rutland, VT: Tuttle Co., 1895.
Bell, Charles Henry. *History of the Town of Exeter, New Hampshire*. Exeter, 1888.
Bentley, William. *The Diary of William Bentley, Pastor of the East Church of Salem, Massachusetts, 1811–1819*. 4 vols. Salem: Essex Institute, 1914.
Benton, E. C. *A History of Guildhall, VT*. Waverly, MA: E. C. Benton, 1886.
Bittinger, Rev. John Quincy. *A History of Haverhill, New Hampshire*. Haverhill, NH: Cohos Steam Press, 1888.
Blackstone, William, and Edward Christianson, ed. *Commentaries on the Laws of England*. 4 vols. Philadelphia, 1825.
Blake, John B. "The Development of American Anatomy Acts." *Journal of Medical Education* 30 (1955): 431–39.
Boston Commercial Gazette. 1824.
Boston Daily Advertiser. 1820.
Bowditch, Henry. *Memoir of Amos Twitchell M.D.* Boston: John Wilson and Son, 1851.
Brattleboro Messenger (Brattleboro, VT). 1831.
Brewer, E. C. *Dictionary of Phrase and Fable*. London: Cassel & Co., 1896.
Bromwell, William Jeremy. *History of Immigration to the United States, Exhibiting the Number, Sex, Age* ... New York: Redfield, 1856.
Brooks, Harry M. *The Olden Times Series, Quaint and Curious Advertisements*. Boston: Ticknor and Co., 1886.
Broussais, François-Joseph-Victor. *Cours de Phrénologie*. Paris: J.B. Bailliere, 1836.
Brown, Samuel G. *The Life of Rufus Choate*. 3rd ed. Boston: Little, Brown, 1879.
Buckminster, Joseph. *A Sermon Preached at the Installation of the Reverend James Thurston, to the Pastoral Charge of the Church of Manchester*. Portsmouth, NH: Oracle Press, 1809.
Burgess, Abiel. "Deposition." March 23, 1823. in Tyler Parsons, *Truth Espoused, Relative to the Difficulties That Existed in the Town of Manchester, Massachusetts*, 65–67. Dedham, MA: M & W M Mann, 1823.
Busey, Samuel Claggett. *Pictures of the City of Washington in the Past*. Washington, D.C.: Wm. Ballard & Sons, 1898.
"A Card," dated 15 January 1824, *Connecticut Herald*, January 20, 1824, 3.
Carey, Francis King. "The Disposition of the Body after Death." *American Law Review* 19 (1855): 251–70.
Cecil Whig (Elkton, MD). 1886.
Cobbett's Weekly Political Register. 16 (April 7, 1832): 15.
Coke, Edward. *Institutes of the Laws of England*. 4 vols. London: M. Flesher, W. Lee, and D. Pakeman, 1644.
Columbian Register (New Haven, CT). 1824, 1833.
Concord Gazette (Concord, NH). 1810.
Connecticut Courant (Hartford, CT). 1824, 1833, 1834.
Connecticut Governor's Foot Guard Company. *A Souvenir of New Haven Connecticut....* 2nd ed. New Haven, CT: Governor's Foot Guard, 1908.
Connecticut Herald (New Haven, CT). 1819, 1824.
Connecticut Mirror (Hartford, CT). 1823, 1824.
Cothren, William. *History of Ancient Woodbury, Connecticut: From the First....* 2 vols. Waterbury, CT: Bronson Brothers, 1854.
Counter Memorial of Sundry Citizens of the District of Columbia praying That a Charter may be granted by Congress to Enable them to Institute a Medical College in the City of Washington, February 20, 1826. U.S. Senate. 19th Congress 1st Session. No. 44. Washington, D.C.: Gab and Seaton, 1826.
Crowell, Robert. *History of the Town of Essex from 1634–1868*. Springfield, MA: Samuel Bowles & Co. 1868.
Crowell, Robert. *Interment of the dead, a dictate of natural affection, sanctioned by the word of God, and the examples of the good in every age: A sermon delivered in Ipswich, Second Parish, July 23, 1818, on the occasion of reinterring the coffins which had been robbed of their contents*. Andover, 1818.
Currier, John M., MD. *Song of Hubbardton Raid: Delivered on the 50 (-1)th anniversary of the citizens of Hubbardton, Vermont, on Castleton Medical College, Held at the Residence of J. Sanford, M.D. Castleton, Vt. November 29, 1879*. Castleton, VT: Tuttle and Co., 1880.
Daggett, John. *A Sketch of the History of Attleborough: From Its Settlement to the Division* ... Boston: Samuel Fisher, 1894.
Daily Richmond Whig (Richmond, VA). 1829.
Dale, R.W. "Impressions of America." *Nineteenth Century* 4 (1878): 713–34.
Dale, William. *The Present State of the Medical Profession in Great Britain and Ireland*. London: A. W. Bennett, 1860.
Dana, Henry S. *History of Woodstock, Vermont*. Boston: Houghton Mifflin. 1889.
Dana, Samuel. [Scribe Ecclesiastical Council]. "To the Ecclesiastical Council Now in Session in Manchester, June 17, 1819." In Tyler Parsons,

Truth Espoused, Relative to the Difficulties That Existed in the Town of Manchester, Massachusetts, 51. Dedham, MA: M & W M Mann, 1823.

Dana, Samuel. "To the Moderator and Gentlemen of the Respectful Council, Now Convened in the Town of Manchester, 17 June 1819." In Tyler Parsons, *Truth Espoused, Relative to the Difficulties That Existed in the Town of Manchester, Massachusetts*, 51–52. Dedham, MA: M & W M Mann, 1823.

Dana, Samuel. "The Committee on the Subject of Remuneration Made Their Report, Which Was Considered Amended, and Filed …" In Tyler Parsons, *Truth Espoused, Relative to the Difficulties That Existed in the Town of Manchester, Massachusetts*, 52–54. Dedham, MA: M & W M Mann, 1823.

D'Arusmont, Frances Wright. *Views of Society and Manners in America: In a Series of Letters from that Country*. London: Longman, Hurst, Rees Orme, and Brown, 1822.

Day, Thomas. *Reports of the Cases Argued and Determined in the Supreme Court of Errors of the State of Connecticut*, Vol. 4. New York: Banks, Gould, and Co., 1848.

Dewey, John, MD. "Deposition," March 13, 1820. In Tyler Parsons, *Truth Espoused, Relative to the Difficulties That Existed in the Town of Manchester, Massachusetts*, 70–71. Dedham, MA: M & W M Mann, 1823.

Dewey, John, MD. "Deposition," April 20, 1820. In Tyler Parsons, *Truth Espoused, Relative to the Difficulties That Existed in the Town of Manchester, Massachusetts*, 72–73. Dedham, MA: M & W M Mann, 1823.

District of Columbia Board of Commissioners. *Fourth Annual Report of the Commissioners of the District of Columbia November 30, 1876, to November 1, 1877*. Washington, D.C.: U.S. Government Printing Office, 1877.

District of Columbia Board of Health. *Third Annual Report of the Board of Health of the District of Columbia, 1874*. Washington, D.C.: Chronicle Publishing Co., 1874.

"Dr. Hun's and Dr. May's Introductory Lectures." *American Medical Intelligencer, April 1, 1839–April 1, 1840*, Vol. 3 (1840): 314–17.

Drake, Daniel. *Practical Essay on Medical Education, and the Medical Profession in the United States*. Cincinnati: Rolfe & Young, 1832.

Duncan, John Morison. *Travels through Part of the United States and Canada in 1818 and…*. 2 vols. Glasgow: Hurst, Robinson & Co., 1823.

Dwight, Thomas. "Anatomy Laws versus Body-snatching." *The Forum* 21 (1896): 494–502.

Ecclesiastical Council. "Council Paper No. 1," June 2, 1819. In Tyler Parsons, *Truth Espoused, Relative to the Difficulties That Existed in the Town of Manchester, Massachusetts*, 50–51. Dedham, MA: M & W M Mann, 1823.

Essex Register (Salem, MA). 1818.

Evening Critic (Washington, DC). 1884.

Evening Star (Washington, DC). 1872, 1873, 1874, 1882, 1884, 1885, 1886.

Felt, Joseph B. *History of Ipswich, Essex, and Hamilton*. Cambridge, MA: Charles Folsom, 1834.

First Congregational Church [Essex, MA]. *Two Centuries of Church History: Celebration of the Two Hundredth Anniversary of the Organization of the Congregational Church and Parish in Essex, Massachusetts, August 19–20, 1883*. Salem, MA: J. H. Choate, and Co., 1884.

Forbes, William S. "History of the First Anatomy Act of Pennsylvania." *Philadelphia Medical Journal* 2 (July–December, 1898): 1131–1136.

Francis, Samuel Ward. *Biographical Sketches of Distinguished Living New York Physicians*. New York: George Putnam & Sons, 1867.

Frothingham, Richard. *Life and Times of Joseph Warren*. Boston: Little, Brown, 1865.

General Court. *Resolves of the General Court of the Commonwealth of Massachusetts*. Boston: Russell and Gardner, 1820.

Georgetown College. *A Catalogue of the Officers and Students of Georgetown University, 1872–1873*. Baltimore: John Murray, 1873.

Georgetown Metropolitan (Washington, DC), 1826.

Girdler, John. "Affidavit," March 9, 1823. In Tyler Parsons, *Truth Espoused, Relative to the Difficulties That Existed in the Town of Manchester, Massachusetts*, 58–64. Dedham, MA: M & W M Mann, 1823.

Gould, Mrs. Sarah. *The Guardian Angels: Or, Friends in Heaven*. Boston: Higgins and Bradley, 1857.

Grant, Ulysses S. *The Papers of Ulysses S. Grant, Digital Edition*. 33 vols. John Y. Simon and John Marszalek, eds. Charlottesville: University of Virginia Press, 2018. https://rotunda.upress.virginia.edu/founders/GRNT.html.

Grant, Ulysses S., to the Secretary of State, May 29, 1873, "Respiting the Execution in the Case of Thomas Wright until the 6th Day of June 1873." Shapell Manuscript Foundation. https://www.shapell.org/manuscript/ulysses-grant-capital-punishment-minorities/.

Great Britain. *The Law Reports: The Public General Statutes … passed in the Fifty Ninth Year and Sixtieth Year of her Majesty Queen Victoria*, Vol. 33. London: William Clowes and Sons Ltd.,1896.

Gross, Samuel D. *Autobiography of Samuel D. Gross, with a Sketch of His …* 2 vols. Philadelphia: George Barrie Publishers, 1887.

Guernsey, R. S. "Ownership of a Corpse." *Central Law Journal* 10 (1880): 303–306, 325–327.

Hale, Charles R. Hale Collection of Connecticut Cemetery Inscriptions. Hartford, Connecticut: Connecticut State Library; Hartford, Connecticut: Connecticut Newspaper Notices, Vol. 17, accessed at Ancestry.com. Connecticut, U.S., Hale Collection of Cemetery Inscriptions and Newspaper Notices, 1629–1934 [database on-line]. Provo, UT, USA.

Hamilton, John B. "Life and Times of Doctor Reuben D. Mussey." *Journal of the American Medical Association* 26 (1896): 649–52.

Hartford Courant (Hartford, CT). 1819.

Hartford Times (Hartford, CT). 1819.

Hartwell, Edward M. "American Anatomy Acts." *Boston Medical Surgical Journal* 103 (1880): 361–63.

Hartwell, Edward M. "The Early American Anatomists and the Legal Status of Anatomy in Massachusetts before 1800." *New England Journal of Medicine* 103 (July–December 1880): 538–41.

Hartwell, Edward M. "The Hindrances to Anatomical Study in the United States, Including a Special Record of the Struggles of Our Early Anatomical Teachers." *Annals of Anatomy and Surgery* 3 (1881): 209–25.

Hartwell, Edward M. "The Present Legal Status of Human Anatomy in the United States." *Annals of Anatomy and Surgery* 4 (1881): 8–14.

Hartwell, Edward M. "The Progress of Anatomical Study in Massachusetts with Remarks upon Its Legal Status." *Annals of Anatomy and Surgery* 3 (1881): 266–273.

Hartwell, Edward M. *The Study of Anatomy, Historically, and Legally Considered.* Boston: Tolman & White, 1881.

Headley, J.T. *The Great Riots of New York, 1712–1873.* New York: E. B. Treat, 1873.

Hemenway, Abby M. *The Vermont Historical Gazetteer: A Magazine, Embracing a History of Each Town, Civil, Ecclesiastical, Biographical, and Military.* 5 vols. Claremont, NH: Claremont Publishing Co., 1867–1891.

Horner, William E. *Necrological Notice of Dr. Philip Syng Physick, Delivered before the American Philosophical Society, May 4, 1838.* Philadelphia: Haswell, 1838.

Houghton, Horace, *Catalogue of the Officers, and Students of the Vermont Academy of Medicine.* Castleton, VT: H.H. Houghton, 1830.

Hun, Thomas. "Introductory Lecture before the Albany Medical College Delivered November 12, 1839." *American Medical Intelligencer, April 1, 1839–April 1, 1840,* Vol. 3 (1840): 314–15.

Hunt, Sanford B. "The Negro as a Soldier." *Anthropological Review* 7 (1869): 40–42.

Hurd, D.H. *History of Bristol County....* Philadelphia: J. W. Lewis, 1883.

Hurd, D. Hamilton. *History of Essex County, Massachusetts.* 2 vols. Philadelphia: J. W. Lewis & Co, 1888.

"John Frederick May Obituary." *Critic and Record,* May 2, 1891.

Jones, John. *Plain Concise Practical Remarks on the Treatment of Wounds and Fractures...* Philadelphia: Robert Bell, 1776.

Kendall, Edward Augustus. *Travels through the Northern Parts of the United States, in the Years 1807 and 1808.* 3 vols. New York: I. Riley, 1809.

Knight, James. *An Eulogium on Nathan Smith Late Professor of the Theory and Practice of Physic and Surgery....* New Haven, CT: Hezekiah Howe, 1829.

Lamson, Darius Francis. *History of the Town of Manchester, Essex County, Massachusetts, 1645–1895.* Published by the Town, 1895.

Literary Cadet and Saturday Evening Bulletin (Providence, RI). 1828.

Locke, John. *A Paraphrase and Notes on the Epistles of St. Paul to the Galatians, First and Second Corinthians, Romans, and Ephesians: To Which Is Prefixed an Essay for the Understanding of St. Paul's Epistles, by Consulting St. Paul Himself.* Cambridge, UK: Brown, Shattuck, and Company, 1832.

Lucke, Jerome B. *History of the New Haven Grays from Sept. 13, 1816, to Sept. 13, 1876.* New Haven, CT: Tuttle Morehouse and Taylor, 1876.

Mackenzie, William. "An Appeal to the Public and to the Legislatures on the necessity of Affording Dead Bodies to the Schools of Anatomy, by Legislative Enactment." *Westminster Review* 2 (1824): 59–97.

Massachusetts. General Court. House of Representatives. Select Committee on Legalizing the Study of Anatomy. "Report 4 of the Select Committee of the House of Representatives On so Much of the Governors Speech, at the June Session, 1830 as it relates to Legalizing the Study of Anatomy." *Massachusetts House of Representatives,* January, 1831, 1-82. Boston, Dutton and Wentworth, 1831.

Massachusetts. *The Public and General Laws of the Commonwealth of Massachusetts: From February 28, 1807, to February 16, 1816.* Boston: Wells and Lilly, for the State, 1816.

May, John F. "An Introductory Lecture, Delivered at the Opening of the Medical Department of Columbian College, November 4, 1839." *American Medical Intelligencer, April 1, 1839-April 1, 1840,* Vol. 3 (1840): 316–17.

McKnight, William J. *Jefferson County Pennsylvania, Her Pioneers and People, 1800–1915.* 2 vols. Chicago: J. H. Beers & Co., 1917.

Mears, J. Ewing, J. D. Bryant, and Thomas Dwight. "Report of the Committee on the Collection and Preservation of Anatomical Material." Report of the Eighth Annual Meeting of the Association of American Anatomists, *Science* 3 (January 17, 1896): 77–86.

"Medical School in Boston." *Boston Medical and Surgical Journal* 35, no. 21 (1846): 417–18.

"Medical Schools in Boston." *Boston Medical and Surgical Journal* 50, no. 14 (1854): 258–62.

Medical Society of the District of Columbia. *History of the Medical Society of the District of Columbia: 1817–1901.* Washington, D.C.: Medical Society of the District of Columbia, 1909.

Memorial of the Professors of the Medical Department of the Columbian College in the District of Columbia, February 13, 1826. 19th Congress, 1st Session, Senate Documents, No. 36, Vol. 2, 1–5. Washington, D.C.: Gab and Seaton, 1826.

Memorial of Sundry Citizens of the District of Columbia Praying That a Charter May Be Granted by Congress to Enable Them to Institute a Medical College, February 13, 1826. 19th Congress 1st Session Senate Documents, No. 35, Vol. 2, 1–4. Washington, D.C.: Gab and Seaton, 1826.

Memorial of Sundry Citizens of the District of Columbia Praying That Another Medical School May Not Be Incorporated in the City of Washington, February 22, 1826. 19th Congress 1st Session, Senate Documents, No. 48, Vol. 2, 1–4. Washington, D.C.: Gab and Seaton, 1826.

Meyer, Jacob C. *Church and State in Massachusetts from 1740–1833.* New York: Russell and Russell, 1930.

Middlesex Gazette (Middletown, CT). 1824.

Morning Advertiser (New York, NY). 1893.

The Morning Times (Washington, DC). 1896

Mulliken, Isaac W. "Letter to the Editor: Popular Feeling Respecting the Anatomy Law." *Boston Medical and Surgical Journal.* 5 (October 31, 1831): 190–191.

Mussey, Dr. Rueben. "Affidavit," March 7, 1820. In Tyler Parsons, *Truth Espoused, Relative to the Difficulties That Existed in the Town of Manchester, Massachusetts,* 69. Dedham, MA: M & W M Mann, 1823.

Mussey, Dr. Reuben. "Letter to Doct. Thomas Sewall. 26 October 1818." In Tyler Parsons, *Truth Espoused, Relative to the Difficulties That Existed in the Town of Manchester, Massachusetts,* 16. Dedham, MA: M & W M Mann, 1823.

National Gazette (Philadelphia, PA). 1831.

National Republican (Washington, DC). 1884.

Newburyport Herald (Newburyport, MA). 1832.

New-England Palladium (Boston, MA). 1818.

New Hampshire General Court. *Laws of New Hampshire: Including public and private acts and resolves and the royal commissions and instructions, with historical and descriptive notes, and an appendix, 1792–1801,* Vol. 6. Concord, NH: Evans Printing Co., 1917.

New Hampshire Sentinel (Keene, NH). 1831.

New London Gazette (New London, CT). 1819, 1823, 1833, 1834.

New York Spectator (New York, NY). 1830.

North, Elisha, MD. *Outlines of the Science of Life: Which Treats Physiologically of Both Body and Mind: Designed Only for Philosophers, and Other Candid Persons, to Which Are Added Essays on Other Subjects.* New York: Collins and Co., 1829.

Norwich Courier (Norwich, CT). 1833.

"Obituary" [Dr. Thomas Sewall]. *Niles' National Register,* May 17, 1845, 164.

Parsons, Tyler. *Truth Espoused, Relative to the Difficulties That Existed in the Town of Manchester, Massachusetts.* Dedham, MA: M & W M Mann, 1823.

Parsons, Tyler, and Richard Allen. "To the Gentlemen of the Committee of the First Baptist Church in Beverly ... , Manchester, 19 April 1819." In Tyler Parsons, *Truth Espoused, Relative to the Difficulties That Existed in the Town of Manchester, Massachusetts,* 40. Dedham, MA: M & W M Mann, 1823.

Peck, Henry. *The New Haven State House with Some Accounts of the Green.* New Haven, CT: Henry Peck and George H. Coe, 1889.

Phelps, Richard H. *Newgate, A History of the Prison: Its Insurrections, Massacres ...* Albany, NY: J. Mussel, 1860.

Philadelphia Inquirer (Philadelphia, PA). 1882, 1883.

Pitkin, Clarence, II, et al. *The Revised Laws of Vermont, 1880, with the Public Acts of the ...* Rutland, VT: Tuttle and Co, 1881.

Public Statutes of the State of Connecticut. Hartford, CT: C. Babcock, 1824.

Poore, Benjamin P. *Congressional Directory.* Washington, D.C.: U.S. Government Printing Office, 1875.

The Portsmouth Journal (Portsmouth, NH). 1824.

Rauch, John. *Report on Medical Education, Medical Colleges ... 1765–1889.* Springfield, IL: H. W. Roker, 1889.

Raymond, Henry. "Editor's Table: The Sacredness of the Human Body." *Harper's New Monthly Magazine* 8 (April 1854): 690–93.

"The Resurrectionists of Old." *Hospital: A Journal of Medical Sciences and Hospital Administration* 21 (1896): 193.

Rutland Daily Herald (Rutland, VT). 1820

Salem Gazette (Salem, MA). 1818, 1824.

San Francisco Bulletin (San Francisco, CA). 1861.

San Francisco Call (San Francisco, CA). 1894.

"Selectman of Manchester to Rev. James Thurston, Manchester, 24 December 1819," In Tyler Parsons, *Truth Espoused, Relative to the Difficulties That Existed in the Town of Manchester, Massachusetts,* 95. Dedham, MA: M & W M Mann, 1823.

Sewall, Thomas. *An Address Delivered before the Washington City Temperance Society, November15, 1830.* Washington, D.C.: Temperance Society, 1830.

Sewall, Thomas. *An Examination of Phrenology: In Two Lectures, Delivered to the Students of Columbian College, District of Columbia, February 1837.* Washington, D.C.: B. Homans Printer, 1837.

Sewall, Thomas. *A Lecture Delivered at the Opening of the Medical Department of the Columbian College in the District of Columbia, March 30, 1825.* Washington, City, 1826.

Sewall, Thomas. *The Pathology of Drunkenness, or the Effects of Alcoholic Drinks, with Drawings of the Drunkard's Stomach.* Albany, NY: C. Van Benthuysen, 1841.

Shipton, Clifford K., and John L. Sibley. *Sibley's Harvard Graduates: Biographical Sketches of Those Who Attended Harvard College ...* , Vol. 17. Boston: Massachusetts Historical Society, 1873–19__.

Smith, Emily Anna. *The Life and Letters of Nathan Smith.* New Haven: Yale University Press, 1914.

Smith, Thomas Southwood. *Use of the Dead to the Living.* London: Craddock and Paternoster Row, 1828.

Sozinsky, T.S. "Grave-Robbing and Dissection." *Penn Monthly* 10 (1879): 206–17.

Spencer, G.D. *A Poem on the Hubbardton Raid*. Rutland, VT: Tuttle and Co., 1880.

Sylvester, Edward. *District of Columbia: A Retrospective of the Police Organization of the Cities of Washington, Georgetown, and the District of Columbia*. Washington, D.C.: Gibson Bros., 1894.

Taylor, Henry Blake. *Chronicles of the New Haven Green from 1638 to 1862*. New Haven, CT: Tuttle, Morehouse, and Taylor Press, 1898.

Thurston, James. "To the Brethren of the Church of Christ, 3 April 1819." In Tyler Parsons, *Truth Espoused, Relative to the Difficulties That Existed in the Town of Manchester, Massachusetts*, 35–36. Dedham, MA: M & W M Mann, 1823. Parsons.

Thurston, James. "To the Brethren of the Church of Christ, 5 April 1819." In Tyler Parsons, *Truth Espoused, Relative to the Difficulties That Existed in the Town of Manchester, Massachusetts*, 38. Dedham, MA: M & W M Mann, 1823.

The Times (Boston, MA). 1807.

Toner, Joseph M. *Anniversary Oration Delivered before the Medical Society of the District of Columbia, September 26, 1866, Medical Society of the District of Columbia, Societies*. Washington, D.C.: Cunningham & McIntosh, 1869.

"Town Meeting Legally Notified and Held at the Meeting House in Manchester on Saturday the 15th Day of May Anno Domini 1819." In Tyler Parsons, *Truth Espoused, Relative to the Difficulties That Existed in the Town of Manchester, Massachusetts*, 42–43. Dedham, MA: M & W M Mann, 1823.

Townsend, George A. *Historic Sketches at Washington*. Hartford, CT: Jas. Betts & Co., 1877.

Townsend, George A. *Washington Outside and Inside: A Picture and a Narrative*. Hartford, CT: James Betts & Co., 1874.

Tracey, Cyrus M. *Standard History of Essex County, Massachusetts*. Boston: Jewett & Co., 1878.

Trout, James Samuel. *Life, Adventures and Anecdotes of "Beau" Hickman: Prince of American Bummers*. Washington: DC, 1879.

United States Army. *Report of the Quartermaster-General to the Secretary of War...* Washington, D.C.: U.S. Government Printing Office, 1872.

United States Bureau of the Census. *Paupers in Almshouses*. Washington, D.C.: U.S. Government Printing Office, 1904.

United States Bureau of the Census. *Tuberculosis in the United States*. Washington, D.C.: U.S. Government Printing Office, 1908.

United States Congress. "An Act for the Promotion of Anatomical Sciences, and to Prevent the Desecration of Graves in the District of Columbia, February 1, 1892." *Congressional Record Containing the Proceedings and Debates of the Fifty Second Congress, First Session*, Vol. 22. Washington, D.C.: U.S. Government Printing Office, 1892.

United States Congress. "An Act for the Promotion of Anatomical Sciences, and to Prevent the Desecration of Graves in the District of Columbia, April 29, 1901." *Public Laws of the United States of America Passed at the First Session of the Fifty-Seventh Congress, 1901–1902*. Washington, D.C.: U.S. Government Printing Office, 1901.

United States Congress. *Congressional Record Containing the Proceedings and Debates of the Fiftieth Congress, First Session*, Vol. 19. Washington, D.C.: U.S. Government Printing Office, 1888.

United States Congress, Senate. "Argument in Support of the Bill (No. 1566) for the Promotion of Anatomical Science, and to Prevent the Desecration of Graves in the District of Colombia, March 7, 1890." *Reports of Committees for the First Session of the Senate of the United States of the Fifty-First Congress 1889–90*, Vol. 2, Rep. 411. Washington, D.C.: U.S. Government Printing Office, 1890.

United States Department of the Treasury. *Annual Report of the Secretary of the Treasury on the State of the Finances*. Washington, D.C.: U.S. Government Printing Office, 1875.

Vermont. *Laws of the State of Vermont: Digested and Compiled ...* Randolph, VT: Printed by Sereno Wright, 1808.

Vermont Journal (Windsor, VT). 1894.

Vickers, George E. *The Fall of Bossism: A History of the Committee of One Hundred and the Reform Movement in Philadelphia*, Vol. 1. Philadelphia: A.C. Bryson, 1883.

Warren, Charles. *A History of the American Bar*. Boston: Little, Brown, 1911.

Warren, Edward. *Life of John Collins Warren, M.D.* 2 vols. Boston: Ticknor and Fields, 1860.

Washingtonian (Windsor, VT). 1811.

Webb, William B. *Centennial History of the City of Washington, D.C.* Dayton, OH: W.J. Shuey, 1892.

Webster, Daniel. *Private Correspondence of Daniel Webster*, 2 vols. Cambridge, MA: John Wilson, and Son, 1826.

Webster, James. *Facts Concerning Anatomical Instruction in Philadelphia*. Philadelphia: n.p., 1833.

Weekly Wanderer (Randolph, VT). 1806.

Weld, Theodore D. *American Slavery as It Is: Testimony of a Thousand Witnesses*. New York: American Slavery Society, 1839.

Wheeling Register (WV). 1883.

Williams, Stephen West. *American Medical Biography: Or, Memoirs of Eminent Physicians; Embracing ...* Greenfield, MA: L. Merriam and Co., 1845.

Wisconsin Democrat (Madison, WI). 1850.

Wisconsin Department of Health and Family Services. *Wisconsin Vital Records Index Pre-1907*, Vol. 1, 4. https://www.wisconsinhistory.org/Records/Article/CS15307.

Wisconsin Enquirer (Madison, WI). 1838.

Wisconsin State Journal (Madison, WI). 1850.

Wolcott, Oliver, *Message of His Excellency Oliver*

Wolcott: To the Senate and House of Representatives of the State of Connecticut, at the Commencement of the Session of the General Assembly, in New-Haven, May, A.D. 1824. Hartford, CT: Joseph Barber, 1924.

Secondary Sources

Abbott, Edith "The Wages of Unskilled Labor in the United States, 1850–1890." *Journal of Political Economy* 13 (1905), 321–67.

Arey, L.B. *Northwestern University Medical School, 1859–1959: A Pioneer in Educational Reform*. Evanston: Northwestern University Medical School, 1959.

"Anatomical Lecture, 1780." American Antiquarian Society, https://www.americanantiquarian.org/Inventories/Revere/anatomical.PDF.

Bean, Willard. *A.B.C. History of Palmyra and the Beginning of Mormonism*. Palmyra,NY: Palmyra Courier Co., 1938.

Beckwith, David H. "History of the Cleveland Homeopathic College." *Cleveland Homeopathic Reporter* 1 (1900): 7–15.

Benedetto, Christopher. "A Most Daring and Sacrilegious Robbery: The Extraordinary Story of Body Snatching at Chebacco Parish in Ipswich, Massachusetts." *New England Ancestors: Newsmagazine of the New England Historical Society* 6 (2005): 31–34, 45.

Berry, Daina Ramey. *The Price for Their Pound of Flesh*. Boston: Beacon, 2017.

Bowman, LeRoy. *The American Funeral: A Study in Guilt*. Washington, D.C.: Public Affairs Press, 1959.

Brockett, Anne O. *Gone but Not Forgotten: Cemeteries in the Nation's Capital*. Washington, D.C.: U.S. Department of the Interior, National Park Service, 2012.

Burrell, Sean, and Geoffrey Gill. "The Liverpool Cholera Epidemic of 1832 and Anatomical Dissection—Medical Mistrust and Civil Unrest." *Journal of the History of Medicine and Allied Sciences* 60 (October 2005): 478–98.

Capen, Edward W. *The Historical Development of the Poor Law of Connecticut*. New York: Columbia University Press, 1905.

Cash, Philip. "The Professionalization of Boston Medicine." *Medicine in Colonial Massachusetts, 1620–1680*, Vol. 57. Boston: The Society, 1980.

Chamberlain, General Joseph L., ed. *Yale University: Its History, Influence, Equipment and Characteristics...* Boston: R. Herndon Company, 1900.

Chapman, Carleton B. *Dartmouth Medical School: The First 175 Years*. Hanover, NH: University Press of New England, 1973.

Churchill, Gardner II. *The Churchill Family in America*. Boston: Gardner Family, 1904.

Clark, Allen, C. "Beau Hickman (Robert S. Hickman)." *Records of the Columbia Historical Society*, Washington, D.C., nos. 40–41 (1940): 79–96.

Cobb, W. Montague. "Surgery and the Negro Physician: Some Parallels in Background." *Journal of the National Medical Association* 43 (1951): 145–52.

Cohen, Samuel Kline, Jr. *Epidemics: Hate and Compassion from the Plague of Athens to AIDS*. Oxford: Oxford University Press, 2018.

Cole, Hubert. *Things for the Surgeon: A History of the Resurrection Men*. London: Heinemann, 1964.

Columb, Seán. *Trading Life: Organ Trafficking, Illicit Networks, and Exploitation*. Stanford: Stanford University Press, 2020.

Cunningham, Charles E. *Timothy Dwight: A Biography, 1752–1817*. New York: Macmillan, 1942.

Darling, Lewis, MD. *Papers, and Proceeding of the Tioga County Historical Society*, Vol. 1. Wellsboro: Agitator, 1906.

Devine, Shauna. *Learning from the Wounded: The Civil War and the Rise of American Medical Science*. Chapel Hill: University of North Carolina Press, 2014.

Dexter, Franklin Bowditch. *Biographical Sketches of the Graduates of Yale College with Annals of the College History*, Vol. 6. New Haven: Yale University Press, 1912.

District of Columbia Board of Commissioners. *Annual Report of the Commissioners of the District of Columbia: Year Ended June 30, 1913*, Vol. 1. Washington, D.C.: Board of Commissioners, 1914.

Dixon, Edward. "Scenes in a Medical Student's Life-Resurrectionizing." *Scalpel: An Entirely Original Quarterly Expositor of the Laws of Health* 7 (1855): 93–100.

"Dr. Almon Lull." Hartland Historical Society (Hartland, VT), https://hartlandhistory.org/?p=1063.

"Dr. Isaac Wood and Dissection Material in the Early Days." *Medical News* 82 (1903): 850–51.

Dumas, Michael O., MD. "The Evolution of Medicine and Surgery." *Journal of the National Medical Association*, Part II, no. 18 (1926): 1–6.

Durey, Michael. *The Return of the Plague: British Society, and the Cholera, 1831–2*. Dublin: Gill and MacMillan, 1979.

Eddy, Hilah Violet. *The Lull Book*. Detroit, 1926.

Edwards, Linden F. "Dr. Frederick C. Waite's Correspondence with Reference to Grave Robbery." *Ohio State Medical Journal* 54 (1958): 600–602.

Edwards, Linden F. "Resurrection Riots during the Heroic Age of Anatomy in America." *Bulletin of the History of Medicine* 25 (1951): 178–84.

Eliot, Llewellin, MD. "Comment on Frank Baker's 'A History of Bodysnatching.'" *Washington Medical Annals* 15 (1916): 247–53.

Ellis, William A., and Granville M. Dodge. *Norwich University, 1819–1911 ...* 3 vols. Montpelier, VT: Capital City Press, 1911.

Faust, Drew Gilpin. *This Republic of Suffering: Death and the American Civil War*. New York: Vintage Books, 2008.

Forman, Samuel A. *Dr. Joseph Warren: The Boston*

Tea Party, Bunker Hill, and the Birth of American Liberty. Gretna, LA: Pelican, 2012.

Foster, H.D. "Some Unpublished Letters of Rufus Choate." *Dartmouth Alumni Magazine* 17, no. 4 (February 1925): 304–309.

"François-Joseph-Victor Broussais." *Encyclopaedia Britannica*, December 13, 2020. https://www.britannica.com/biography/Francois-Joseph-Victor-Broussais (Accessed 6 July 2021).

"Francois Magendie" *World Biographical Encyclopedia.* https://prabook.com/web/francois.magendie/2446583.

Freedman, David L. "Practicing on the Newly Dead: Is a Corpse Considered Property?" *ED Legal Letter*, February 1, 2000. https://www.reliasmedia.com/articles/44628-practicing-on-the-newly-dead-is-a-corpse-considered-property.

Fry, Gladys-Marie. *Night Riders in Black Folk History.* Chapel Hill: University of North Carolina Press, 1975.

Goodwin, Michele. *The Global Body Market: Altruism's Limits.* Cambridge: Cambridge University Press, 2013.

Greenberg, Kenneth. "Name, Face, Body." In *Nat Turner: A Slave Rebellion in History and Memory*, ed. Kenneth Greenberg. New York: Oxford University Press, 2003.

Greenberg, Kenneth, ed. *Nat Turner: A Slave Rebellion in History and Memory.* New York: Oxford University Press, 2003.

Guerrasio, Venetia M. "Dissecting the Pennsylvania Anatomy Act: Laws, Bodies, and Science, 1880–1960." PhD dissertation, University of New Hampshire Scholars Repository, https://scholars.unh.edu/cgi/viewcontent.cgi?article=1375&context=.

Guttmacher, Alan F. "Bootlegging Bodies: A History of Body Snatching." *Bulletin of the Society of Medical History of Chicago* 4 (1935): 353–402.

Halperin, Edward C. "The Poor, the Black, and the Marginalized as the Source of Cadavers in United States Anatomical Education." *Clinical Anatomy* 20 (2007): 489–95.

Hamlin, Hannibal. "The Dissection Riot of 1824 and the Connecticut Anatomical Law." *Yale Journal of Biology and Medicine* 7 (1934–1935): 275–89.

Handlin, Oscar. *Boston's Immigrants: A Study in Acculturation.* Cambridge: Harvard University Press, 1991.

Harrington, Thomas Francis. *The Harvard Medical School.* 3 vols. New York: Lewis Publishing, 1905.

Havemeyer, Loomis. *Out of Yale's Past: A Story of Undergraduate Traditions.* New Haven, CT: n.p. 1960.

Hay, Douglas, et al. *Albion's Fatal Tree: Crime and Society in Eighteenth-Century England.* New York: Pantheon Books, 1975.

Hayward, Oliver S., and Constance E. Putnam. *Improve, Perfect, & Perpetuate: Nathan Smith and Early American Medical Education.* Hanover, NH: University Press of New England, 1998.

Hoffmann, Frederick L. *Pauper Burials and the Interment of the Dead in Large Cities.* Newark, NJ: Prudential Press, 1919.

Humphrey, David C. "Dissection and Discrimination: The Social Origins of Cadavers in America, 1760–1915." *Bulletin of the New York Academy of Medicine* 49 (1973): 819–27.

Hurd, Charles. *Washington Cavalcade.* New York: E.P. Dutton, 1948.

Jenkins, George B. "The Legal Status of Dissecting." *Anatomical Record* 7 (1913): 387–99.

Kayser, Elmer L. *A Medical Center: The Institutional Development of the Medical Education in George Washington University.* Washington, D.C.: George Washington University Press, 1973.

Keen, William. *Addresses and Other Papers.* Philadelphia: W.B. Saunders, 1905.

Klaver, Elizabeth. *Sites of Autopsy in Contemporary Culture.* Albany: State University of New York Press, 2005.

Knott, John. "Popular Attitudes to Death and Dissection in Early Nineteenth Century Britain: The Anatomy Act and the Poor." *Labour History: A Journal of Labour and Social History*, no. 49 (1985): 1–18.

Ladenheim, J.C. "The Doctors Mob of 1788." *Journal of the History of Medicine and Allied Sciences* 5 (1950): 23–43.

Lassek, Arthur M. *Human Dissection: Its Drama and Struggle.* Springfield, IL: Charles C. Thomas, 1958.

LeBlond, S. "Les Anatomists et les Résurrectionistes aux Etat-Unis." *Canadian Medical Association Journal* 101 (1969): 216–22.

Lee, Max. "Long before Prohibition, D.C. Had a Brief Ban on Liquor." Boundary Stones, October 11, 2016. https://boundarystones.weta.org/2016/10/11/long-prohibition-dc-had-brief-ban-liquor#footnote-2.

Linebaugh, P. "The Tyburn Riot against Surgeons." In *Albion's Fatal Tree: Crime and Society in Eighteenth-Century England*, ed. Douglas Hay et al. New York: Pantheon Books, 1975.

Lovejoy, Bess. *Rest in Pieces: The Curious Fates of Famous Corpses.* London: Duckworth, 2021.

Macfarlane, A.D.J. *Witchcraft in Tudor and Stuart England.* New York: Harper Torchbooks, 1970.

Malinowski, Bronisław. *Magic, Science and Religion, and Other Essays.* Boston: Beacon, 1948.

Mall, Franklin P. "Anatomical Material: Its Collection and Its Preservation at the Johns Hopkins Anatomical Laboratory." *Bulletin of the Johns Hopkins Hospital* 16, no. 167 (February 1905): 38–42.

Mansel, R.E., David J.T. Webster, and H.M. Sweetland. *Hughes, Mansel & Webster's Benign Disorders and Diseases of the Breast.* New York: Elsevier, 2009.

Maxwell, Will J. *General Register of Georgetown University.* Washington, D.C.: Georgetown University, 1916.

McLeary, Erin. "The Curious Case of Body Snatching at Lebanon Cemetery." Hidden City, April 13, 2015. https://hiddencityphila.org/2015/04/the-curious-case-of-body-snatching-at-lebanon-cemetery/.

Medical Society of the District of Columbia. *History of the Medical Society of the District of Columbia, 1817–1909.* Washington, D.C.: The Society, 1909.

Melish, Joanne Pope. *Disowning Slavery: Gradual Emancipation and "Race" in New England, 1780–1860.* Ithaca: Cornell University Press, 2016.

Montgomery, Horace. "A Body Snatcher Sponsors Pennsylvania's Anatomy Act." *Journal of the History of Medicine and Allied Sciences* 21, no. 4 (1966): 374–93.

Morris, R.J. *Cholera 1832: The Social Response to an Epidemic.* New York: Holmes and Meier, 1976.

Morse, Jarvis Means. *A Neglected Period of Connecticut's History, 1818–1850.* New York: Octagon Books, [1933] 1979.

Mt. Lebanon Fiftieth Anniversary, 1912–1962. Mt. Lebanon, PA: Mt. Lebanon News, 1912.

Nola, Mike F. "Paul Revere and Forensic Dentistry." *Military Medicine* 181, no. 7 (July 2016): 714–15.

Phelps, Isaac Newton. *The Iconography of Manhattan Island, 1498–1909: Compiled from Original Sources and Illustrated by Photo-Intaglio Reproductions of Important Maps, Plans, Views, and Documents in Public and Private Collections.* 6 vols. New York: Robert H. Dodd, 1915.

Polleys, Maidee P. "Robbed the Graveyard." RootsWeb. http://sites.rootsweb.com/~macessex/cemetery/ref3.html (accessed August 29, 2021).

Richardson, Ruth. *Death Dissection and the Destitute.* Chicago: University of Chicago Press, 2000.

Riegel, Robert E. "American Father of Birth Control." *New England Quarterly* 6 (1937): 470–90.

Riznik, Barnes. "The Professional Lives of Early Nineteenth Century New England Doctors." *Journal of the History of Medicine and Allied Sciences* 19 (1964): 1–16.

Roach, Mary. *Stiff: The Curious Lives of Human Cadavers.* New York: Norton, 2004.

Rosner, Lisa. *The Anatomy Murders.* Philadelphia: University of Pennsylvania Press, 2010.

Ross, Richard S., III. *Before Salem: Witch Hunting in the Connecticut River Valley, 1647–1663.* Jefferson, NC: McFarland, 2017.

Ross, Richard S., III. *Contagion in Prussia, 1831: The Cholera Epidemic and the Threat of the Polish Uprising.* Jefferson, NC: McFarland, 2015.

Rothstein, William G. *American Medical Schools and the Practice of Medicine: A History.* New York: Oxford University Press, 1987.

Saldago, Catherine. "Uncovered HHS Docs Reveal Federal Funding the Harvest Human Fetal Organs." *National Pulse,* August 5, 2021. https://thenationalpulse.com/breaking/uncovered-hhs-docs-reveal-federal-funding-to-harvest-human-fetal-organs/.

Sappol, Michael. "The Odd Case of Charles Knowlton: Anatomical Performance, Medical Narrative, and Narrative Identity in Antebellum America." *Bulletin of the History of Medicine* 83 (2009): 460–98.

Sappol, Michael. *A Traffic of Dead Bodies.* Princeton: Princeton University Press, 2002.

Schantz, Mark S. *Awaiting the Heavenly Country: The Civil War and America's Culture of Death.* Ithaca: Cornell University Press, 2011.

Shultz, Suzanne. *Body Snatching: The Robbing of Graves for the Education of Physicians in Early Nineteenth Century America.* Jefferson, NC: McFarland, 1992.

Sievers, Harry J. *The Harrison Horror.* Fort Wayne, IN: Public Library of Fort Wayne and Allen County, 1956.

Smith, Nathan. Letter to Governor John Langdon, June 19, 1806. In John Waite, "The Doctor, the Murderer, and the Governor." *The New Antiquarian, the Blog of the Antiquarian Booksellers of America,* February 9, 2015. https://www.abaa.org/blog/post/the-doctor-the-murderer-and-the-governor.

Sondergeld, Donald R. *History of Hubbardton, Vermont.* Collierville, TN: Instant Publisher, 2005.

Spalding, James A., MD. "The Friendship of Dr. Nathan Smith and Dr. Lyman Spalding." *Bulletin of the American Academy of Medicine* 7, no. 10 (1906): 714–34.

Spalding, James Alfred. *Dr. Lyman Spalding: The Originator of the United States Pharmacopoeia.* Boston: W.M. Leonard, 1916.

Starr, Paul. *The Social Transformation of American Medicine: The Rise of a Sovereign Profession and the Making of a Vast Industry.* New York: Basic Books, 1982.

Stevens, Rosemary. *American Medicine and the Public Interest.* Berkeley: University of California Press, 1998.

Stone, Bingham H. "One Hundred Years of Medicine in Vermont." *Vermont Medical Monthly* 19 (1913): 235–45.

Thorpe, Walter. *History of Wallingford Vermont.* Rutland, VT: Tuttle Co., 1911.

United States Congress, House Committee on Ways and Means. *Subcommittee on Health: Panel Discussions on National Health Insurance.* Washington, D.C.: U.S. Government Printing Office, 1975.

"Vermont Vital Records through 1870." Ancestry. https://www.ancestry.com/discoveryui- content/view/487590:4661?tid=&pid=&queryId=a9ab-6384d8a4a2d9a0f3c68dbb7cf74b&_phsrc=oMP5711&_phstart=successSource.

Vital Records of Ipswich, Massachusetts: Marriages and Deaths to the End of 1849. 3 vols. Salem, MA: Essex Institute, 1910.

Waite, Frederick C. "The Development of Anatomical Laws in the States of New England." *New England Journal of Medicine* 233 (1945): 716–26.

Waite, Frederick C. "An Episode in Massachusetts

in 1818 Related to Teaching of Anatomy." *New England Journal of Medicine* 220 (1939): 221–27.

Waite, Frederick C. *The First Medical College in Vermont: Castleton, 1818–1862.* Montpelier, VT: Vermont Historical Society, 1949.

Waite, Frederick C. "Grave Robbing in New England." *Bulletin of the Medical Library Association* 33 (1945): 272–94.

Walsh, James. *The History of Medicine in New York.* 5 vols. New York: National Americana Society, J.J. Little, and Ives, 1919.

Washington, Harriet. *Medical Apartheid: The Dark History of Medical Experimentation on Blacks.* New York: Harlem, Moon, 2006.

Whitcher, Willliam F., ed. *Josiah Burnham his trial and execution for murder with sermon preached at Haverhill, N.H. by the Rev. David Sutherland at time and place of execution August 12, 1806.* Woodsville, NH: New Books and Job Print, 1909.

Wigglesworth, William C. "Surgery in Massachusetts, 1620–1800." In *Medicine in Colonial Massachusetts, 1620–1820.* 215–48. Boston: The Society, 1980.

Wilder, Craig Steven. *Ebony and Ivy: Race, Slavery, and the Troubled History of American Universities.* New York: Bloomsbury, 2013.

Wilf, Steven. "Anatomy and Punishment in Late Eighteenth Century New York." *Journal of Social History* 2 (1989): 507–30.

Wilf, Steven. *Law's Imagined Republic: Popular Politics and Criminal Justice in Revolutionary America.* New York: Cambridge University Press, 2010.

Woodruff, A.W., and S. Bell. *Synopsis of Infectious Tropical Diseases.* Baltimore: Williams and Wilkins, 1987.

Yale University. *Catalogue of Officers and Graduates of Yale University.* New Haven: Tuttle, Morehouse, and Taylor, 1910.

Yale University, School of Medicine. *Memorial of the Centennial of the Yale Medical School.* New Haven: Yale University Press, 1915.

Index

Numbers in ***bold italics*** indicate pages with illustrations

www.ingramcontent.com/pod-product-compliance
Ingram Content Group UK Ltd.
Pitfield, Milton Keynes, MK11 3LW, UK
UKHW051930100926
8556IPUK00022B/1466

9 781476 695013